Current Clinical Psychiatry

Series editor

Jerrold F. Rosenbaum
Boston, MA, USA

More information about this series at http://www.springer.com/series/7634

Ana-Maria Vranceanu • Joseph A. Greer
Steven A. Safren

Editors

The Massachusetts General Hospital Handbook of Behavioral Medicine

A Clinician's Guide to Evidence-based
Psychosocial Interventions for Individuals
with Medical Illness

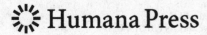 Humana Press

Editors
Ana-Maria Vranceanu, Ph.D.
Behavioral Medicine Service
Department of Psychiatry
Institute of Brain Health
Massachusetts General Hospital
Boston, MA, USA

Joseph A. Greer, Ph.D.
Center for Psychiatric Oncology &
    Behavioral Sciences
Massachusetts General Hospital
    Cancer Center
Boston, MA, USA

Steven A. Safren, Ph.D.
Department of Psychology
University of Miami
Coral Gables, FL, USA

Current Clinical Psychiatry
ISBN 978-3-319-29292-2   ISBN 978-3-319-29294-6   (eBook)
DOI 10.1007/978-3-319-29294-6

Library of Congress Control Number: 2016958583

Printed on acid-free paper

This Humana Press imprint is published by Springer Nature
The registered company is Springer Science+Business Media LLC
The registered company address is: 233 Spring Street, New York, NY 10013, U.S.A.

Contents

Contributors

Nicole Amoyal Behavioral Medicine Service, Department of Psychiatry, Massachusetts General Hospital, Harvard Medical School, Boston, MA, USA

C. Andres Bedoya, Ph.D. Behavioral Medicine Service, Department of Psychiatry, Massachusetts General Hospital, Harvard Medical School, Boston, MA, USA

Aaron Blashill Department of Psychology, San Diego State University, San Diego, CA, USA

Jennifer A. Burbridge, Ph.D. Behavioral Medicine Service, Department of Psychiatry, Massachusetts General Hospital, Harvard Medical School, Boston, MA, USA

Trina E. Chang, M.D., M.P.H. Depression Clinical and Research Program, Department of Psychiatry, Massachusetts General Hospital, Boston, MA, USA

Sannisha K. Dale Behavioral Medicine Service, Department of Psychiatry, Massachusetts General Hospital, Harvard Medical School, Boston, MA, USA

Peter P. Ehlinger Behavioral Medicine Service, Department of Psychiatry, Massachusetts General Hospital, Harvard Medical School, Boston, MA, USA

Jeffrey S. Gonzalez, Ph.D. Ferkauf Graduate School of Psychology, Yeshiva University, Bronx, NY, USA

Diabetes Research Center, Albert Einstein College of Medicine, Yeshiva University, Bronx, NY, USA

Mark J. Gorman, Ph.D. Department of Psychiatry, Massachusetts General Hospital Weight Center, Boston, MA, USA

Hetta Gouse, Ph.D. Department of Psychiatry and Mental Health, University of Cape Town, Cape Town, South Africa

Joseph A. Greer, Ph.D. Center for Psychiatric Oncology & Behavioral Sciences, Massachusetts General Hospital Cancer Center, Boston, MA, USA

Rebecca Hicks Behavioral Medicine, Department of Psychiatry, Massachusetts General Hospital, Boston, MA, USA

Jeff C. Huffman, M.D. Department of Psychiatry, Massachusetts General Hospital, Boston, MA, USA

Vicki A. Jackson Massachusetts General Hospital Cancer Center, Harvard Medical School, Boston, MA, USA

Jamie M. Jacobs, Ph.D. Massachusetts General Hospital, Boston, MA, USA

Juliet C. Jacobsen Massachusetts General Hospital Cancer Center, Harvard Medical School, Boston, MA, USA

Jonathan Jampel The Fenway Institute, Fenway Health, Boston, MA, USA

Naomi S. Kane, M.A. Ferkauf Graduate School of Psychology, Yeshiva University, Bronx, NY, USA

John F. Kelly, Ph.D. Department of Psychiatry, Harvard Medical School, Massachusetts General Hospital, Boston, MA, USA

Department of Psychiatry, Center for Addiction Medicine, Massachusetts General Hospital, Boston, MA, USA

Ronald Kulich Pain Medicine and Anesthesia, Harvard Medical School, Massachusetts General Hospital, Boston, MA, USA

Allison K. Labbe, Ph.D. Behavioral Medicine Service, Department of Psychiatry, Massachusetts General Hospital, Harvard Medical School, Boston, MA, USA

Jonathan A. Lerner, Ph.D. Behavioral Medicine Service, Department of Psychiatry, Massachusetts General Hospital, Harvard Medical School, Boston, MA, USA

Catherine L. Leveroni, Ph.D. Behavioral Medicine Service, Department of Psychiatry, Massachusetts General Hospital, Harvard Medical School, Boston, MA, USA

Christina M. Luberto Behavioral Medicine Service, Department of Psychiatry, Massachusetts General Hospital, Harvard Medical School, Boston, MA, USA

Jessica F. Magidson, Ph.D. Behavioral Medicine Service, Department of Psychiatry, Massachusetts General Hospital, Harvard Medical School, Boston, MA, USA

Rachel A. Millstein, Ph.D., M.H.S. Behavioral Medicine Service, Department of Psychiatry, Massachusetts General Hospital, Harvard Medical School, Boston, MA, USA

Conall O'Cleirigh Behavioral Medicine Service, Department of Psychiatry, Massachusetts General Hospital, Harvard Medical School, Boston, MA, USA

Elyse R. Park, Ph.D., M.P.H. Behavioral Medicine Service, Department of Psychiatry, Massachusetts General Hospital, Harvard Medical School, Boston, MA, USA

Giselle K. Perez Behavioral Medicine Service, Department of Psychiatry, Massachusetts General Hospital, Harvard Medical School, Boston, MA, USA

G. Perez-Lougee, Ph.D. Massachusetts General Hospital, Boston, MA, USA

William F. Pirl Massachusetts General Hospital Cancer Center, Harvard Medical School, Boston, MA, USA

Christina Psaros, Ph.D. Behavioral Medicine Service, Department of Psychiatry, Massachusetts General Hospital, Harvard Medical School, Boston, MA, USA

Noreen A. Reilly-Harrington, Ph.D. Department of Psychiatry, Massachusetts General Hospital Weight Center, Boston, MA, USA

Jocelyn E. Remmert Behavioral Medicine Service, Department of Psychiatry, Massachusetts General Hospital, Harvard Medical School, Boston, MA, USA

Steven A. Safren, Ph.D. Department of Psychology, University of Miami, Coral Gables, FL, USA

Stephanie S. Sogg, Ph.D., M.G.H. Department of Psychiatry, Massachusetts General Hospital Weight Center, Harvard Medical School, Boston, MA, USA

Melissa Stone Pain Medicine and Anesthesia, Harvard Medical School, Massachusetts General Hospital, Boston, MA, USA

Jennifer S. Temel Massachusetts General Hospital Cancer Center, Harvard Medical School, Boston, MA, USA

Lara Traeger, Ph.D. Behavioral Medicine Service, Department of Psychiatry, Massachusetts General Hospital, Harvard Medical School, Boston, MA, USA

Ana-Maria Vranceanu, Ph.D. Behavioral Medicine Service, Department of Psychiatry, Institute of Brain Health, Massachusetts General Hospital, Boston, MA, USA

Tim Wallace Behavioral Medicine Service, Department of Psychiatry, Massachusetts General Hospital, Harvard Medical School, Boston, MA, USA

Julianne G. Wilner, M.A. Behavioral Medicine Service, Department of Psychiatry, Massachusetts General Hospital, Harvard Medical School, Boston, MA, USA

Julie Yeterian, M.A. Department of Psychiatry, Center for Addiction Medicine, Massachusetts General Hospital, Boston, MA, USA

Chapter 1
Introduction to the MGH Handbook of Behavioral Medicine

Ana-Maria Vranceanu, Joseph A. Greer, and Steven A. Safren

Over the last few decades, a large body of research has clearly demonstrated that the traditional disease-focused, biomedical approach to illness management is less effective than a biopsychosocial, evidence-based, patient-centered approach. The utility of this more comprehensive approach has been evident for both a variety of chronic illnesses and, more recently, acute medical conditions. In contrast to the traditional biomedical model of illness, which typically reduces illness to a pathophysiologic disease process, a biopsychosocial approach accounts for the complex interaction among biologic, psychological, social, and behavioral factors [1].

The field of Behavioral Medicine developed in response to the transition toward a biopsychosocial model and ever-growing evidence documenting the importance of psychosocial factors in the etiology, progression and outcomes of illness. Indeed, psychological factors influence adherence to medical regimens (e.g., [2–6, 16], success of medical procedures (e.g., [7, 8]), physical functioning (e.g., [9]), mortality (e.g., [10, 11, 17]), recovery after injury [12], and overall quality of life (e.g., [13]). Psychosocial factors are also associated with increased service utilization and health care costs (e.g. [14]).

A.-M. Vranceanu, Ph.D. (✉)
Behavioral Medicine Service, Department of Psychiatry, Institute of Brain Health,
Massachusetts General Hospital, Boston, MA 02174, USA
e-mail: avranceanu@mgh.harvard.edu

J.A. Greer, Ph.D.
Center for Psychiatric Oncology & Behavioral Sciences, Massachusetts General Hospital
Cancer Center, Yawkey Suite 10B, 55 Fruit Street, Boston, MA 02114, USA
e-mail: jgreer2@mgh.harvard.edu

S.A. Safren, Ph.D.
Department of Psychology, University of Miami, 5665 Ponce de Leon Blvd., Coral Gables,
FL 33124, USA
e-mail: ssafren@miami.edu

The large body of research supporting the biopsychosocial model has led to the development of behavioral medicine interventions delivered as adjunct to medical treatment. Due to increased reliance on evidenced-based outcomes focused on cost and patient satisfaction, as well as on clinical efficacy and effectiveness, behavioral medicine interventions integrate the best available scientific evidence with clinician expertise in order to help patients prevent and cope with disease. Interventions are also patient centered, accounting for individual patient preferences, needs and values, while customizing treatments on the basis of informed, shared decision making, development of patient knowledge, enhancement of skills needed for self-management of illness and engagement in preventive behaviors.

The field of behavioral medicine has grown and expended over the last few decades to include treatments delivered in outpatient psychiatry departments by clinical psychologists as well as treatments integrated within inpatient or outpatient medical practices by clinical psychologists, social workers, other mental health professionals, and sometimes medical staff such as nurses or physician assistants. The field of behavioral medicine is malleable and aims to accommodate developments and changes within the larger health care system. Currently behavioral medicine interventions are delivered not only face to face, but also through videoconferencing, or over the telephone. Nurses and other medical providers are becoming more involved in the delivery of behavioral medicine interventions, sometimes with training from clinical psychologists or other behavioral health professionals. With the current emphasis on population-based medicine and developing "medical homes" focused on continuity and coordination of care for medical patients through multidisciplinary teams, it is expected that the field of behavioral medicine will continue growing, changing and expanding in years to come [15].

The Behavioral Medicine Service at Massachusetts General Hospital was developed by Dr. Steven Safren in 2004. After working for several years in the Cognitive Behavioral Therapy (CBT) program, which predominately supported the Department of Psychiatry, and treating many patients with comorbid psychological and medical conditions, Dr. Safren noticed that it would be important to meet the needs of the primary care and specialty practices in our system through a specialized Behavioral Medicine Service with clinicians trained specifically in addressing the psychological needs of medical patients. Dr. Safren had been conducting research and providing clinical care with the MGH HIV service, in which patient adherence to potentially life-saving medications was essential to optimal disease management. Additionally, many of the referrals that came through to the CBT program from the Infectious Disease Unit were for patients whose mental health or substance use problems interfered with them achieving their optimal disease-management self-care goals. Dr. Joseph Greer was the first postdoctoral fellow within the department in 2004, while Dr. Ana-Maria Vranceanu was the first Behavioral Medicine clinical fellow (pre-doctoral intern) in 2005. Over the years, Drs. Greer and Vranceanu advanced through the MGH and Harvard system, developing their own clinical and research programs within the Behavioral Medicine Program, specializing in psycho-oncology and pain management, behavioral health integration in specialty clinics, respectively. Dr. Greer is currently Program Director of the Center for Psychiatric

Oncology & Behavioral Sciences. Dr. Vranceanu is currently Assistant Director of Behavioral Health Integration within Behavioral Medicine, and Executive Director of Comprehensive Care for the Institute of Brain Health. Under the direction of Dr. Safren from its inception 2004 until 2015, the department has grown considerably and now encompasses 18 core clinical psychologists, two postdoctoral fellows and two pre-doctoral interns yearly. The department is currently led by Dr. Conall O'Cleirigh.

The Massachusetts General Hospital's Behavioral Medicine Service has the primary goal of addressing the psychosocial needs of medical outpatients and fostering multidisciplinary collaborations to improve the clinical care of patients with medical illness. Consistent with the biopsychosocial model, the treatment philosophy assumes the presence of a physical problem that can be influenced by behavioral and psychological factors. Treatment seeks to identify, control and limit the potentially negative influence these factors can have on a patient's medical problem. To this end, a variety of evidence-based behavioral and cognitive-behavioral treatments and techniques are used within a general CBT framework. Treatments are time-limited, problem-focused, directly linked to the medical need, and actively involve the patient in his or her own treatment. Engaging individual patients in treatment occurs in at least two ways. First, the patient monitors the status of the presenting concern in between sessions. Second, the patient learns and practices evidence-based techniques that modify and limit the negative effects of certain cognitive and behavioral factors. These techniques may include problem-solving training, relaxation training, cognitive restructuring, communication skills, contingency management, motivational enhancement, and behavioral assessment and modification. Regular communication with medical team is essential to this approach.

The MGH Handbook of Behavioral Medicine outlines the importance of biopsychosocial factors in improving medical care and illustrates evidence-based, state-of-the-art interventions for patients with a variety of medical conditions. Each chapter is focused on a particular health concern or illness, which is described both in terms of prevalence and frequent psychological and psychiatric comorbidities that may present to clinicians working with these populations. Unified by a focus on the biopsychosocial model, each health concern has unique challenges, which are addressed in each chapter. Consistent with an evidence-based approach to care, relevant research on the efficacy of the various treatments is presented, to support their continued use and dissemination. To accommodate the needs of clinicians, we describe population-specific approaches to treatment, including goal setting, therapeutic interventions, as well as strategies to assess and monitor progress. To facilitate learning, each chapter contains one or more case examples that explicate the interventions and illustrate patient improvement within a behavioral medicine protocol. Each chapter also includes resources in the form of books and websites to gain additional knowledge and detail as needed. We have selected authors who are either currently part of the Behavioral Medicine Service at MGH, or who have trained within our department–and are now practicing in other settings. Either the first or senior author on each chapter is an expert in the specific topic of the chapter, ensuring that the information presented is recent and of high quality.

The book is organized into three main parts. The first part is concerned with health-risk behaviors that directly impact physical and/or psychological functioning, including chapters focused on smoking cessation, obesity/weight conditions, and substance abuse. The second part addresses the treatment of chronic conditions and includes chapters on chronic pain, diabetes, HIV, cardiovascular issues, cancer, epilepsy/other neurological conditions, and gastro-intestinal conditions. The third and final part includes more recent developments in the field of behavioral medicine, with chapters focused on women's health, palliative care and end-of-life concerns, cultural considerations, and the delivery of behavioral medicine interventions in resource poor global settings.

We believe that this handbook will be of equal relevance to clinicians, researchers, academicians and graduate students in clinical psychology. The detailed presentation should facilitate the ability of clinicians and other mental health providers to treat diverse populations with health-risk concerns and chronic illnesses more effectively. Moreover, the specific elements of the presented treatments may inform investigators about salient clinical issues in need of empirical testing and support. Lastly, the detailed explanations of the research and various behavioral medicine interventions targeting health-risk behaviors and chronic illnesses make this handbook an ideal teaching tool for clinical psychology graduate programs.

References

1. Engel GL. The need for a new medical model: a challenge for biomedicine. Science. 1977;196:129–36. doi:10.1126/science.847460. ISSN 0036-8075 (print)/ISSN 1095-9203 (web).
2. DiMatteo MR, Lepper HS, Croghan TW. Depression is a risk factor for noncompliance with medical treatment: meta-analysis of the effects of anxiety and depression on patient adherence. Arch Intern Med. 2000;160(14):2101–7.
3. Gonzalez JS, Peyrot M, McCarl LA, Collins EM, Serpa L, Mimiaga MJ, Safren SA. Depression and diabetes treatment nonadherence: a meta-analysis. Diabetes Care. 2008;31(12):2398–403.
4. Greer JA, Pirl WF, Park ER, Lynch TJ, Temel JS. Behavioral and psychological predictors of chemotherapy adherence in patients with advanced non-small cell lung cancer. J Psychosom Res. 2008;65(6):549–52.
5. Mitchell AJ, Chan M, Bhatti H, Halton M, Grassi L, Johansen C, Meader N. Prevalence of depression, anxiety, and adjustment disorder in oncological, haematological, and palliative-care settings: a meta-analysis of 94 interview-based studies. Lancet Oncol. 2011;12(2):160–74.
6. Traeger L, Greer JA, Fernandez-Robles C, Temel JS, Pirl WF. Evidence-based treatment of anxiety in patients with cancer. J Clin Oncol. 2012;30(11):1197–205.
7. Adogwa O, Parker SL, Shau DN, Mendenhall SK, Aaronson O, Cheng JS, Devin CJ, McGirt MJ. Cost per quality-adjusted life year gained of revision neural decompression and instrumented fusion for same-level recurrent lumbar stenosis: defining the value of surgical intervention. J Neurosurg Spine. 2012;16:135–40.
8. Vranceanu AM, Ring D. Predictors of disability after minor hand surgery. J Bone Joint Surg. 2010;12:123–45.

9. Stegenga BT, Geerlings MI, Torres-González F, Xavier M, Svab I, Penninx BW, Nazareth I, King M. Risk factors for onset of multiple or long major depressive episodes versus single and short episodes. Soc Psychiatry Psychiatr Epidemiol. 2013;48(7):1067–75.
10. Cook JA, Grey D, Burke J, Cohen MH, Gurtman AC, Richardson JL, Hessol NA. Depressive symptoms and AIDS-related mortality among a multisite cohort of HIV-positive women. Am J Public Health. 2004;94(7):1133–40.
11. Pirl WF, Temel JS, Billings A, Dahlin C, Jackson V, Prigerson HG, Greer J, Lynch TJ. Depression after diagnosis of advanced non-small cell lung cancer and survival: a pilot study. Psychosomatics. 2008;49(3):218–24.
12. Vranceanu AM, Hageman M, Strooker J, ter Meulen D, Vrahas M, Ring D. A preliminary RCT of a mind body intervention in patients with acute trauma at risk for chronic pain and disability. Injury. 2015;46(4):552–7.
13. Rapaport MH, Clary C, Fayyad R, Endicott J. Quality-of-life impairment in depressive and anxiety disorders. Am J Psychiatr. 2005;162(6):1171–8.
14. McLaughlin TP, Khandker RK, Kruzikas DT, Tummala R. Overlap of anxiety and depression in a managed care population: prevalence and association with resource utilization. J Clin Psychiatry. 2006;67(8):1187–93.
15. Keefe FJ. Behavioral medicine: a voyage to the future. Ann Behav Med. 2011;41(2):141–51.
16. Kronish IM, Rieckmann N, Halm EA, Shimbo D, Vorchheimer D, Haas DC, Davidson KW. Persistent depression affects adherence to secondary prevention behaviors after acute coronary syndromes. Journal of General Internal Medicine. 2006;21:1178–1183. doi:10.1111/j.1525-1497.2006.00586.x.
17. Katon WJ, Von Korff M, Lin EH, et al. The Pathways Study: a randomized trial of collaborative care in patients with diabetes and depression. Arch Gen Psychiatry. 2004;61:1042–1049.

Part I
Health Risk Behaviors

Chapter 2
Smoking Cessation

Elyse R. Park, Christina M. Luberto, Conall O'Cleirigh, Giselle K. Perez, and Julianne G. Wilner

2.1 Introduction

2.1.1 Prevalence of Smoking

Despite its negative health effects, smoking remains the leading cause of preventable death and disability in the United States [1]. Smoking accounts for 1 in 5 deaths and $193 billion in healthcare costs each year [1–3]. Although there was a decline in smoking rates following the release of the Surgeon General's report in 1965, prevalence rates have remained relatively stable over the past 20 years [4, 5]. Currently, approximately 18% of adults in the USA are regular cigarette smokers [6]. Prevalence rates are higher among males (20.5%) compared to females (15.8%), and American Indians/Alaska Natives (21.8%) compared to Whites (19.7%), African-Americans (18.1%), and Asians (10.7%; [6]). Of importance to note, individuals with less education and lower incomes are particularly vulnerable to smoking. From a treatment perspective, it is key to emphasize that the majority of current smokers want to quit, and approximately half of all smokers try to quit each year; however, fewer than 6% will achieve long-term quitting [7, 8].

E.R. Park, Ph.D., M.P.H. (✉) • C.M. Luberto • C. O'Cleirigh
G.K. Perez • J.G. Wilner, M.A.
Behavioral Medicine Service, Department of Psychiatry,
Massachusetts General Hospital, Harvard Medical School,
Boston, MA, USA
e-mail: epark@mgh.harvard.edu; gperez@mgh.harvard.edu; jgwilner@mgh.harvard.edu

© Springer Science+Business Media New York 2017
A.-M. Vranceanu et al. (eds.), *The Massachusetts General Hospital Handbook of Behavioral Medicine*, Current Clinical Psychiatry, DOI 10.1007/978-3-319-29294-6_2

2.2   Psychological Comorbidities and the Role of Stress and Negative Affect

Psychological factors play a central role in smoking behavior. As a group, smokers have higher rates of mental illness and report greater levels of negative affect than nonsmokers [9, 10]. Smoking is also more common among individuals with mental illness, with an overall prevalence rate of 41 % across psychiatric disorders [6]. Rates of smoking among individuals with severe mental illness are even higher; for example, 60–80 % of patients with schizophrenia smoke [11]. Smokers consistently cite reduction or regulation of negative emotions, as well as coping with emotional distress, as primary reasons for smoking [12, 13]. The high levels of negative affect among smokers contribute to sustained smoking behavior and complicate smoking cessation efforts. Given that negative affect is a salient symptom of nicotine withdrawal, smokers who are unable to tolerate distress without the use of cigarettes experience greater difficulties with smoking cessation, including greater perceived barriers to quitting [14], shorter time to smoking relapse [15], and lower rates of participation in tobacco treatment programs [16].

2.3   Treatment Delivery

Smoking cessation treatment may be delivered individually or in a group setting. Individual treatment provides patient-centered care and may be more logistically feasible. Group treatment provides an opportunity for enhanced social support and shared learning of quitting techniques. Other modalities may be used as an adjunct or primary behavioral treatment, such as telephone counseling, text message programs, or phone applications. Telephone counseling can be provided (1) proactively, in which calls to smokers are initiated by a counselor according to a prearranged time and (2) reactively, such as via a quitline, in which patients initiate calls. A meta-analysis conducted in 2013 found that proactive telephone counseling is more effective than reactive counseling [17]. Web-based smoking treatments can also help patients to quit smoking, particularly if the programs are individualized and interactive [18]. Mobile phone text messaging smoking treatments may consist of automated personalized support messages; several trials have found that text messaging is effective in promoting smoking abstinence [19, 20]. Phone apps have yet to be rigorously studied [20]; however, a 2011 review of the 47 iPhone smoking cessation apps determined that there was low adherence to evidence-based practice guidelines [21].

2.4   Smoking Cessation Medications and Adherence

Seven first-line medications are recommended by the 2008 Clinical Practice Guidelines to increase long-term smoking abstinence rates. These include the following five nicotine replacement therapies: patch, gum, inhaler, lozenge, and nasal spray. The patch is long-acting and provides slow delivery. Short acting therapies with faster onset include the gum, inhaler (nicotine vapor that is absorbed through the mouth), lozenge, and nasal spray (rapid release delivery). Nicotine replacement therapies involve nicotine substitutes to assist with nicotine withdrawal symptoms and are dosed based on a patient's level of smoking. The side effects vary by nicotine delivery method, and it is essential that smokers are trained in proper use of each product. Bupropion SR (Zyban, Wellbutrin SR) is an antidepressant that inhibits reuptake of dopamine and norepinephrine, which can reduce craving for tobacco. Varenicline (Chantix) is a non-nicotine medication which interferes with nicotine receptors; it has both agonist and antagonist function and thus simultaneously reduces pleasure gained from smoking as well as withdrawal symptoms. In 2009, the FDA published a public health advisory on the neuropsychiatric side effects of varenicline and bupropion, specifically, stating that "[Varenicline] or [bupropion] has been associated with reports of changes in behavior such as hostility, agitation, depressed mood, and suicidal thoughts or actions." A patient's psychiatric stability should therefore be considered when considering varenicline. However, of importance is that recent trials have supported the safety of varenicline and bupropion, even among schizophrenic and depressed patients [22–24]. When patients stop smoking they often, albeit temporarily, experience nicotine withdrawal symptoms (e.g., depressed mood, anxiety, and irritability) and thus should be monitored closely around the time of quitting.

The nicotine replacement products and bupropion have been shown to approximately double quit rates, compared to unassisted attempts, and there is evidence that the use of varenicline can triple quit rates [25]. A Cochrane Database review of 12 trials testing these pharmacological options found that varenicline and combination NRT were superior to single forms of NRT or bupropion [26]. Moreover, the combination of counseling and medications is more effective than either alone. Specifically, studies have shown that the use of smoking cessation medications doubles abstinence rates when combined with evidence-based behavioral treatment [27, 28]. In fact, a series of meta-analyses report abstinence rates to be 1.5–2.27 times higher among smokers who use pharmacological intervention vs. placebo to aid quitting efforts, with rates reportedly higher for patients who use Varenicline [29–32]. Accordingly, the USDHHS Public Health Service guidelines recommend combined medication and behavioral approaches to tobacco treatment [25, 33]. Furthermore, smoking cessation medications have been shown to be effective even amongst smokers with varying levels of quit motivation [34], engendering successful quit attempts in those intending to cut back. While there is evidence that using smoking cessation medications prior to quitting and for extended periods of time may increase the likelihood of achieving better outcomes [35, 36], findings are inconsistent regarding the benefits of long-term consumption [37].

Despite their documented benefit, the use of smoking cessation medications amongst individuals remains suboptimal. Studies conducted in the general population of smokers document low rates of medication use [38] and adherence [39, 40]. In fact, only 25 % of smokers who have made a quit attempt using a pharmacologic agent to assist cessation efforts [37]. Further, among smokers who choose to initiate pharmaco-therapy, a substantial proportion has been shown to discontinue treatment prematurely and to use inadequate, and often, ineffective doses [36]. For instance, a recent survey of 1219 adult smokers in four countries determined that a little over half of the sample (55%) discontinued NRT use altogether after only 4 weeks [41]. Similar patterns of early treatment withdrawal have been reported for Varenicline [39] and bupropion [42]. These findings are disconcerting, as adherence to smoking cessation medications is central to optimizing cessation outcomes [35, 43].

Given the important role medication adherence has in promoting abstinence, researchers have endeavored to develop a profile of smokers who are likely to have difficulty adhering to cessation medications. Several key factors have been associ-ated with medication discontinuation. In general, studies have found that smokers who are female, younger, and less educated are more likely to demonstrate abrupt and early discontinuation of stop smoking medications [36, 43]. Factors associated with nonadherence to pharmacotherapy guidelines include forgetting, perceived unhelpfulness, relapse, negative attitudes toward medication, distrust in the effec-tiveness of medication, other substance use (e.g., alcohol), psychiatric history, low quit self-efficacy, and greater smoking rate [35, 41, 44].

In light of this evidence, a focal point of tobacco treatment should include encouraging pharmacotherapy use and adherence amongst smokers intending to quit or reduce cigarette use. Adherence to smoking cessation medication regimens should also be monitored closely; patients often need strategies to decrease, and cope with, side effects. Primary emphasis should be placed on providing psycho-education regarding the value of smoking cessation medications, their functional-ity and limitations, and the import of taking them as instructed in efforts to maximize their therapeutic effect [36]. Special attention should be placed on gath-ering a thorough medical, psychiatric, and smoking history to determine the most effective medication and therapeutic dose. Efforts should be made to help patients develop a medication schedule, which may include assisting patients in identifying and problem-solving barriers to adherence, implementing cue-control strategies to remind them to take their medication and adhere to their regimen, and managing potential side effects [35]. In these endeavors, clinicians can aid patients with developing a medication calendar to monitor use, which the provider can review and provide feedback during each visit. As adherence tends to be strongest during the early stages of treatment and tends to decrease with time, providers should engage patients in ongoing discussion about their medication, noting any changes in medication beliefs, attitudes, and motivation [45]. Use of motivational inter-viewing and standard cognitive-behavioral approaches will help clinicians in increasing their patients' quitting motivation and self-efficacy as well as modify negative thoughts or beliefs that may dissuade patients from complying with treat-ment recommendations [35].

2.5   Electronic Cigarettes

Electronic cigarettes are electronic devices which deliver a nicotine vapor, sometimes referred to as e-cigs, e-cigarettes, e-hookah, or personal vaporizers. E-cigs are not FDA regulated as a device or drug product, but they are becoming increasingly used in the USA. Smokers are using them purportedly to try to quit and/or in places where smoking is prohibited. However, it is unclear whether, indeed, e-cigs should be used as a substitute for combustible tobacco use or they provide value as harm reduction devices or quitting assistance. The content of e-cigs, as well as how much nicotine is delivered, is relatively unknown. Research is needed on the efficacy of e-cigs to help smokers cut down and/or quit as well as long-term effects.

2.6   Assessments

A comprehensive assessment of a smoker is an integral starting point to smoking cessation treatment. Smoking history, including age of initiation, quit attempts, and current medical history, in particular comorbid smoking-related medical conditions, should be obtained.

Information should be gathered on cognitive determinants of behavior change, including motivation/readiness to quit, self confidence and importance to quit smoking, perceived severity and risks of smoking. In past quit attempts, triggers to smoking, including individual factors (cravings and withdrawal symptoms) and social/environmental factors (quitting support, smoking policy in household), should be assessed. In addition, a smoker's emotional status, such as psychiatric diagnoses, as well as level of emotional distress, and symptoms of depression and anxiety, should be assessed. Lastly, as many smokers experience shame and self-directed stigma for smoking, such constructs should be assessed.

2.7   Behavioral Treatments: Cognitive-Behavioral Therapy Approaches

Effective counseling programs generally use cognitive-behavioral techniques (CBT; changing maladaptive thinking patterns and associated behaviors) to help patients to identify and cope with triggers that may tempt smoking. Cognitive-behavioral interventions for nicotine dependence that also aim to reduce negative affect or improve emotion regulation are therefore particularly important. Social support is also an important treatment component to reinforce a smoker's confidence in his or her ability to quit [25, 46]. Key CBT strategies to achieving and maintaining abstinence include:

Cutting Back/Tapering: This involves restricting periods of time or places where one smokes, or limiting the number of daily cigarettes smoked. It is helpful to set up, and record, a weekly tapering structure.

Tracking: This is the process of recording one's smoking. Tracking can be used, initially, to help a smoker understand his/her smoking patterns and motivations. It is an integral part of the tapering process; setting up a monitoring system is a concrete way for a smoker to document progress.

Creating a Smoke-Free Environment: An often helpful initial step towards quitting involves creating smoke-free environments, particularly in smokers' homes and cars. The less exposure one has to others' smoking, the better it is for the smoker trying to achieve abstinence. One can begin this process by first creating smoke-free areas in the home and then progress toward the goal of eliminating any smoking in the home or car.

Setting Up Coping Strategies: Inevitably, and particularly during the initial couple of weeks following a quit attempt, smokers may experience withdrawal symptoms such as irritability, restlessness, and feelings of anxiety and depression. It is important to assess what types of withdrawal symptoms smokers are concerned about, and which he/she has experienced in previous quit attempts. It is also crucial for a smoker to anticipate and prepare for how to cope with these symptoms. ACE (Avoid, Change, and Escape) is a helpful pneumonic to learn and practice, in anticipation of confronting a trigger. Avoid ("What can you do to avoid triggers?") Change ("What can you do to change the situation to make smoking less tempting?") Escape ("What would it be like to leave?").

Overcoming Cravings: Often smokers experience cravings, and urges to smoke, intermittently, for a period of time following a quit attempt. It is important to reinforce that cravings are often fleeting, lasting a minute or two. Mini relaxation exercises (e.g., repeating, "This will pass," visualizing a place which feels restful) can help a smoker pass this experience. The "4Ds" are helpful to remember and implement when experiencing cravings. Delay—pause a few moments; Drink—a glass of water; Distraction—do something else; and Deep breathing.

Stress Management and Relaxation Strategies: Stress management strategies such as breath awareness, deep breathing, guided imagery, body scanning, progressive muscle relaxation, brief meditation, or stretching can help one be aware of stressful sensations and decrease the experiences of stress. These strategies can be practiced on an ongoing basis as well as used when confronting a smoking trigger.

Relapse Prevention: It is important for a smoker to be taught to differentiate between a slip (e.g., a puff or a cigarette) vs. a relapse (return to previous rate of smoking) and to anticipate how to handle a slip or relapse. Preparation can be important in determining whether a slip remains a slip or converts into a relapse. If a relapse occurs, a smoker should resume the quitting process, as soon as he/she is ready.

2.8 Motivational Interviewing

Motivational interviewing (MI) is a skillful and empathic clinical style for eliciting from patients their own good motivations for making behavior change in the interest of their health [47]. It posits that, through trained strategic questioning and listening, a clinician can help patients resolve their ambivalence about behavior change, such as quitting smoking. The main goal of MI is to elicit one's own reasons for change—to create and amplify the discrepancy between a patient's behavior and broader goals. Discrepancy is developed through a skillful delivery of questions such as: Why do you want to quit smoking? What are you currently doing? What stops you from becoming smoke-free?

While MI is influenced by the Stages of Change Theory, Rogerian Patient Centered Therapy and cognitive-behavioral therapy, it is distinct in a number of ways. MI differs from the Stages of Change theory in that it conceptualizes motivation as a continuously fluctuating, nonlinear state. MI is akin to Rogerian therapy in its patient-centered approach, but differs in that it is directive, indeed, clinician directed. MI is also very goal-directed, with an ultimate goal to be attained, through negotiations with the clinicians and patient. During times of elevated motivation, CBT skills may be integrated with MI treatment, to apply action goals, such as cutting back on the number of cigarettes per day, or to target barriers to achieving smoking cessation goals, such as stress management practices to alleviate stress-related smoking triggers.

The theory underlying MI is that (1) Motivation is a fluctuating state, (2) The clinician style can determine patient success, (3) Ambivalence is an important part of change, and (4) Everyone has a potential for change. Through use of MI, a clinician uses a series of directive and nondirective approaches. MI aims to (1) build a patient's intrinsic motivation to change (e.g., quit smoking) and (2) resolve ambivalence about change (i.e., the goal of MI is to create and amplify the discrepancy between the patient's present behavior and broader goals). Simply put, to contrast where a patient is (e.g., nicotine dependent) and where a patient wants to be (e.g., nonsmoker). The four MI principles are: (1) Express Empathy (Skillful reflective listening is fundamental); (2) Develop Discrepancy (The patient should present the arguments for change); (3) Roll with Resistance (Avoid arguing for change); and (4) Support Self-Efficacy (The patient's own belief in his/her ability to change becomes a self-fulfilling prophecy). At each MI session, an assessment should be conducted of a patient's motivation and confidence (0–10), as well as the pros and cons to quitting and continuing to smoke. A 2010 meta-analysis was conducted to determine the effects of MI in promoting smoking cessation. Fourteen studies compared MI to brief advice or usual care for smoking cessation and concluded that MI yielded an increase in quitting (RR = 1.27; CI = 1.14–1.42 [48]). The effects of MI, compared with other treatments, however, are mixed.

2.9   Anxiety and Smoking

Anxiety disorders are significantly more prevalent among smokers than in the general population [10, 49]. Reported rates of smoking were highest among individuals with panic-related disorders (i.e., panic attacks, panic disorder, and agoraphobia) and other anxiety disorders in which panic attacks often occur (e.g., social anxiety disorder, posttraumatic stress disorder [PTSD], generalized anxiety disorder; [10]). There is also mounting evidence to suggest that the presence of anxiety disorders can interfere with one's ability to reap the benefit of smoking cessation programs and reduce the odds successful quitting [50]. In addition to diagnosable anxiety disorders, Anxiety Sensitivity, a cognitive risk factor for anxiety, has been associated with worse cessation outcomes [51]. These findings suggest that integrated treatment programs capable of addressing smoking cessation in the presence of co-occurring anxiety disorders or high levels of anxiety sensitivity may allow for improved cessation outcomes and a recent case report provides some preliminary evidence supporting this approach [52].

2.10   Mindfulness and Mind-Body Approaches

Mindfulness involves the self-regulation of attention toward, and nonjudgmental awareness of, present moment experiences [53]. It is most commonly defined as "paying attention in a particular way: on purpose, in the present moment, and non-judgmentally" [54]. Mindfulness involves several related but distinct skills, including the ability to (1) observe internal and external events as they occur in the present moment; (2) describe or label these events objectively; (3) act with awareness of the present moment; (4) accept present moment events without judgment; and (5) refrain from reacting impulsively to events. Mindfulness-based interventions help patients cultivate these skills through regular practice in formal (e.g., mindful sitting meditation, body scan meditation) and informal (e.g., mindful walking, mindful eating) mindfulness exercises.

One primary goal of mindfulness-based treatments for nicotine dependence is to increase awareness and acceptance of smoking cues as they occur in the moment. This awareness helps smokers tolerate smoking triggers and choose goal-directed behaviors (e.g., going for a walk vs. automatically smoking a cigarette when upset). Initially, the goal of mindfulness training is simply to become more aware of internal and external events. After bringing these events into conscious awareness, the goal becomes learning to relate to these experiences with openness, non-judgment, and curiosity. Treatment ultimately aims to teach patients to then "de-center" from these experiences by learning to view them as transient aspects of their awareness that may or may not need to be acted upon. For tobacco treatment, this de-centering process means learning to experience smoking triggers without automatically responding to them by smoking.

Mindfulness-based interventions generally take a cognitive-behavioral approach. However, they differ from standard cognitive-behavioral therapies in a few key ways. For example, mindfulness-based interventions aim to change the process of responding to smoking cues, rather than the content of the cues themselves. Additionally, mindfulness-based approaches incorporate a heavy focus on experiential learning in which a clinician helps the patient internalize important lessons from mindfulness or exposure exercises by reflecting key observations back to them (e.g., that a craving naturally subsided on its own during the meditation).

The structure of different mindfulness interventions can vary, though the content remains largely the same. Across interventions, the focus is generally on the role of negative affect and automatic thoughts in smoking, and how to use mindfulness skills to manage these experiences. Treatment typically begins by providing psychoeducation about the nature of addiction, the concept of mindfulness, and how mindful attention can interrupt addiction cycles. Formal meditations are often included in the first session. Over time, mindfulness exercises expand to include a focus on thoughts and emotions, and how they perpetuate smoking behavior. Techniques for applying mindfulness skills to smoking triggers are then highlighted throughout the treatment. For example, the Mindfulness Training for Smoking Cessation program utilizes the acronym RAIN (Recognize, Accept, Investigate, and Note cravings) to help smokers refrain from smoking in response to cravings [55].

2.10.1 Research Evidence Base for Mind-Body Interventions

Research supports the use of mind-body interventions. Previous studies have involved the application of standard mindfulness-based interventions for nicotine dependence (e.g., Mindfulness-Based Stress Reduction; [54]) and the development of smoking-specific mindfulness treatments (e.g., [55, 56]). Two studies comparing mindfulness training to the American Lung Association's (ALA) Freedom from Smoking (FFS) program [57] found similar abstinence rates immediately post-treatment but significantly higher abstinence rates in the mindfulness group at longer-term follow-ups [58]. A study comparing nicotine replacement therapy (NRT) to combination NRT and Acceptance and Commitment Therapy (ACT)—a behavioral intervention incorporating elements of mindfulness and acceptance—found no significant differences post-intervention, but significantly higher abstinence rates at 1-year follow-up in the NRT/ACT group [59]. Mindfulness training might provide unique benefits for relapse prevention.

Improvements in emotional outcomes may serve as mechanisms by which mindfulness training improves smoking outcomes. One study found that levels of acceptance post-treatment significantly mediated the effect of mindfulness training on smoking status at 1-year follow-up [60]. Several other studies have found that mindfulness training weakens or eliminates the relationship between negative affect and smoking urges [61, 62], as well as the relationship between cravings and smoking behavior [63]. These findings suggest that mindfulness training helps smokers break associations between aversive internal experiences and smoking, which likely contributes to decreased smoking behavior.

2.11 Specific Populations of Concern

2.11.1 Asthma

Cigarette smoking and asthma commonly co-occur. Prevalence rates of smoking have been shown to be higher among individuals with asthma as compared to those without, particularly for female smokers [64, 65]. For example, 35 % of asthma patients presenting to the emergency department for asthma problems were shown to be current smokers [66], which is substantially higher than the 22 % rate of the general population at that time [6]. Bidirectional associations between smoking and asthma also exist, with smoking serving as a risk factor for the later development of asthma [67]. Smoking among asthma patients is associated with a range of poor asthma outcomes, including decreased asthma control, increased asthma attacks and exacerbations, and increased risk of mortality [67]. Smoking cessation, however, can afford improvements in lung function and asthma symptoms [68, 69].

Smokers with asthma may differ from smokers without asthma in ways that are relevant to tobacco prevention and intervention efforts. There is some research to suggest that smokers with asthma have different risk factors for smoking, including different reasons for smoking and different expectations about what smoking will do for them [67]. For example, adolescents with asthma are more likely than adolescents without asthma to begin smoking due to peer pressure, and continue smoking for weight control reasons [70]. Among smokers, those with asthma have also been found to begin smoking at an earlier age, make more quit attempts, and be motivated to quit smoking in order to develop greater self-control [71].

Anxiety-related factors have been shown to play an important role in asthma-smoking associations. In general, lifetime prevalence rates for anxiety disorders are higher among individuals with asthma compared to those without (e.g., 24 % vs. 10 %, respectively; [72]), and higher among smokers compared to nonsmokers (e.g., 68 % vs. 5 %, respectively; [10]). Recent research suggests that these anxiety-related problems may actually be one of the key mechanisms by which asthma and smoking co-occur. For example, recent findings have shown that anxiety sensitivity mediates the relationship between an asthma diagnosis and smoking status [73]. Taken together, these findings highlight the importance of developing targeted tobacco treatments for asthma patients, and suggest that these treatments include a focus on anxiety-related problems.

2.11.2 Cancer Patients and Survivors

Tobacco use following a cancer diagnosis is prevalent and compromises treatment outcomes. About 10–30 % of cancer patients are smoking at the time of diagnosis [74–79]. Quitting smoking upon cancer diagnosis may improve cancer treatment effectiveness, reducing risk of recurrence and of developing new primary tumors [10–12, 19–22], and may improve chances of survival [75, 80, 81]. Continuing to smoke upon cancer diagnosis may result in diminished quality of life (e.g., elevated pain, shortness of breath; [75, 82]); cancer treatment delays; and increased complications from surgery, radiation, and chemotherapy [83–85]. Adverse effects from smoking at the time of surgery include complications from general anesthesia, increased risk of pulmonary complications, and impaired wound healing. Complications from smoking while undergoing radiation therapy include reduced cancer treatment efficacy and increased toxicity. Smoking while receiving chemotherapy exacerbates drug toxicity side effects and increases the incidence of infection [76, 86–92]. Continued smoking increases patients' vulnerability to subsequent smoking-related diseases following chest radiation [93, 94].

Cancer patients who smoke have socioeconomic, biologic, and psychosocial vulnerabilities. Individuals with lower incomes and education have much higher prevalence of smoking [7, 95]. One study in particular found that Cancer Care Outcomes Research and Surveillance Consortium (CanCORS) participants who were smoking at cancer diagnosis were less likely to have completed high school and more likely to be covered by public health insurance ($p < 0.001$; [78]). Low socioeconomic status increases an individual's risk for smoking initiation and continuation [96]. Moreover, cancer patients face increasing financial hardship [97]. Cancer patients who report current smoking at diagnosis are highly dependent smokers who need comprehensive tobacco treatment to successfully quit smoking. A pilot smoking cessation study of lung cancer patients at a large, city-based hospital found that, 77 % of smokers recruited from lung cancer clinics were nicotine dependent [98]. Furthermore, among CanCORS participants, the heaviest smokers were the most likely to continue smoking following diagnosis [78]. Cancer patients who continue to smoke after diagnosis are vulnerable to internalized stigma for causing their disease [99, 100]; in turn, these smokers who perceive high stigma are less likely to disclose their smoking status.

2.11.3 HIV/AIDS and Smoking

Smoking rates among people living with HIV are considerably higher than the smoking rates observed in the general population (i.e., 21 %; [101]). In fact, Niaura et al. [102] reported that over 70 % of HIV+ outpatients smoked on a daily basis. Prior to the widespread availability of protease inhibitors, smoking had been repeatedly related to poorer health outcomes in HIV, including significantly reduced survival [103], increased clinical progression to AIDS through more rapid development of pneumocystis carinii pneumonia [104], and increased likelihood of AIDS-related conditions such as community-acquired pneumonia, oral candidiasis, oral hairy leukoplakia, and AIDS-related dementia [105, 106]. The success of antiretroviral therapy in containing HIV viral replication, delaying symptom onset and clinical progression of HIV disease has resulted in an increase in chronic non-AIDS outcomes for patients managing HIV. Accordingly, smoking is playing an increasingly important role in the morbidity and mortality in people living with HIV [107]. For example, among patients living with HIV in San Francisco, smoking was associated with nearly a threefold increase in hazard ratio for death [108]. Similarly, studies have documented an increased risk of bacterial pneumonia, chronic obstructive pulmonary disease (COPD), cardiovascular disease, non-AIDS cancer, and mortality among HIV-infected smokers relative to HIV-infected nonsmokers [109–112]. The relationship between pneumonia and smoking in HIV is evident across the variety of risk groups. For example, among HIV-infected women with a history of IV drug use, smoking doubled the risk of bacterial pneumonia [113]. Similarly, among HIV-infected patients admitted to hospitals, smokers were three times more likely to have pneumocystis carinii pneumonia (PCP) and twice as likely to have bacterial pneumonia than nonsmokers [114]. Importantly, Benard, Mercie, Alioum et al. [115] found that smoking cessation dramatically reduced the risk of bacterial pneumonia regardless of HIV disease stage in HIV+ patients followed longitudinally for 5 years. There also is emerging evidence in diverse samples to suggest that HIV-infected smokers are less adherent to ART than nonsmokers [116, 117]. In a longitudinal study that followed over 900 HIV-infected women for up to 7.9 years, smoking was predictive of poorer medication adherence [118]. This study also found that smokers had poorer viral and immunologic response to highly active antiretroviral therapy (HAART), a greater risk of virologic rebound, and more frequent immunologic failure. More recent work by the same team identified the biological pathways associated with this impaired response to HAART demonstrating the adverse effects of smoking over and above poor adherence.

2.11.3.1 Smoking Cessation and HIV

To date, only a small number of randomized controlled trials examining the efficacy of smoking cessation interventions among HIV-infected adults have been conducted [119–122]. Vidrine and colleagues compared a combination of NRT plus eight sessions of counseling delivered via cell phone to usual care (NRT, self-help materials, physician advice to quit) in 95 HIV+ smokers. The cell phone intervention condition utilized cognitive-behavioral therapy principles (e.g., problem-solving, coping, and social support utilization) aiming to meet the needs if HIV-infected smokers, particularly anticipating HIV-related stressors. At 3 months post-quit date, abstinent rates were 36.8 % in the cell phone intervention condition relative to 10.3 % in the control condition, representing a significant difference. Lloyd-Richardson and colleagues randomized 444 participants to receive either standard care (SC, 2 brief sessions with a health educator)+NRT, or motivationally enhanced (ME) treatment (four sessions tailored to the needs of HIV+ individuals)+NRT. Abstinence rates at 2-, 4-, and 6-month follow-up ranged from 9 to 12% for the ME+NRT condition relative to 10–13% for the SC+NRT condition, indicating no significant difference. Ingersoll and colleagues also failed to detect significant differences between ME+NRT and standard care in 40 HIV-infected smokers; 22% of the full sample reported abstinence at 3-month follow-up. Collectively, these findings suggest that: (1) motivational interventions do not contribute significantly to the efficacy of NRT among HIV+ individuals; (2) there may be some benefit to targeting HIV-related stressors and related negative affect as part of smoking cessation programs for HIV+ individuals; and (3) there is a need for the development of interventions [123] that can yield durable positive smoking cessation outcomes in people living with HIV (see also PA-08-253: Unique Interactions Between Tobacco Use and HIV/AIDS).

2.11.4 Smoking Among Ethnic and Racial Minority Patients

Although the prevalence of tobacco use is lower among most racial and ethnic minority groups, blacks and Hispanics are at elevated risk of experiencing the negative health effects of smoking [124]. Specifically, blacks are disproportionally burdened by most of the tobacco-related cancers, including colon, breast, uterine, lung, and prostate cancers, compared to other racial and ethnic groups [124]. Similarly, cancer and heart disease remain two of the leading causes of death for Hispanics [125, 126]. While researchers speculate these disparities may be partially due to environmental and socioeconomic influences, blacks and Hispanics present with a distinctive behavioral profile that may increase their susceptibility for greater smoking-related morbidity and mortality. For instance, although blacks initiate smoking later, have fewer mean-pack years, and smoke fewer cigarettes per day compared to whites [127, 128], they have been shown to take longer and deeper puffs when smoking. In fact, the amount of nicotine and carcinogens consumed per cigarette has been shown to be 30% higher among blacks [129, 130]. In addition, blacks are more likely to smoke mentholated cigarettes, which also have higher levels of nicotine and carbon monoxide [131]. There is also emerging evidence that blacks may metabolize nicotine at a slower rate, thereby increasing the amount and length of time nicotine is in the body [132]. Hispanics share similar characteristics as blacks, often engaging in light or intermittent smoking. Importantly, although the overall smoking prevalence is typically low, smoking rates vary widely across this heterogeneous group [125]. For instance, Puerto Ricans and more acculturated Hispanics are more likely to resemble white smokers in terms of smoking prevalence and patterns of use [133].

While quitting smoking is a substantial challenge for most smokers, Hispanics and blacks are at increased risk for continued smoking. In particular, despite demonstrating greater intentions, confidence, and more attempts to quit, black and Hispanic smokers are less likely to receive quit advice and assistance from providers [125, 137]. They are also less likely to initiate, participate in, comply with tobacco treatment, and maintain abstinence after quitting [125, 134–137]. Among treatment-seekers, many refuse to utilize pharmacologic agents to assist cessation efforts as a result of fear, distrust, or misconceptions regarding the efficacy, utility, and safety of the medications [138–140]. In fact, a recent study by Fu and colleagues [136] determined that blacks were less likely to report ever having used NRT during a quit attempt (34 % of blacks vs. 50 % of whites). Treatment adherence is particularly difficult for Hispanics, who demonstrate low rates of compliance with treatment recommendations for other chronic illnesses [125]. Additional challenges that may interfere with treatment include the role of risk perceptions. Blacks and Hispanics have been evidenced to have lower knowledge about the risks associated with smoking and the benefits of smoking cessation [141, 142]; accordingly, they may not be motivated to quit as they may not be identified as a smoker.

Given these trends, providers engaging blacks and Hispanics in tobacco treatment will need to account for these racial and ethnic-specific factors in efforts to promote optimal cessation outcomes in these vulnerable groups. Important treatment targets should include psychoeducation around the risks associated with light smoking and the utility of smoking cessation medications. Motivational interviewing strategies will also be advantageous in helping identify and address their reasons for quitting, particularly since other factors, such as their family and children's health, may be driving their motivation to quit. Also, in light of evidence suggesting that blacks are more likely to live with a smoker and to be exposed to secondhand smoking, it may be important to assist them with providing cessation support to their partners.

2.11.5   Case Illustration

Below is a description of a telephone-based motivational treatment to assist cancer patients to quit smoking. The behavioral treatment was delivered in conjunction with FDA-approved smoking cessation medication, over a 6-month period. The treatment was delivered in a motivational style and included CBT and relaxation strategies. The patient completed all recommended sessions, within the allotted time period: four weekly sessions, followed by 4 biweekly sessions, with a final 3 monthly sessions. The initial session lasted for over 40 min; subsequent sessions were 20–30 min.

Patient Description at Intake. Evelyn is a 63-year-old married retired woman, who had smoked for 41 years. She had been diagnosed 3 weeks prior, with stage three lung cancer. At the start of treatment, she was smoking close to 20 ciga-rettes, or one pack of cigarettes, per day. She began her day by smoking, within 30 min of waking, which is a marker for nicotine addiction. She was in the "Contemplation" stage of quitting, but she reported that it was very important (10 on a scale of 0–10) for her to quit smoking. Her confidence to quit smoking was very low (2 on a scale of 0–10). In addition to smoking cigarettes, she had recently tried using e-cigs to help her quit. She, like most Americans who smoke, had tried to quit several times in the past. Her longest quit occurred 10 years prior and lasted for many months, but she relapsed due to work stressors. She was not cur-rently using any smoking cessation medications. Her husband was a former smoker, and there was a no smoking policy in their household and home; no one was allowed to smoke anywhere in their home or car. This was encouraging, as a smoke-free environment can help facilitate staying quit.

Evelyn was aware of some of the benefits of quitting (e.g., to decrease treatment complications) but was unaware of other potential benefits, such as protection from recurrence. She denied that her oncology providers had asked about or intervened upon her smoking. She described perceiving moderate (3 on a 1–5 scale of support) social support. She reported very low levels of psychological and physical symp-toms (distress, pain, fatigue, nausea) and mild levels of depression and anxiety (PHQ-9 = 8; GAD-7 = 5). However, she rated very high on illness stigma (e.g., "I feel others think I am to blame for my illness").

2.12 First Four Weekly Sessions

Initial Treatment Session (Importance to quit = 10; Confidence to quit = 2; Distress score = 8). Prior to the session, the counselor reviewed the patient's electronic medi-cal chart. She was just about to begin radiation treatment, and the uncertainty of the procedure and anticipatory pain made her very distressed. Her recent cancer diag-nosis made quitting of highest importance, but she was not confident that she could quit, since she had not made any recent smoking behavior changes. Evelyn and the tobacco counselor reviewed her past and current smoking behaviors and FDA approved smoking cessation medications (varenicline, bupropion, and combination NRT). She was not interested in taking additional oral medications and thus selected combination NRT (patch plus lozenge); given her current level of smoking, a 21 mg patch and 4 mg lozenge was dispensed. The clinician also reviewed the benefits of quitting at diagnosis and the potential harms of continued smoking. Pros and cons of continued smoking were elicited. Pros included a perceived calming effect and boredom; cons were the smell, shortness of breath, and health concerns. Barriers to quitting included having no other form of stress or boredom release. Benefits of quitting were to be and feel healthier and stronger.

Goal=Taper down 1 cigarette per day (CPD) and record CPD activity.

Session 2. (Importance to quit=10; Confidence to quit=2; Distress score=5). Evelyn had begun radiation treatment, and thus some of her anticipatory distress had diminished, and had tapered to 15 cigarettes per day but had not yet started the nicotine patches. She noticed a slight improvement in her shortness of breath. The health benefits for cancer patients quitting smoking were again discussed. She shared some negative self-talk ("I might not have the strength to do this too.") and concerns regarding her quitting goals.

Goal=Taper to 12 CPD, by limiting the number of CPD, and begin NRT.

Session 3: (Importance to quit=10; Confidence to quit=4; Distress score=4). Evelyn had completed her first round of radiation treatment. She was smoking 8–12 CPD and is entering the "Preparation" stage of quitting. She attributed her increase in confidence to her success at beginning to cut back; however, she was experiencing some back pain. She began using the patch and lozenge (as needed); the counselor discussed patient's concerns about "too much nicotine." Evelyn reported feeling itchy and obtained hydrocortisone cream. The clinician reviewed the ACE (Avoid, Change and Escape) strategies for dealing with triggers, which included taking a walk after meals, to break the end-of-meal pairing with cigarette and decreasing contact with people who caused stress. Evelyn reflected upon her social support; her husband was her primary source of emotional support and quitting support (e.g., "He does not nag me."); her sister, who once smoked herself, was also a strong source of quitting support.

Goal=Continue on patch and decrease to 9 cpd. Practice ACE. Quit date set for 2 weeks.

Session 4: (Importance to quit=10; Confidence to quit=2; Distress score=6). Evelyn was smoking 10–15 CPD. Her confidence to quit had decreased, since she had not been able to maintain her previous week's reduced smoking rate. Her distress had increased, as she had acclimated to the routine, and support, of ongoing cancer center visits, which was now absent, and waiting a month until her next scan was distressing. The clinician discussed the importance of decreasing to 10 CPD if her patch use were to continue in the same dosage. The importance of proper patch use and adherence was reviewed. The clinician emphasized the importance of decreasing to a 14 mg patch to decrease total nicotine intake and discussed increasing lozenge use if needed to cope with craving. Evelyn had continued to use the patch but itching persisted; she rotated the patch location to decrease itching. She discussed an increasing awareness of her cravings; the counselor and she reviewed how to apply Delay and Distraction techniques (from the 4Ds) to help with her cravings. In addition, the clinician introduced the topic of MINI relaxation exercises (Park et al., Psychosomatics), and Evelyn practiced a few of these.

Goal: Decrease to CPD and switch to 14 mg patch with PRN lozenges. Practice mini. Quit date postponed.

2.13 Four Biweekly Sessions

Session 5: (Importance to quit=10; Confidence to quit=4; Distress score=5). Evelyn was smoking 8–12 CPD. She used the 14 mg patch for a few days but was off of the patch at the time of session. She and the clinician reviewed self-management strategies from previous session, and Evelyn reported that the MINIS were very helpful. The clinician checked in to confirm that her house and car were still smoke-free and reinforced importance of maintaining a smoke-free environment. The counselor asked Evelyn about her beliefs on nicotine and addiction and reinforced importance of medication adherence. They discussed if Evelyn was experiencing any negative self-talk, particularly around quitting; the counselor reinforced the importance of continued positive self-talk. A Values Clarification exercise was introduced, in which the counselor elicited Evelyn's highest priorities; Evelyn identified being considerate of others among her priorities; she and the counselor discussed how becoming smoke-free (e.g., no exposing others to second or thirdhand smoke) was concordant with this perspective.

Goal: Taper to <10 cpd, consistently, every day.

Session 6: (Importance to quit=8; Confidence to quit=7; Distress score=2). The session began with an Appreciation exercise, in which Evelyn shared a few things which she was appreciative of for that week. Evelyn was smoking 12 CPD and is not using any NRT. She was feeling physically well and shared that her follow-up with a mammogram was in one more month. She attributed her slight decrease in importance in not being able to have quit yet, and the clinician elicited confident statements by reviewing her past accomplishments. Evelyn was using cutting back strategies to delay time between cigarettes, which the clinician encouraged her to continue to do. The clinician checked in on expressed smoking-related stigma and negative self-talk; Evelyn's negative talk was that she was not demanding enough of herself. She and the counselor constructed an "Energy Battery," which delineated her "drains" and "charges." Evelyn cited that her negative thoughts were drains and that practicing daily Appreciations and decreases in shortness of breath as charges. Evelyn was particularly appreciative of being able to attend a close friend's daughter's communion. She was not using alternative forms of tobacco or nicotine, but the dangers of light smoking were reviewed. The counselor emphasized the importance of utilizing social support and stress management strategies.

Goal=<10 CPD and work on positive self-talk.

Session 7: (Importance to quit=8; Confidence to quit=7; Distress score=2). Evelyn was still smoking 12 CPD. Her Appreciations included feeling productive, which she also identified as a charge on her energy battery. She and her counselor reviewed her social support, post-treatment support, and compared this to her support during treatment (i.e., her oncology team was very supportive). Now that treatment is finished, Evelyn expressed the need to find a senior group or other avenues of additional social interaction. She reported that her sleep is often disrupted by awakening due to coughing and breathing, which she identified as a drain on her energy battery. Reducing her cough and improving her breathing are big quit motivators.

Goal = <10 CPD and quit date set.

Session 8. (Importance to quit = 10; Confidence to quit = 6; Distress score = 4). Evelyn was still smoking 12 CPD and was not using any NRT patch or lozenge. Her clinician revisited the health benefits of quitting (decreased shortness of breath and coughing). Evelyn's Appreciation was her health; her mammogram results had been good. She and her counselor discussed the importance of tangible rewards to help with quitting efforts (computer games, creating a nice meal, track improved breathing). They discussed fear of cancer recurrence as a possible trigger to smoke and practiced MINI exercises.

Goal = set quit date with patch use.

2.14 Monthly Sessions

Session 9: (Importance to quit = 10; Confidence to quit/stay quit = 6; Distress score = 3). Evelyn was no longer smoking and had been quit for 2 weeks. She was using the 14 mg patch with no side effects. Her Appreciations included living in a smoke-free beautiful home and having social support. She reported noticeable improvements in her breathing, coughing, and sleep. The counselor conducted a didactic on differentiating smoking slips vs. relapses and normalization of slips. Evelyn expressed concerns about relapsing, and she and the counselor reviewed her ACE strategies for coping with triggers.

Goal = Stay smoke-free and reduce to 7 mg patch.

Session 10: (Importance to quit = 10; Confidence to quit = 10; Distress score = 3). Evelyn was smoke-free and no longer smoking or using the patch. She reported feeling healthier being smoke-free. She had no slips over the past month and described how she utilized her social support to help maintain her smoke-free status. She and the counselor reviewed coping strategies to deal with cravings and relapses.

Goal: Stay smoke-free.

Session 11: (Importance to quit = 10; Confidence to quit = 10; Distress score = 2). Evelyn remained smoke-free and feeling good. She reported minimal cravings and had not had a slip in the past month. Her confidence had increased and she was very proud of her work. She had joined a senior group and she takes time out during the week to prepare some special meals. She and the counselor reviewed the strategies that she had learned throughout the treatment and discussed continued utilization of relapse prevention strategies; Evelyn continued to her ACE, stress management skills, and accesses her support as needed.

References

1. U.S. Department of Health and Human Services. The health consequences of smoking—50 years of progress: a report of the surgeon general. Atlanta: U.S.: Department of Health and Human Services, Centers for Disease Control and Prevention, National Center for Chronic Disease Prevention and Health Promotion, Office on Smoking and Health; 2014.
2. Centers for Disease Control and Prevention. Prevalence of current smoking among adults aged 18 years and over: United States, 1997–June 2008. Atlanta: CDC; 2008.
3. Centers for Disease Control and Prevention. Annual smoking-attributable mortality, years of potential life lost, and productivity losses—United States, 2000–2004 (No. 57). Atlanta: CDC; 2008. p. 1226–8.
4. Centers for Disease Control and Prevention. History of the surgeon general's reports on smoking and health. Atlanta: Office on Smoking and Health, National Center for Chronic Disease Prevention and Health Promotion; 2009.
5. Pleis J, Lucas J, Ward B. Summary health statistics for U.S. adults: National Health Interview Survey, 2008. Vital Health Stat 10. 2009;242:1–157.
6. Centers for Disease Control and Prevention. Current cigarette smoking among adults—United States, 2005–2012 (No. 63). Atlanta: CDC; 2014. p. 29–34.
7. Centers for Disease Control and Prevention (CDC). Current cigarette smoking prevalence among working adults—United States, 2004–2010. MMWR Morb Mortal Wkly Rep. 2011;60(38):1305–9.
8. Centers for Disease Control and Prevention (CDC). Quitting smoking among adults—United States, 2001–2010. MMWR Morb Mortal Wkly Rep. 2011;60(44):1513–9.
9. Kassel JD, Stroud LR, Paronis CA. Smoking, stress, and negative affect: correlation, causation, and context across stages of smoking. Psychol Bull. 2003;129(2):270–304.
10. Lasser K, Boyd JW, Woolhandler S, Himmelstein DU, McCormick D, Bor DH. Smoking and mental illness: a population-based prevalence study. JAMA. 2000;284(20):2606–10.
11. Lawrence D, Hancock KJ, Kisely S. The gap in life expectancy from preventable physical illness in psychiatric patients in Western Australia: retrospective analysis of population based registers. BMJ. 2013;346:f2539.
12. Copeland AL, Brandon TH, Quinn EP. The smoking consequences questionnaire-adult: measurement of smoking outcome expectancies of experienced smokers. Psychol Assess. 1995;7(4):484–94. http://doi.org/10.1037/1040-3590.7.4.484.
13. Piper ME, Piasecki TM, Federman EB, Bolt DM, Smith SS, Fiore MC, Baker TB. A multiple motives approach to tobacco dependence: the Wisconsin Inventory of Smoking Dependence Motives (WISDM-68). J Consult Clin Psychol. 2004;72(2):139–54. http://doi.org/10.1037/0022-006X.72.2.139.
14. Kraemer KM, McLeish AC, Jeffries ER, Avallone KM, Luberto CM. Distress tolerance and perceived barriers to smoking cessation. Subst Abus. 2013;34(3):277–82. http://doi.org/10.1080/08897077.2013.771597.
15. Brown RA, Lejuez CW, Strong DR, Kahler CW, Zvolensky MJ, Carpenter LL, Niaura R, Price LH. A prospective examination of distress tolerance and early smoking lapse in adult self-quitters. Nicotine Tob Res. 2009;11(5):493–502. http://doi.org/10.1093/ntr/ntp041.
16. MacPherson L, Stipelman BA, Duplinsky M, Brown RA, Lejuez CW. Distress tolerance and pre-smoking treatment attrition: examination of moderating relationships. Addict Behav. 2008;33(11):1385–93. http://doi.org/10.1016/j.addbeh.2008.07.001.
17. Stead LF, Hartmann-Boyce J, Perera R, Lancaster T. Telephone counselling for smoking cessation. Cochrane Database Syst Rev. 2013;8, CD002850. http://doi.org/10.1002/14651858.CD002850.pub3.
18. Civljak M, Stead LF, Hartmann-Boyce J, Sheikh A, Car J. Internet-based interventions for smoking cessation. Cochrane Database Syst Rev. 2013;7, CD007078. http://doi.org/10.1002/14651858.CD007078.pub4.
19. Free C, Knight R, Robertson S, Whittaker R, Edwards P, Zhou W, Rodgers A, Cairns J, Kenward MG, Roberts I. Smoking cessation support delivered via mobile phone text messag-

ing (txt2stop): a single-blind, randomised trial. Lancet. 2011;378(9785):49–55. http://doi. org/10.1016/S0140-6736(11)60701-0.

20. Whittaker R, Borland R, Bullen C, Lin RB, McRobbie H, Rodgers A. Mobile phone-based interventions for smoking cessation. Cochrane Database Syst Rev. 2009;4, CD006611. http:// doi.org/10.1002/14651858.CD006611.pub2.

21. Abroms LC, Padmanabhan N, Thaweethai L, Phillips T. iPhone apps for smoking cessation: a content analysis. Am J Prev Med. 2011;40(3):279–85. http://doi.org/10.1016/j. amepre.2010.10.032.

22. Anthenelli RM, Morris C, Ramey TS, Dubrava SJ, Tsilkos K, Russ C, Yunis C. Effects of varenicline on smoking cessation in adults with stably treated current or past major depression: a randomized trial. Ann Intern Med. 2013;159(6):390–400. http://doi. org/10.7326/0003-4819-159-6-201309170-00005.

23. Thomas KH, Martin RM, Davies NM, Metcalfe C, Windmeijer F, Gunnell D. Smoking cessation treatment and risk of depression, suicide, and self harm in the Clinical Practice Research Datalink: prospective cohort study. BMJ. 2013;347:f5704.

24. Williams JM, Anthenelli RM, Morris CD, Treadow J, Thompson JR, Yunis C, George TP. A randomized, double-blind, placebo-controlled study evaluating the safety and efficacy of varenicline for smoking cessation in patients with schizophrenia or schizoaffective disorder. J Clin Psychiatry. 2012;73(5):654–60. http://doi.org/10.4088/JCP.11m07522.

25. Fiore M. Treating tobacco use and dependence: 2008 update: clinical practice guideline. Darby: DIANE Publishing; 2008.

26. Cahill K, Stevens S, Perera R, Lancaster T. Pharmacological interventions for smoking cessation: an overview and network meta-analysis. Cochrane Database Syst Rev. 2013;5, CD009329. http://doi.org/10.1002/14651858.CD009329.pub2.

27. Buller DB, Halperin A, Severson HH, Borland R, Slater MD, Bettinghaus EP, Tinkelman D, Cutter GR, Woodall WG. Effect of nicotine replacement therapy on quitting by young adults in a trial comparing cessation services. J Public Health Manag Pract. 2014;20(2):E7–15. http://doi.org/10.1097/PHH.0b013e3182a0b8c7.

28. Fiore MC, Baker TB. Stealing a march in the 21st century: accelerating progress in the 100-year war against tobacco addiction in the United States. Am J Public Health. 2009;99(7):1170–5. http://doi.org/10.2105/AJPH.2008.154559.

29. Cahill K, Stead LF, Lancaster T. Nicotine receptor partial agonists for smoking cessation. Cochrane Database Syst Rev. 2012;4, CD006103. http://doi.org/10.1002/14651858. CD006103.pub6.

30. Lundahl, B. The effectiveness and applicability of motivational interviewing: a practice-friendly review of four meta-analyses. Journal of Clinical Psychology. 2009; 65:1232.

31. Stead LF, Lancaster T. Behavioural interventions as adjuncts to pharmacotherapy for smoking cessation. Cochrane Database Syst Rev. 2012;12, CD009670. http://onlinelibrary.wiley. com/doi/10.1002/14651858.CD009670.pub2/abstract.

32. Stead LF, Lancaster T. Combined pharmacotherapy and behavioural interventions for smoking cessation. Cochrane Database Syst Rev. 2012;10, CD008286. http://doi. org/10.1002/14651858.CD008286.pub2.

33. U.S. Department of Health and Human Services. The health benefits of smoking cessation (No. DHHS Publication No. (CDC) 90-8416). U.S. Department of Health and Human Services. Public Health Service, Centers for Disease Control, Center for Chronic Disease Prevention and Health Promotion, Office on Smoking and Health. 1990.

34. Jardin BF, Cropsey KL, Wahlquist AE, Gray KM, Silvestri GA, Cummings KM, Carpenter MJ. Evaluating the effect of access to free medication to quit smoking: a clinical trial testing the role of motivation. Nicotine Tob Res. 2014;16(7):992–9. http://doi.org/10.1093/ntr/ ntu025.

35. Catz SL, Jack LM, McClure JB, Javitz HS, Deprey M, Zbikowski SM, McAfee T, Richards J, Swan GE. Adherence to varenicline in the COMPASS smoking cessation intervention trial. Nicotine Tob Res. 2011;13(5):361–8. http://doi.org/10.1093/ntr/ntr003.

36. Raupach T, Brown J, Herbec A, Brose L, West R. A systematic review of studies assessing the association between adherence to smoking cessation medication and treatment success. Addiction. 2014;109(1):35–43. http://doi.org/10.1111/add.12319.

37. Foulds J, Schmelzer AC, Steinberg MB. Treating tobacco dependence as a chronic illness and a key modifiable predictor of disease. Int J Clin Pract. 2010;64(2):142–6. http://doi.org/10.1111/j.1742-1241.2009.02243.x.

38. Schnoll RA, Engstrom PF. Tobacco control in the physician's office: a matter of adequate training and resources. J Natl Cancer Inst. 2004;96(8):573–5.

39. Liberman JN, Lichtenfeld MJ, Galaznik A, Mastey V, Harnett J, Zou KH, Leader JB, Kirchner HL. Adherence to varenicline and associated smoking cessation in a community-based patient setting. J Manag Care Pharm. 2013;19(2):125–31.

40. Smith SS, Keller PA, Kobinsky KH, Baker TB, Fraser DL, Bush T, Magnusson B, Zbikowski SM, McAfee TA, Fiore MC. Enhancing tobacco quitline effectiveness: identifying a superior pharmacotherapy adjuvant. Nicotine Tob Res. 2013;15(3):718–28. http://doi.org/10.1093/ntr/nts186.

41. Balmford J, Borland R, Hammond D, Cummings KM. Adherence to and reasons for premature discontinuation from stop-smoking medications: data from the ITC Four-Country Survey. Nicotine Tob Res. 2011;13(2):94–102. http://doi.org/10.1093/ntr/ntq215.

42. Nollen NL, Mayo MS, Ahluwalia JS, Tyndale RF, Benowitz NL, Faseru B, Buchanan TS, Cox LS. Factors associated with discontinuation of bupropion and counseling among African American light smokers in a randomized clinical trial. Ann Behav Med. 2013;46(3):336–48. http://doi.org/10.1007/s12160-013-9510-x.

43. Hays JT, Leischow SJ, Lawrence D, Lee TC. Adherence to treatment for tobacco dependence: association with smoking abstinence and predictors of adherence. Nicotine Tob Res. 2010;12(6):574–81. http://doi.org/10.1093/ntr/ntq047.

44. Berg CJ, Ahluwalia JS, Cropsey K. Predictors of adherence to behavioral counseling and medication among female prisoners enrolled in a smoking cessation trial. J Correct Health Care. 2013;19(4):236–47. http://doi.org/10.1177/1078345813499307.

45. Fucito LM, Toll BA, Salovey P, O'Malley SS. Beliefs and attitudes about bupropion: implications for medication adherence and smoking cessation treatment. Psychol Addict Behav. 2009;23(2):373–9. http://doi.org/10.1037/a0015695.

46. Stead LF, Lancaster T. Group behaviour therapy programmes for smoking cessation. Cochrane Database Syst Rev;(2), CD001007. http://doi.org/10.1002/14651858.CD001007.pub2.

47. Rollnick S, Miller WR, Butler CC, Aloia MS. Motivational interviewing in health care: helping patients change behavior. J Chron Obstruct Pulmon Dis. 2008;5(3):203. http://doi.org/10.1080/15412550802093108.

48. Lai DT, Cahill K, Qin Y, Tang J-L. Motivational interviewing for smoking cessation. Cochrane Database SystRev. 2010;(1):CD006936. http://onlinelibrary.wiley.com/doi/10.1002/14651858.CD006936.pub2/abstract.

49. Ziedonis DM, Hitsman B, Beckham JC, Zvolensky MJ, Adler LE, Audrain-McGovern J, et al. Tobacco use and cessation in psychiatric disorders: National Institute of Mental Health report. Nicotine Tob Res. 2008;10(12):1691–715.

50. Piper ME, Smith SS, Schlam TR, Fleming MF, Bittrich AA, Brown JL, et al. Psychiatric disorders in smokers seeking treatment for tobacco dependence: relations with tobacco dependence and cessation. J Consult Clin Psychol. 2010;78(1):13–23.

51. Pomerleau OF, Pomerleau CS, Marks JL. Abstinence effects and reactivity to nicotine during 11 days of smoking deprivation. Nicotine Tob Res. 2000;2(2):149–57.

52. Labbe AK, Wilner JG, Kosiba JD, Gonzalez A, Smits JA, Zvolensky MJ, Norton PJ, O'Cleirigh C. Demonstration of an integrated treatment for smoking cessation and anxiety symptoms in people with HIV: a clinical case study. Cogn Behav Pract. In Press.

53. Bishop SR, Lau M, Shapiro S, Carlson L, Anderson ND, Carmody J, Segal ZV, Abbey S, Speca M, Velting D, Devins G. Mindfulness: a proposed operational definition. Clin Psychol Sci Pract. 2004;11(3):230–41. http://doi.org/10.1093/clipsy.bph077.

54. Kabat-Zinn J. An outpatient program in behavioral medicine for chronic pain patients based on the practice of mindfulness meditation: theoretical considerations and preliminary results. Gen Hosp Psychiatry. 1982;4(1):33–47.

55. Brewer JA, Mallik S, Babuscio TA, Nich C, Johnson HE, Deleone CM, Minnix-Cotton CA, Byrne SA, Kober H, Weinstein AJ, Carroll KM, Rounsaville BJ. Mindfulness training for smoking cessation: results from a randomized controlled trial. Drug Alcohol Depend. 2011;119(1–2):72–80. http://doi.org/10.1016/j.drugalcdep.2011.05.027.

56. Davis JM, Mills DM, Stankevitz KA, Manley AR, Majeskie MR, Smith SS. Pilot randomized trial on mindfulness training for smokers in young adult binge drinkers. BMC Complement Altern Med. 2013;13:215. http://doi.org/10.1186/1472-6882-13-215.

57. American Lung Association. Freedom from smoking. 2010. http://www.lung.org/stop-smoking/how-to-quit/freedom-from-smoking/. Accessed 23 Jul 2015.

58. Davis JM, Manley AR, Goldberg SB, Smith SS, Jorenby DE. Randomized trial comparing mindfulness training for smokers to a matched control. J Subst Abuse Treat. 2014;47(3):213–21. http://doi.org/10.1016/j.jsat.2014.04.005.

59. Gifford EV, Kohlenberg BS, Hayes SC, Antonuccio DO, Piasecki MM, Rasmussen-Hall ML, Palm KM. Acceptance-based treatment for smoking cessation. Behav Ther. 2004;35(4):689–705. http://doi.org/10.1016/S0005-7894(04)80015-7.

60. Gifford EV, Kohlenberg BS, Hayes SC, Pierson HM, Piasecki MP, Antonuccio DO, Palm KM. Does acceptance and relationship focused behavior therapy contribute to bupropion outcomes? A randomized controlled trial of functional analytic psychotherapy and acceptance and commitment therapy for smoking cessation. Behav Ther. 2011;42(4):700–15. http://doi.org/10.1016/j.beth.2011.03.002.

61. Adams CE, Benitez L, Kinsaul J, Apperson McVay M, Barbry A, Thibodeaux A, Copeland AL. Effects of brief mindfulness instructions on reactions to body image stimuli among female smokers: an experimental study. Nicotine Tob Res. 2013;15(2):376–84. http://doi.org/10.1093/ntr/nts133.

62. Bowen S, Marlatt A. Surfing the urge: brief mindfulness-based intervention for college student smokers. Psychol Addict Behav. 2009;23(4):666–71. http://doi.org/10.1037/a0017127.

63. Elwafi HM, Witkiewitz K, Mallik S, Thornhill TA, Brewer JA. Mindfulness training for smoking cessation: moderation of the relationship between craving and cigarette use. Drug Alcohol Depend. 2013;130(1–3):222–9. http://doi.org/10.1016/j.drugalcdep.2012.11.015.

64. Backer V, Nepper-Christensen S, Ulrik CS, von Linstow M-L, Porsbjerg C. Factors associated with asthma in young Danish adults. Ann Allergy Asthma Immunol. 2002;89(2):148–54. http://doi.org/10.1016/S1081-1206(10)61930-8.

65. Langhammer A, Johnsen R, Holmen J, Gulsvik A, Bjermer L. Cigarette smoking gives more respiratory symptoms among women than among men. The Nord-Trondelag Health Study (HUNT). J Epidemiol Community Health. 2000;54(12):917–22.

66. Silverman RA, Boudreaux ED, Woodruff PG, Clark S, Camargo CA. Cigarette smoking among asthmatic adults presenting to 64 emergency departments. Chest. 2003;123(5):1472–9.

67. McLeish AC, Zvolensky MJ. Asthma and cigarette smoking: a review of the empirical literature. J Asthma. 2010;47(4):345–61. http://doi.org/10.3109/02770900903556413.

68. Chaudhuri R, Livingston E, McMahon AD, Lafferty J, Fraser I, Spears M, McSharry CP, Thomson NC. Effects of smoking cessation on lung function and airway inflammation in smokers with asthma. Am J Respir Crit Care Med. 2006;174(2):127–33. http://doi.org/10.1164/rccm.200510-1589OC.

69. Holm M, Omenaas E, Gíslason T, Svanes C, Jögi R, Norrman E, Janson C, Torén K, RHINE Study Group. Remission of asthma: a prospective longitudinal study from northern Europe (RHINE study). Eur Respir J. 2007;30(1):62–5. http://doi.org/10.1183/09031936.00121705.

70. Precht DH, Keiding L, Nielsen GA, Madsen M. Smoking among upper secondary pupils with asthma: reasons for their smoking behavior: a population-based study. J Adolesc Health. 2006;39(1):141–3. http://doi.org/10.1016/j.jadohealth.2005.10.012.

71. Avallone KM, McLeish AC, Zvolensky M, Kraemer KM, Luberto CM, Jeffries ER. Asthma and its relation to smoking behavior and cessation motives among adult daily smokers. J Health Psychol. 2012;1359105312456322. http://doi.org/10.1177/1359105312456322.

72. Strine TW, Mokdad AH, Balluz LS, Berry JT, Gonzalez O. Impact of depression and anxiety on quality of life, health behaviors, and asthma control among adults in the United States with asthma, 2006. J Asthma. 2008;45(2):123–33. http://doi.org/10.1080/02770900701840238.

73. Avallone KM, McLeish AC. Anxiety sensitivity as a mediator of the association between asthma and smoking. J Asthma. 2014;52(5):498–504. http://doi.org/10.3109/02770903.2014.984845.

74. Bellizzi KM, Rowland JH, Jeffery DD, McNeel T. Health behaviors of cancer survivors: examining opportunities for cancer control intervention. J Clin Oncol. 2005;23(34):8884–93. http://doi.org/10.1200/JCO.2005.02.2343.

75. Garces YI, Yang P, Parkinson J, Zhao X, Wampfler JA, Ebbert JO, Sloan JA. The relationship between cigarette smoking and quality of life after lung cancer diagnosis. Chest. 2004;126(6):1733–41. http://doi.org/10.1378/chest.126.6.1733.

76. Gritz E. Rationale for treating tobacco dependence in the cancer setting. Presented at the Treating Tobacco Dependence at the National Cancer Institute's Cancer Centers, Bethesda 2009.

77. Nishihara R, Morikawa T, Kuchiba A, Lochhead P, Yamauchi M, Liao X, Imamura Y, Nosho K, Shima K, Kawachi I, Qian ZR, Fuchs CS, Chan AT, Giovannucci E, Ogino S. A prospective study of duration of smoking cessation and colorectal cancer risk by epigenetics-related tumor classification. Am J Epidemiol. 2013;178(1):84–100. http://doi.org/10.1093/aje/kws431.

78. Park ER, Japuntich SJ, Rigotti NA, Traeger L, He Y, Wallace RB, Malin JL, Zallen JP, Keating NL. A snapshot of smokers after lung and colorectal cancer diagnosis. Cancer. 2012;118(12):3153–64. http://doi.org/10.1002/cncr.26545.

79. Yang H-K, Shin D-W, Park J-H, Kim S-Y, Eom C-S, Kam S, Choi JH, Cho BL, Seo H-G. The association between perceived social support and continued smoking in cancer survivors. Jpn J Clin Oncol. 2013;43(1):45–54. http://doi.org/10.1093/jjco/hys182.

80. Gritz ER, Fingeret MC, Vidrine DJ, Lazev AB, Mehta NV, Reece GP. Successes and failures of the teachable moment: smoking cessation in cancer patients. Cancer. 2006;106(1):17–27. http://doi.org/10.1002/cncr.21598.

81. Parsons AC, Shraim M, Inglis J, Aveyard P, Hajek P. Interventions for preventing weight gain after smoking cessation. Cochrane Database Syst Rev. 2009;(1): CD006219. http://doi.org/10.1002/14651858.CD006219.pub2.

82. Daniel M, Keefe FJ, Lyna P, Peterson B, Garst J, Kelley M, Bepler G, Bastian LA. Persistent smoking after a diagnosis of lung cancer is associated with higher reported pain levels. J Pain. 2009;10(3):323–8. http://doi.org/10.1016/j.jpain.2008.10.006.

83. Chen AM, Chen LM, Vaughan A, Sreeraman R, Farwell DG, Luu Q, Lau DH, Stuart K, Purdy JA, Vijayakumar S. Tobacco smoking during radiation therapy for head-and-neck cancer is associated with unfavorable outcome. Int J Radiat Oncol Biol Phys. 2011;79(2):414–9. http://doi.org/10.1016/j.ijrobp.2009.10.050.

84. Dresler CM. Is it more important to quit smoking than which chemotherapy is used? Lung Cancer. 2003;39(2):119–24.

85. Shen T, Le W, Yee A, Kamdar O, Hwang PH, Upadhyay D. Nicotine induces resistance to chemotherapy in nasal epithelial cancer. Am J Rhinol Allergy. 2010;24(2):e73–7. http://doi.org/10.2500/ajra.2010.24.3456.

86. Gritz ER, Dresler C, Sarna L. Smoking, the missing drug interaction in clinical trials: ignoring the obvious. Cancer Epidemiol Biomarkers Prev. 2005;14(10):2287–93. http://doi.org/10.1158/1055-9965.EPI-05-0224.

87. McBride CM, Ostroff JS. Teachable moments for promoting smoking cessation: the context of cancer care and survivorship. Cancer Control. 2003;10(4):325–33.

88. Tsurutani J, Castillo SS, Brognard J, Granville CA, Zhang C, Gills JJ, Sayyah J, Dennis PA. Tobacco components stimulate Akt-dependent proliferation and NFkappaB-dependent survival in lung cancer cells. Carcinogenesis. 2005;26(7):1182–95. http://doi.org/10.1093/carcin/bgi072.

89. Vaporciyan AA, Merriman KW, Ece F, Roth JA, Smythe WR, Swisher SG, Walsh GL, Nesbitt JC, Putnam JB. Incidence of major pulmonary morbidity after pneumonectomy: association with timing of smoking cessation. Ann Thorac Surg. 2002;73(2):420–5; discussion 425–426.

90. Xu J, Huang H, Pan C, Zhang B, Liu X, Zhang L. Nicotine inhibits apoptosis induced by cisplatin in human oral cancer cells. Int J Oral Maxillofac Surg. 2007;36(8):739–44. http://doi.org/10.1016/j.ijom.2007.05.016.

91. Zevallos JP, Mallen MJ, Lam CY, Karam-Hage M, Blalock J, Wetter DW, Garden AS, Sturgis EM, Cinciripini PM. Complications of radiotherapy in laryngopharyngeal cancer: effects of a prospective smoking cessation program. Cancer. 2009;115(19):4636–44. http://doi.org/10.1002/cncr.24499.

92. Zhang J, Kamdar O, Le W, Rosen GD, Upadhyay D. Nicotine induces resistance to chemotherapy by modulating mitochondrial signaling in lung cancer. Am J Respir Cell Mol Biol. 2009;40(2):135–46. http://doi.org/10.1165/rcmb.2007-0277OC.

93. Adams MJ, Lipshultz SE, Schwartz C, Fajardo LF, Coen V, Constine LS. Radiation-associated cardiovascular disease: manifestations and management. Semin Radiat Oncol. 2003;13(3):346–56. http://doi.org/10.1016/S1053-4296(03)00026-2.

94. Clemak A, Li S, Marur S, Zhao W, Westra W, Chung C, et al. E1308: Reduced-dose IMRT in human papilloma virus (HPV)-associated resectable oropharyngeal squamous carcinomas (OPSCC) after clinical complete response (cCR) to induction chemotherapy (IC). Oral Presentation presented at the 50th Annual Meeting of the ASCO. 2014.

95. Hiscock R, Bauld L, Amos A, Fidler JA, Munafò M. Socioeconomic status and smoking: a review.AnnNYAcadSci.2012;1248(1):107–23.http://doi.org/10.1111/j.1749-6632.2011.06202.x.

96. Kanjilal S, Gregg EW, Cheng YJ, Zhang P, Nelson DE, Mensah G, Beckles GLA. Socioeconomic status and trends in disparities in 4 major risk factors for cardiovascular disease among US adults, 1971–2002. Arch Intern Med. 2006;166(21):2348–55. http://doi.org/10.1001/archinte.166.21.2348.

97. Collins LG, Wender R, Altshuler M. An opportunity for coordinated cancer care: intersection of health care reform, primary care providers, and cancer patients. Cancer J. 2010;16(6):593–9. http://doi.org/10.1097/PPO.0b013e3181feee9a.

98. Park ER, Japuntich S, Temel J, Lanuti M, Pandiscio J, Hilgenberg J, Davies D, Dresler C, Rigotti NA. A smoking cessation intervention for thoracic surgery and oncology clinics: a pilot trial. J Thorac Oncol. 2011;6(6):1059–65. http://doi.org/10.1097/JTO.0b013e318215a4dc.

99. Chapple A, Ziebland S, McPherson A. Stigma, shame, and blame experienced by patients with lung cancer: qualitative study. BMJ. 2004;328(7454):1470. http://doi.org/10.1136/bmj.38111.639734.7C.

100. Else-Quest NM, LoConte NK, Schiller JH, Hyde JS. Perceived stigma, self-blame, and adjustment among lung, breast and prostate cancer patients. Psychol Health. 2009;24(8):949–64. http://doi.org/10.1080/08870440802074664.

101. Centers for Disease Control and Prevention (CDC). Cigarette smoking among adults-United States, 2006. MMWR Morb Mortal Wkly Rep. 2007;56(44):1157.

102. Niaura RS, Shadel WG, Morrow K, Tashima K, Flanigan T, Abrams DB, et al. Human immunodeficiency virus infection, AIDS, and smoking cessation: the time is now. Clin Infect Dis. 2000;31(3):808–12.

103. Page-Shafer K, Delorenze GN, Satariano WA, Winkelstein W. Comorbidity and survival in HIV-infected men in the San Francisco Men's Health Survey. Ann Epidemiol. 1996;6(5):420–30.

104. Nieman RB, Fleming J, Coker RJ, Harris JR, Mitchell DM. The effect of cigarette smoking on the development of AIDS in HIV-1-seropositive individuals. AIDS. 1993;7(5):705–10.

105. Burns DN, Hillman D, Neaton JD, Sherer R, Mitchell T, Capps L, et al. Cigarette smoking, bacterial pneumonia, and other clinical outcomes in HIV-1 infection. J Acquir Immune Defic Syndr Hum Retrovirol. 1996;13(4):374–83.

106. Conley LJ, Bush TJ, Buchbinder SP, Penley KA, Judson FN, Holmberg SD, et al. The association between cigarette smoking and selected HIV-related medical conditions. AIDS. 1996;10(10):1121–6.

107. Marshall MM, McCormack MC, Kirk GD. Effect of cigarette smoking on HIV acquisition, progression, and mortality. AIDS Educ Prev. 2009;21(3 Suppl):28–39.
108. Cockerham L, Scherzer R, Zolopa A. Association of HIV infection, demographic and cardio-vascular risk factors with all-cause mortality in the recent HAART Era. JAIDS. 2010;53(1):102–6.
109. Crothers K, Goulet JL, Rodriguez-Barradas MC, Gibert CL, Oursler KA, Goetz MB, et al. Impact of cigarette smoking on mortality in HIV-positive and HIV-negative veterans. AIDS Educ Prev. 2009;21(3 Suppl):40–53.
110. Crothers K, Griffith TA, McGinnis KA, Rodriguez-Barradas MC, Leaf DA, Weissman S, et al. The impact of cigarette smoking on mortality, quality of life, and comorbid illness among HIV-positive veterans. J Gen Intern Med. 2005;20(12):1142–5.
111. Cui Q, Carruthers S, McIvor A, Smaill F, Thabane L, Smieja M, et al. Effect of smoking on lung function, respiratory symptoms and respiratory diseases amongst HIV-positive subjects: a cross-sectional study. AIDS Res Ther. 2010;7:6.
112. Lifson AR, Neuhas J, Arribas JR, Van der Berg-Wolf M, Labriola AM, Read TR, INSIGH SMART Study Group. Smoking-related health risks among persons with HIV in the strate-gies or management of antiretroviral therapy clinical trial. Am J Public Health. 2010;100:1896–902.
113. Kohli R, Lo Y, Homel P, Flanigan T, Gardner LI, Howard AA, et al. Bacterial pneumonia, HIV therapy, and disease progression among HIV-infected women in the HIV epidemiologic research (HER) study. Clin Infect Dis. 2006;43(1):90–8.
114. Miguez-Burbano MJ, Flores M, Ashkin D, Rodriguez A, Granada AM, Quintero N, Pitchenik A. Non-tuberculous mycobacteria disease as a cause of hospitalization in HIV-infected sub-jects. Int J Infect Dis. 2006;10(1):47–55.
115. Bénard A, Mercié P, Alioum A, Bonnet F, Lazaro E, Dupon M, et al. Bacterial pneumonia among HIV-infected patients: decreased risk after tobacco smoking cessation. ANRS CO3 Aquitaine Cohort, 2000–2007. PLoS One. 2010;5(1):e8896.
116. Shuter J, Bernstein S. Cigarette smoking is an independent predictor of nonadherence in HIV-infected individuals receiving highly active antiretroviral therapy. Nicotine Tob Res. 2008;10(4):731–6.
117. Webb MS, Vanable PA, Carey MP, Blair DC. Cigarette smoking among HIV+ men and women: examining health, substance use, and psychosocial correlates across the smoking spectrum. J Behav Med. 2007;30(5):371–83.
118. Feldman JG, Minkoff H, Schneider MF, Gange SJ, Cohen MH, Watts DH, et al. Association of cigarette smoking with HIV prognosis among women in the HAART era: a report from the women's interagency HIV study. Am J Public Health. 2006;96(6):1060–5.
119. Ingersoll KS, Cropsey KL, Heckman CJ. A test of motivational plus nicotine replacement interventions for HIV positive smokers. AIDS Behav. 2009;13(3):545–54.
120. Lloyd-Richardson EE, Stanton CA, Papandonatos GD, Shadel WG, Stein MB, Tashima K, et al. Motivation and patch treatment for HIV+ smokers: a randomized controlled trial. Addiction. 2009;104(11):1891–900.
121. Vidrine DJ, Arduino RC, Lazev AB, Gritz ER. A randomized trial of a proactive cellular telephone intervention for smokers living with HIV/AIDS. AIDS. 2006;20(2):253–60.
122. Stanton CA, Papandonatos GD, Shuter J, Bicki A, Lloyd-Richardson EE, de Dios MA, Morrow KM, Makgoeng SB, Tashima KT, Niaura RS. Outcomes of a tailored intervention for cigarette smoking cessation among Latinos living with HIV/AIDS. Nicotine Tob Res. 2015;17(8):975–82.
123. Harris JK. Connecting discovery and delivery: the need for more evidence on effective smok-ing cessation strategies for people living with HIV/AIDS. Am J Public Health. 2010;100(7):1245–9.
124. American Cancer Society. Cancer facts and figures 2013. 2013. http://www.cancer.org/research/cancerfactsfigures/cancerfactsfigures/cancer-facts-figures-2013. Accessed 23 Jul 2015.

125. de Dios MA, Anderson BJ, Stanton C, Audet DA, Stein M. Project impact: a pharmacotherapy pilot trial investigating the abstinence and treatment adherence of Latino light smokers. J Subst Abuse Treat. 2012;43(3):322–30. http://doi.org/10.1016/j.jsat.2012.01.004.
126. Park E. Overestimation and underestimation: adolescents' weight perception in comparison to BMI-based weight status and how it varies across socio-demographic factors. J Sch Health. 2011;81(2):57–64. http://doi.org/10.1111/j.1746-1561.2010.00561.x.
127. Finkenauer R, Pomerleau CS, Snedecor SM, Pomerleau OF. Race differences in factors relating to smoking initiation. Addict Behav. 2009;34(12):1056–9. http://doi.org/10.1016/j.addbeh.2009.06.006.
128. Trinidad DR, Gilpin EA, Lee L, Pierce JP. Has there been a delay in the age of regular smoking onset among African Americans? Ann Behav Med. 2004;28(3):152–7. http://doi.org/10.1207/s15324796abm2803_2.
129. Rubinstein ML, Shiffman S, Rait MA, Benowitz NL. Race, gender, and nicotine metabolism in adolescent smokers. Nicotine Tob Res. 2013;15(7):1311–5. http://doi.org/10.1093/ntr/nts272.
130. Trinidad DR, Pérez-Stable EJ, Emery SL, White MM, Grana RA, Messer KS. Intermittent and light daily smoking across racial/ethnic groups in the United States. Nicotine Tob Res. 2009;11(2):203–10. http://doi.org/10.1093/ntr/ntn018.
131. Williams JM, Gandhi KK, Steinberg ML, Foulds J, Ziedonis DM, Benowitz NL. Higher nicotine and carbon monoxide levels in menthol cigarette smokers with and without schizophrenia. Nicotine Tob Res. 2007;9(8):873–81. http://doi.org/10.1080/14622200701484995.
132. Benowitz NL, Herrera B, Jacob P. Mentholated cigarette smoking inhibits nicotine metabolism. J Pharmacol Exp Ther. 2004;310(3):1208–15. http://doi.org/10.1124/jpet.104.066902.
133. Covey LS, Botello-Harbaum M, Glassman AH, Masmela J, LoDuca C, Salzman V, Fried J. Smokers' response to combination bupropion, nicotine patch, and counseling treatment by race/ethnicity. Ethn Dis. 2008;18(1):59–64.
134. Cokkinides VE, Halpern MT, Barbeau EM, Ward E, Thun MJ. Racial and ethnic disparities in smoking-cessation interventions: analysis of the 2005 National Health Interview Survey. Am J Prev Med. 2008;34(5):404–12. http://doi.org/10.1016/j.amepre.2008.02.003.
135. Croghan IT, Hurt RD, Ebbert JO, Croghan GA, Polk OD, Stella PJ, Novotny PJ, Sloan J, Loprinzi CL. Racial differences in smoking abstinence rates in a multicenter, randomized, open-label trial in the United States. Z Gesundh Wiss. 2010;18(1):59–68. http://doi.org/10.1007/s10389-009-0277-2.
136. Fu SS, Sherman SE, Yano EM, van Ryn M, Lanto AB, Joseph AM. Ethnic disparities in the use of nicotine replacement therapy for smoking cessation in an equal access health care system. Am J Health Promot. 2005;20(2):108–16. http://doi.org/10.4278/0890-1171-20.2.108.
137. Park ER, Japuntich SJ, Traeger L, Cannon S, Pajolek H. Disparities between blacks and whites in tobacco and lung cancer treatment. Oncologist. 2011;16(10):1428–34. http://doi.org/10.1634/theoncologist.2011-0114.
138. Carpenter MJ, Ford ME, Cartmell K, Alberg AJ. Misperceptions of nicotine replacement therapy within racially and ethnically diverse smokers. J Natl Med Assoc. 2011;103(9–10):885–94.
139. Ryan KK, Garrett-Mayer E, Alberg AJ, Cartmell KB, Carpenter MJ. Predictors of cessation pharmacotherapy use among black and non-Hispanic white smokers. Nicotine Tob Res. 2011;13(8):646–52. http://doi.org/10.1093/ntr/ntr051.
140. Yerger VB, Wertz M, McGruder C, Froelicher ES, Malone RE. Nicotine replacement therapy: perceptions of African-American smokers seeking to quit. J Natl Med Assoc. 2008;100(2):230–6.
141. Honda K, Neugut AI. Associations between perceived cancer risk and established risk factors in a national community sample. Cancer Detect Prev. 2004;28(1):1–7. http://doi.org/10.1016/j.cdp.2003.12.001.
142. Lyna P, McBride C, Samsa G, Pollak KI. Exploring the association between perceived risks of smoking and benefits to quitting: who does not see the link? Addict Behav. 2002;27(2):293–307.

Resources

Websites

www.lung.org/stop-smoking
www.cancer.gov/cancertopics/tobacco
Smokefree.gov
www.cancer.gov/cancertopics/factsheet/Tobacco/symptoms-triggers-quitting
www.quitnet.com
Smokefree.gov/quit-plan

Chapter 3
Cognitive-Behavioral Management of Obesity

Noreen A. Reilly-Harrington, Stephanie S. Sogg, Rachel A. Millstein, and Mark J. Gorman

3.1 Introduction

3.1.1 Prevalence and Definition of Obesity

Approximately 69 % of adults in the United States meet criteria for being either overweight or obese, with approximately 35 % meeting criteria for obesity [1]. There is evidence that the epidemic of obesity is steadily and globally spreading [2]. Obesity is a multifactorial disease with a complex interplay of genetic, environmental, and behavioral causes. An increasingly large body of empirical evidence demonstrates that there are strong biological influences implicated in the development of obesity. Obesity has been called "among the most heritable of human traits" [3], with an estimated 45–75 % of individual differences in body mass index (BMI) attributable to heritable factors, as genetic factors have been found to influence multiple and varied determinants of body weight [3]. Behavioral factors, of course, play a substantial role in determining body weight, but even ostensibly volitional behaviors related to weight are driven by a variety of underlying biological substrates [3–5].

N.A. Reilly-Harrington, Ph.D. (✉) • S.S. Sogg, Ph.D. • M.J. Gorman, Ph.D.
Department of Psychiatry, Massachusetts General Hospital Weight Center,
50 Staniford Street, 4th Floor, Boston, MA 02114, USA
e-mail: Nharrington11@mgh.harvard.edu; nhreilly@partners.org; ssogg@partners.org

R.A. Millstein, Ph.D., M.H.S.
Behavioral Medicine Service, Department of Psychiatry, Massachusetts General Hospital,
Harvard Medical School, Boston, MA, USA
e-mail: ramillstein@mgh.harvard.edu

© Springer Science+Business Media New York 2017
A.-M. Vranceanu et al. (eds.), *The Massachusetts General Hospital
Handbook of Behavioral Medicine*, Current Clinical Psychiatry,
DOI 10.1007/978-3-319-29294-6_3

The BMI, which is calculated as weight (kg) divided by height $(m)^2$, serves as a proxy for body fat and related health risks [6]. A BMI of 18.5–24.9 kg/m^2 is considered to be in the "healthy" range. "Overweight" is defined as a BMI from 25 to 29.9 kg/m^2 and "obesity" is defined as a BMI of 30 kg/m^2 or greater. Obesity severity can be further categorized into the following subclasses: Class I: BMI 30.0–34.9, Class II: BMI 35.0–39.9, Class III: BMI $\geq$ 40, with each class progressively carrying higher disease risk.

3.1.2 Medical and Psychosocial Comorbidities

Obesity has an impact on nearly every system in the human body. Obesity raises the risk of hypertension, dyslipidemia, type 2 diabetes mellitus, coronary heart disease, stroke, gallbladder disease, osteoarthritis, sleep apnea and respiratory problems, and some cancers [7]. For every 5 unit increase in BMI beyond a BMI of 25 kg/m^2, there is a 29 % increase in all-cause mortality, a 41 % increase in vascular-related mortality, and a 200 % increase in mortality related to diabetes [8]. However, BMI alone may not be the most accurate predictor of adiposity-related risk, since it is not as sensitive an index of visceral adiposity, which is a more direct threat to health, than are, for instance, waist circumference (WC) or waist-to-hip ratio (WHR) [9]. For instance, central adiposity is also a predictor of all-cause mortality, independent of the influence of BMI [8].

Patients with severe obesity have been found to endorse higher rates of psychopathology than individuals with healthy weight or those with milder obesity [10, 11]. Specifically, higher current and lifetime rates of mood disorders (e.g., unipolar depression and bipolar disorder) and anxiety disorders (e.g., PTSD, social phobia, panic disorder) have been reported in those with severe obesity [10]. Additionally, patients seeking treatment for obesity tend to have higher rates of psychopathology than individuals with obesity in community samples [10, 12]. In particular, the highest rates of psychopathology are found in patients seeking medical treatments for obesity (e.g., surgery or pharmacotherapy), as compared to those patients seeking behavioral treatment for obesity [13]. The etiological pathways between obesity and psychopathology have been most thoroughly studied for depression. Longitudinal studies suggest that the causal pathways are bidirectional; that is, depression appears to increase the risk for subsequent development of obesity, and obesity increases the risk for the onset of depression [14]. Depression and obesity also each affect the course of the other condition—for instance, weight loss tends to be associated with a decrease in depression, while current depression is associated with poorer outcomes in weight loss treatment [14]. These causal pathways are likely multifactorial. Symptoms of various psychiatric disorders (low energy, anhedonia, changes in appetite) may lead to behaviors that contribute to weight gain or pose barriers to weight loss, and many psychotropic medications are weight promoting. Animal studies suggest that a high-fat diet may increase depression and anxiety symptoms [15]. Conversely, obesity may promote psychopathological symptoms through its impact on pain, poor health, impaired functioning, weight-related discrimination and stigma, and poor body image, and/or through the perturbation of hormonal pathways [16].

Individuals from lower socioeconomic groups are disproportionately affected by obesity, [17] as well as those from certain racial and ethnic minority groups. For example, African American and Mexican American women have a higher prevalence of obesity than Caucasian women or than men of any ethnic background [7]. There is also some evidence that individuals from certain ethnic minority groups, such as African American women, may lose less weight when participating in behavioral weight loss interventions, particularly when such programs lack specific cultural adaptations [18].

This chapter provides an overview of cognitive-behavioral strategies for weight management, as well as tools for treating binge and emotional eating. Cognitive and behavioral strategies will be a main focus of this chapter, given the strong evidence base that supports the use of these techniques in weight loss and management [19]. As obesity has complex, multifactorial causes, the importance of a thorough initial assessment is discussed. Specific treatment concerns based on demographics and comorbid medical conditions are presented. Finally, a case example will be included to illustrate the use of the techniques described.

3.2 Treatment

3.2.1 Overview and Empirical Evidence for the Role of CBT in the Treatment of Obesity

Obesity can be viewed as a chronic, treatment-resistant condition. Given the strong biological etiology of obesity, even "gold-standard" behavioral weight loss approaches, delivered to highly selected participants in an academic medical center tend to achieve a mean short-term weight loss of approximately 10 % of initial body weight, with weight regain commonly observed at longer term follow-up [20]. However, while cognitive behavioral interventions may not realistically be expected to "cure" obesity, even a reduction of as little as 5 % of initial body weight is helpful in reducing health risks [21]. Further, given the progressive nature of obesity, even an intervention that is effective in halting further weight gain is of significant value to the patient's health [22]. In addition, cognitive-behavioral approaches are of great value in addressing a number of factors that either contribute to, or result from obesity. Thus, the goals of cognitive-behavioral intervention for patients with obesity include not only weight loss per se but also focus on normalizing and regulating eating behaviors, addressing body image issues, preventing weight gain, and improving overall health by facilitating behavior change.

3.2.2   Assessment

Because obesity is an extremely complex, multifactorial condition, a detailed bio-psychosocial assessment is an essential first step, in order to identify potential domains for intervention (see Table 3.1). This type of multidisciplinary, multifaceted assessment would include professionals from medical, psychological, nutrition, and potentially social work fields. There are barriers and facilitators to treatment at each level of the biopsychosocial model. We will review each level in more depth and describe the necessary domains for a thorough assessment. Genetic factors, medical comorbidities, and family history are basic considerations at the biological level. At the psychological level, clinicians would assess for subclinical and higher levels of mental health symptoms both precipitating or resulting from excess weight. Preceding any psychosocial treatment for obesity, there must also be a detailed assessment of what the current barriers may be to making and sustaining behavior change. These barriers may range from practical or logistical issues to interpersonal, emotional, or psychological factors. As social-level factors also play important roles in maintaining behavior or facilitating change, clinicians would want to assess social support, availability of healthy foods and activity spaces, and social norms around eating and exercise. Interventions are more likely to be effective when they are tailored to address the particular factors that are contributing to an individual's obesity. Following we summarize the main domains of assessment for patients with obesity presenting to weight loss programs.

Eating-related factors are significant contributors to obesity in many cases, and these can range from simple maladaptive eating habits to eating disorder symptoms. Patients entering treatment for weight loss should be assessed for both eating disorder symptoms as well as a variety of weight-promoting eating patterns, such as meal-skipping, unstructured and frequent snacking, consuming large portions, obtaining many meals/snacks outside the home, and choosing unhealthy types of food. These patterns are often best addressed with a behavioral problem-solving approach, with a particular focus on the barriers preventing patients from engaging in more healthy eating behaviors. However, some patients with obesity engage in "emotional eating," or eating as a way of coping with negative emotions. Some patients with obesity present with eating disorder symptoms, with binge eating (BE) and binge eating disorder (BED) being the most common eating disorder symptoms among people with obesity [43]. These patterns may be most effectively addressed with an intervention designed specifically to improve coping skills and directly target binge eating.

Physical activity patterns also play an important role in weight regulation. Assessment of physical activity includes both the patient's past and current patterns of structured physical activity (e.g., going to the gym, taking walks, etc.), and the unstructured activity that occurs as part of daily living and/or on the job (e.g., walking to the train as part of one's commute). As noted earlier in the discussion of eating behaviors, it is also crucial to examine the nature of any current barriers to engaging in consistent physical activity, particularly since physical activity has consistently been found to be associated with better weight control both at short- and long-term follow-up [44].

Table 3.1 A multidisciplinary approach to obesity assessment within a biopsychosocial framework

Domain	Constructs of interest	Example measures (general and disorder specific)
Biological	Current weight	• Weight, BMI
	Weight history/trajectory	• Blood pressure, cardiac screening
	Personal medical history, comorbidities	• Blood tests (cholesterol, lipids, endocrine function)
	Family weight and medical history	
Psychological, including weight and eating concerns	Depression, anxiety/PTSD	• Structured clinical interview (i.e., SCID, MINI) [23] • Depression: Patient Health Questionnaire (PHQ-9) [24] • Beck Depression Inventory (BDI)-II [25] • Anxiety: Beck Anxiety Inventory [26] • Stress: Depression Anxiety and Stress Scale (DASS-21) [27], • Perceived Stress Scale (PSS) [28] • PTSD: PTSD Checklist-Civilian (PCL-C) [29]
	Dieting history, current eating patterns	• Food frequency questionnaires (examples can be found at http://appliedresearch.cancer.gov/diet/shortreg/register.php) • Dietary recalls/food diaries (examples can be found at https://fnic.nal.usda.gov/surveys-reports-and-research/research-tools/dietary-assessment-instruments-research)
	Body image	• Multidimensional Body-Self Relations Questionnaire (MBSRQ) [30]
	Disordered eating (including anorexia nervosa, bulimia nervosa, binge eating disorder, eating disorder NOS)	• Eating Attitudes Test (EAT-26) [31] • Eating Disorder Inventory (EDI-3) [32]
	Current and past physical activity habits	• Physical Activity Readiness Questionnaire (PAR-Q) [33] • International Physical Activity Questionnaire (IPAQ) [34]
	Weight loss readiness/motivation	• Weight loss readiness test-II [35]
	Pain	• PROMIS Pain interference short-form [36] • Brief pain inventory [37]

(continued)

Table 3.1 (continued)

Domain	Constructs of interest	Example measures (general and disorder specific)
Social environment	Family structure	• Social support (general) (ESSI) [38]
	Social support (general)	• Social support for diet, exercise [39]
	Social support for healthy eating/exercise	
	Social group norms around eating/exercise	
Built environment	Neighborhood food pricing/availability	• Healthy food checklist [40]
	Neighborhood walkability, safety	• Neighborhood Environment Measures Survey in Stores (NEMS-S) [41]
	Accessibility of physical activity and recreational facilities	• Neighborhood Environment Walkability Scale (NEWS) [42]
	Transportation options	

Motivation for treatment is particularly important in achieving success with treatment goals. While many patients with obesity enumerate multiple ways in which their weight dramatically and adversely affects their lives, and thus almost universally express a strong desire to lose weight, patients present with varying levels of motivation for making and sustaining behavioral changes. Further, patients may be quite motivated to change certain behaviors while simultaneously being less motivated to change others. Thus, it is essential to make a distinction between behavior changes that a patient does not feel motivated or willing to make, and desired changes that are difficult to make because of specific barriers to doing so, as this will directly affect the choice of intervention.

Psychosocial correlates of obesity should also be incorporated within the assessment. As a chronic, often-disabling, and highly stigmatized condition, obesity may engender a number of psychosocial sequelae, and assessment should include this domain as well. Individuals with obesity may experience significant distress around their body image, occasionally to the extent that it has a significant impact on their activities, social functioning, and mood. It is therefore important to assess mood symptoms in order to address overt psychological or psychiatric disorders, or to otherwise incorporate mood management into the treatment plan. Obesity may also have a significant impact on a patient's interpersonal relationships and interactions, and this should also be explored in the initial assessment.

While as noted earlier, cognitive-behavioral therapy alone may not be sufficient to effect a "cure" for obesity, CBT techniques can be effectively employed to address each of the domains described earlier to effectively improve behavioral patterns, health and fitness, psychological distress, and overall well-being.

3.2.3 Cognitive and Behavioral Strategies for Weight Management

Cognitive behavioral therapy for weight management, also referred to as lifestyle modification or behavioral weight control, includes three core strategies: dietary changes, increased physical activity, and behavior modification to support healthy habits [45]. Dietary changes typically involve calorie reduction and making food substitutions (i.e., reduced fat dairy products) or additions (i.e., more fruits and vegetables) that facilitate such calorie reduction. Increasing physical activity typically occurs gradually, by helping patients find activities they will enjoy and be able to sustain. Aerobic and strength-based exercises are encouraged, in line with national recommendations from the Center for Disease Control [46]. The cornerstones of behavioral weight management are self-monitoring, goal setting, and problem-solving. When these strategies are employed, research has found that cognitive and behavioral treatment can result in up to 8–10 % of initial body weight lost in the first 6 months [47].

Behavioral weight management programs typically last for 16–26 weeks, with 60–90-min group meetings. Groups usually include 10–20 patients and are led by dieticians, psychologists, exercise physiologists, social workers, or other qualified professionals. The group format is generally preferable to individual meetings, with research finding increased patient satisfaction and better weight and cost outcomes [48]. Group cohesion and support, in addition to elements of competition among members, appear to be beneficial. The curriculum of group treatment sessions is often based upon evidence from the protocol used in the Diabetes Prevention Program (DPP) [49] and the LEARN Program for Weight Control (LEARN) [50]. Self-monitoring of food intake, physical activity, and weight are central to behavioral weight control programs and represent a cornerstone of group discussion and problem-solving. Homework is assigned weekly, and patients weigh themselves on a regular (weekly) schedule. Regular weight self-monitoring has been shown to be associated with improved short- and long-term weight loss outcomes [51–53]. Group sessions typically consist of reviewing patients' food and physical activity logs and instruction in strategies to help patients overcome barriers to healthy eating and physical activity. Group members are expected to set individual goals at each session.

Generally, participants can be expected to lose 1–2 lb/week in a behavioral weight loss paradigm, with a combination of reduced caloric intake and increased physical activity [54]. One pound of weight loss per week requires a deficit of 3500 cal or 500 cal/day. Reduced caloric intake through dietary changes is the primary driver of weight loss.

3.2.4 Physical Activity Module

Physical activity has been shown to be a consistent predictor of weight loss maintenance and contributes to overall calorie deficit in weight loss. Recommendations for weight loss for healthy adults are 150–250 min/week of moderate intensity physical activity, or more for greater benefit [55], or about 60 min/day, plus strength training. However, physical activity alone is generally not sufficient to produce clinically meaningful weight loss given the high intensity and duration of exercise required [45, 47].

3.2.5 Dietary Module

There are several different types of diets that are typically recommended in behavioral weight control programs, the most common being low fat/high carbohydrate (i.e., fruits, vegetables, and whole grains). Other prescribed diets include preportioned foods or liquid meal replacements, which tend to result in greater initial weight losses but poorer maintenance. In particular, the completion of daily food records has been found to be the most consistent predictor of initial weight loss and maintenance [56]. "The more you write down, the more you lose" is a helpful mnemonic for patients and counselors.

3.2.6 Behavior Modification Module

In addition to diet and physical activity changes, behavior modification strategies employing fundamentals of behavioral learning theory include using functional analysis, or the identification of "behavior chains," to help patients recognize antecedents or cues for overeating, develop alternate coping strategies for managing cravings, restructure their environments to reduce temptation (stimulus control), and reinforce healthy behaviors (contingency management) [47].

SMART goals and cognitive distortions. Goal setting is another key behavioral strategy. Goals for eating and exercise should be SMART: specific, measurable, attainable, realistic, and time bound (achievable within a specified time frame) [57]. Such a system can help patients meet their goals by anticipating barriers and setting up small goals along the way to larger ones, as smaller behaviors are more likely to be achievable and maintainable, and therefore reinforce continued success [47]. Negative cognitions often arise for most weight loss patients at some point on their journey. Some common cognitive distortions include "all-or-nothing" thinking, such as, "I already ruined my diet today, so I may as well finish the box of cookies." Or, "I only have 15 min for exercise today. What's the point in doing such a small amount?" Another common distortion would be the fortune-telling error in the face of a weight loss "plateau": "That's it, what I'm doing is of no use, I'm never going to lose the rest of the weight." Cognitive restructuring in this setting involves helping patients evaluate the evidence for and against cognitive errors, understand and set realistic goals, critically evaluate their eating and physical activity choices, and see weight control as a long-term lifestyle change [47]. Lifestyle modification requires ongoing planning; portion control; healthy food choices; and ongoing self-monitoring of diet, physical activity, and weight.

3.2.7 Motivational Interviewing (MI)

Using Motivational Interviewing (MI) as an adjunct to CBT for weight management has been shown to enhance outcomes [22]. In this context, MI is used to explore discrepancies between patients' current beliefs/behaviors and their goals. In the MI framework, clinicians use active listening and an empathic style to bring attention to these discrepancies and help patients' problem solve barriers. MI basics include using open-ended questions, affirmations, reflective listening, and summaries (OARS). Using MI leads to increased patient self-efficacy and commitment to behavioral goals (i.e., improved diet, increased physical activity) [58]. In service of assessing ambivalence about weight, clinicians might ask questions such as, "How ready do you feel to change your eating patterns or lifestyle behaviors? How is your current weight affecting your life? What have you done in the past to change your eating? Some people talk about part of them wanting to change their eating patterns, and part of them not really wanting to change; is this true for you? How would your life be different if you lost weight and adopted a healthier lifestyle?" [59]. Clinicians using MI also spend a good deal of time using such open-ended questions to assess readiness, importance of goals, confidence around behavior change, barriers, and the pros/cons of changing vs. not changing. Patients' perceptions of the importance of each goal, and his or her confidence in the likelihood of achieving them, can be gauged using "rulers" — verbal or visual scales ranging from 0 (not ready to make changes to your eating or physical activity habits/change is not important) to 10 (very ready/very important to make changes). "Change talk" can be elicited by inquiring: "You gave yourself a score of X, why are you an X and not ___ (a lower number)? Why are you an X and not ___ (a higher number)? What would it take for you to move up to (a higher number)?" A useful mnemonic for the MI clinician is the FRAMES acronym, provide Feedback respectfully, emphasize the patient's Responsibility and autonomy, provide Advice about lifestyle change, offer a Menu of options for successful ways to change, respond and reflect with Empathy, and enhance Self-efficacy and optimism [60].

3.2.8 Behavioral Problem-Solving

A detailed evaluation should yield information about the specific behaviors (or absence of certain healthy behaviors) that may be contributing to a patient's weight. With its emphasis on functional analysis, CBT is an ideal intervention for individuals who need assistance in creating and maintaining healthy behavioral habits. As noted earlier, one of the more important aspects of the initial evaluation of patients presenting with obesity is the identification of barriers to healthy eating and consistent physical activity. Once such barriers have been identified, many of them can be addressed using a behavioral problem-solving approach.

In our current obesogenic environment, with its hyper-availability of highly caloric, convenient, and tempting foods, it is difficult for most individuals to maintain healthy eating without some degree of structure and planning. By the same token, given most people's very busy schedules, it is often very difficult for patients to initiate and maintain a regimen of consistent physical activity. Many patients with obesity are psychologically healthy, well-adjusted individuals who nevertheless stand to benefit greatly from assistance with the organizational skills and strategies necessary for maintaining healthy eating and physical activity over the long term. This is even more the case for patients who have some executive functioning deficits, such as ADHD. In fact, increasing numbers of studies are linking ADHD with a higher risk of obesity [61], and individuals with ADHD may have less successful outcomes following weight loss treatment [62]. Maintaining healthy eating requires a number of basic but crucial elements in one's eating "infrastructure," including meal planning, maintaining a consistent routine for food shopping, creating a daily regimen for eating small meals on a regular basis, finding efficient and sustainable ways to make physical activity part of one's daily or weekly schedule, and planning ahead for times when one's routine is altered, such as during holidays or on vacations. Functional analysis and behavioral problem-solving can be effectively employed to facilitate the development and maintenance of healthy habits. For instance, for some patients, the tendency to obtain many meals outside of the home is a significant contributor to weight gain and/or a barrier to weight loss. Functional analysis may reveal that the patient's busy work schedule makes it difficult to find time for home cooking. An appropriate intervention in such a case would be to help the patient to create an efficient system for regular grocery shopping, cooking "in bulk" over the weekends, and freezing meals for convenient consumption during the work week so that he or she does not have to rely on restaurants or unhealthy convenience foods.

3.2.9 Communication Skills

In examining contributors to weight and unhealthy behaviors, or barriers to behavior change, it may transpire that interpersonal factors are at play. For instance, some patients report that while they are motivated to make behavioral changes, others in their environment are not supportive of these changes, or are actively offering unhealthy foods, interfering with patients' attempts to make time to be active, etc. In these situations, patients may benefit from a brief communication skills intervention. Patients may find that interpersonal barriers to behavior change are more easily surmounted when they have the proper tools to communicate their needs effectively and assertively with the people in their home and/or work environments.

3.3 Related Considerations in the Cognitive-Behavioral Treatment of Obesity

3.3.1 Binge and Emotional Eating

A good deal of research has demonstrated that CBT is an effective treatment for binge eating disorder [63]. There is some evidence that there are differing phenotypes of BED, with binge eating in one phenotype being predominantly related to irregular meal patterns and meal skipping, and another phenotype in which binge eating represents an effort to cope with negative emotions [64]. It appears that the former phenotype often responds well to basic behavioral weight management techniques, without specific focus on binge eating; this type of treatment tends to produce a decrease in both binge eating and weight [65]. The second phenotype may be the most appropriate for focused psychological input, as it appears to be better suited for CBT that specifically targets the connection between binge eating and emotions [66]. The techniques employed here can also be employed in addressing emotionally triggered eating that contributes to obesity but does not necessarily take the form of eating binges, since the focus on self-monitoring, behavioral regulation, and coping skills is applicable to both patterns.

CBT for BED typically begins with establishing a habit of self-monitoring one's intake, and next moves on to establishing a consistent, planned eating structure to regulate intake patterns. The last phase of treatment focuses on identifying specific triggers for eating episodes, which are often emotional in nature, and building coping skills for managing these triggers without eating [67]. Throughout the treatment of binge- or emotional eating, cognitive restructuring plays a central role. A number of types of cognitive distortions contribute to and maintain these eating patterns, and addressing these directly enhances the efficacy of treatment and reduces distress. For instance, an almost universal feature of individuals who engage in binge or emotional eating is a tendency to engage in dichotomous thinking: foods are considered either "good" or "bad," and efforts are made to completely avoid eating the "bad" foods. However, because this is not a realistic goal, these efforts are more or less doomed to failure, and when the "bad" foods are eventually eaten, individuals often feel that they have "blown it" and abandon their efforts to eat healthfully. Binges may be triggered in this process. A more effective and psychologically adaptive approach is to help the patients to think in terms of overall dietary balance, acknowledging that no foods are completely "off limits," and that even highly caloric foods can be consumed in moderation without one's efforts to lose weight being irreparably "destroyed." Research suggests that a "flexible" style of cognitive control over eating is related to a lower body mass index (BMI) and better weight loss than a "rigid" style [68], and cognitive restructuring can help patients achieve a more adaptive way of thinking about food and eating. Another contributor to the cycle of binge- or emotional eating is a marked and relatively ubiquitous tendency for patients to have extremely self-punitive cognitions when they commit perceived deviations from their intended diets. Rather than helping patients to return to and maintain healthier eating, self-punitive thinking, and the negative emotions that it engenders, tends to put patients at risk for further unhealthy eating, feelings of discouragement, and abandoning efforts to sustain healthy eating patterns [69]. Restructuring of guilt-inducing food-related cognitions is an important component of CBT for binge- and emotional eating. Cognitive restructuring can be employed in an informal manner throughout therapy sessions as instances of maladaptive cognitive patterns arise; in addition, specific tools such as thought records or other structured protocols for cognitive restructuring may be used.

While cognitive-behavioral treatment is effective in treating binge and emotional eating, it must be noted that, compared to addressing binge eating with standard, non-binge-specific, behavioral weight management interventions, CBT for BED does not tend to produce significant weight loss. Nevertheless, effective psychological treatment of binge- or emotional eating decreases emotional distress, engenders healthier eating attitudes and patterns, and affords individuals a sense of control over their eating and their health [63].

3.3.2 Body Image Disturbance

Obesity and overweight are associated with poor body image and decreased quality of life [70]. Body image, or the subjective experience of evaluations of the appearance of one's body, is a central component of emotional well-being and self-perception, and is directly related to behaviors that influence weight and efforts to lose weight [71]. The term "body image" refers to one's estimated size, while "body size satisfaction" is the attitudinal component of body image, reflecting one's subjective feelings about one's body [72]. Degree of body image satisfaction is associated with self-esteem and health-related behaviors, such as smoking, nutrition patterns, and engaging in physical activity [73]. Understanding the factors related to perceptions about body image, including cognitive distortions, can assist with weight loss and maintenance behaviors, as well as overall well-being.

Several studies of US adults have assessed body size satisfaction and related sociodemographic factors. Lower BMI, increasing age, and better health are generally associated with greater body size satisfaction among women [74]. Women typically view themselves as heavier than they actually are and desire a thinner figure, reporting dissatisfaction with their body at a lower BMI than men [74]. While most women who are overweight or obese desire to lose weight, some report acceptance or satisfaction with their body size. This has particularly been found among Black, and, to a lesser extent, among Hispanic women [74, 75]. White women tend to express greater body size dissatisfaction and at lower BMIs than do their African American or Hispanic peers, although this pattern may be mediated by social class [76]. Men are generally less aware of being overweight and are less likely to attempt weight loss if they are overweight or obese. Men appear to ascribe less importance to their body size than do women, which may account for the observed gender discrepancies in body image and weight-control behaviors [77]. Men who are dissatisfied with their size or weight tend to wish to gain muscle, as the culturally ideal male body type is lean and muscular [77].

Body image disturbance (BID) can range from mild feelings of distress over one's body image to intense preoccupation with an imagined or slight "defect" of one's body. BID underlies body dysmorphic disorder (BDD) and eating disorders (EDs) [78]. Recent research has suggested that "BID should be conceptualized as a dynamic failure to integrate subjective experiences of one's own body appearance with an objective appraisal of the body." [79]. BID has been shown to respond well to CBT in group and individual therapy settings [80]. Techniques include: understanding the causes of BID, relaxation strategies and imaginal exposure/body image desensitization, uncovering underlying assumptions, cognitive distortions, and body image judgments that perpetuate BID, challenging assumptions and distortions, stopping ritualistic (i.e., over-grooming) or avoidant behaviors (i.e., avoiding feared situations), improving self-care (i.e., healthy eating, physical activity), and relapse prevention [80, 81].

Cognitive restructuring within BID can be applied to several common distortions or assumptions underlying BID [81]. Distortions such as overgeneralization, jumping to conclusions, labeling, magnification/minimization, personalization, and mental filter may often be used by BID patients. Example cognitive assumptions include, "Good looking people are better off," "If I could look how I want, my life would be much happier," and "My appearance is responsible for much of what has happened in my life."

Therapists can assist patients using Socratic questioning and asking patients to generate alternative cognitions. Some examples might be, "Attractive people are not always happier and have their own insecurities," "Looks don't matter to everyone," "So what if someone notices I look like _____, I have plenty of wonderful qualities," and "Is it possible that I am making this a bigger problem than it really is?" [81].

A promising area of research and practice in this domain involves using the principles of Acceptance and Commitment Therapy (ACT) [82]. ACT aims to bring about greater psychological flexibility and reduced avoidance of one's internal experiences. It is values based and encourages increased participation in valued activities. Patients with BID may benefit from gaining distance from their negative cognitions (seeing thoughts only as thoughts, without judgment) and pursuing valued actions in spite of negative body image cognitions. A core component of ACT is mindfulness and mindful eating involves a nonjudgmental awareness of the physical and emotional sensations involved with eating. Mindfulness strategies can help patients to recognize and respond to satiety, to differentiate between appropriate and inappropriate cues for eating, and to develop greater self-acceptance.

3.3.3   Weight Loss Surgery

Weight loss surgery (WLS) is an option for individuals with severe obesity (BMI of ≥40 or BMI of 35.0–39.9 with at least one severe medical comorbidity). Cognitive-behavioral interventions play an important role in helping patients prepare for WLS and maintain the necessary lifelong lifestyle changes required to sustain weight loss. While a detailed review of the available surgical procedures, risks, and side effects is beyond the scope of this chapter, it is important to note that there is substantial empirical evidence that weight loss surgery results in significantly greater, and more durable, weight loss than do behavioral or pharmacological weight loss interventions, and is highly effective in promoting the improvement or remission of many obesity-related health conditions, including diabetes, sleep apnea, fatty liver disease, etc. [83]. Although WLS is arguably the most effective treatment for severe obesity and its related medical consequences, not all patients achieve optimal initial weight loss, and substantial regain is possible in the long term, particularly if the patient does not engage in healthy behaviors, such as maintaining a nutritious diet and engaging in consistent physical activity [84]. While it has been challenging to identify preoperative psychosocial factors that consistently predict long-term WLS outcomes, there is fairly solid empirical consensus that patients who experience mood or eating disorder symptoms after surgery are at risk for poorer long-term weight outcomes [85–87].

Therefore, long-term behavioral and psychosocial monitoring and support is crucial for WLS patients. Research suggests that bariatric patients who receive behavioral/lifestyle interventions, and/or participate in postoperative support groups, demonstrate better weight loss outcomes than those who do not have or use such resources [88–92]. There is some limited data to support family-based approaches to postoperative lifestyle modifications for patients with bariatric surgery as well [93].

3.4   Special Population Concerns

3.4.1   Children and the Elderly

Obesity is an ever growing concern within the child and adolescent population as well. A recent review of the National Health and Nutrition Examination Survey (NHANES) data indicates that in 2011–2012, 18 % of children and adolescents (age 2–18) were defined as obese (based upon waist circumference), and 33 % of children and adolescents (age 6–18) were considered obese (based upon waist-to-hip ratio: WHR) [94]. Higher WHR has been shown to be correlated with indicators for increased risk of metabolic syndrome not only in adults, but in children and adolescents as well [95].

Adolescents with severe obesity experience many of the serious medical comorbidities seen in adults with obesity (e.g., dyslipidemia, chronic pain, obstructive sleep apnea) and report significant impairment in weight-related quality of life [96, 97]. In addition, as noted earlier, studies have shown a link between obesity and ADHD [61, 98].

The care of children and adolescents with obesity has historically fallen to their pediatricians; however, there has been a recent increase in the number of specialized obesity medicine centers treating children and adolescents. Treatment options include behavioral intervention/nutrition education, pharmacotherapy, and surgical intervention for weight loss, though the latter two options are approved for adolescents only.

While much is known of obesity in the adult literature, there is considerably less literature focusing on obesity in the elderly, and literature regarding behavioral treatment of obesity in the elderly is sparse. Although research suggests that being in the overweight range may confer a slight advantage for survival in older men, in general obesity in midlife is associated with an elevated risk of mortality [99]. Although caloric intake tends to decrease as individuals enter older age, the prevalence of obesity is increasing in the elderly [100]. Obesity may be a more potent risk factor in elderly individuals, to the extent that by virtue of their age, they may have experienced a longer "exposure" to obesity and its attendant metabolic risks.

3.4.2   Socioeconomic Factors and Ethnicity

Among US adults, obesity disproportionately affects African Americans and Hispanics [101] and low-income women (but not men) [102]. Socioeconomic associations are difficult to disentangle from racial associations because many people living in low-income areas in the U.S. are African Americans, Hispanics, or other racial/ethnic minorities. Interest has grown substantially in recent years in examining the interpersonal, social, and neighborhood-level characteristics that may impact the previously identified risk factors for the development of obesity and chronic diseases [103]. Some explanations for this increased risk in predominantly racial/ ethnic minority and low-income areas include increased stress, cultural norms regarding food choices, taste, and body size preferences, limited access to medical care and preventive education, access to healthy foods, and disadvantages in the built environment for walkability [104]. These factors can affect physical activity and diet, and thus, obesity.

Research has shown that the local food environment, as defined by the presence of different types of food stores and restaurants, as well as food prices, can play a strong role in peoples' diets and weight [105–107]. Individuals from ethnic minorities disproportionately reside in low-income and/or urban areas, and these areas tend to have reduced access to healthy foods and greater access to fast food or energy-dense foods [107]. Residing in a neighborhood where whole grains, fruits, vegetables, and low-fat dairy foods are available is a strong predictor of meeting dietary recommendations, putting individuals in low-income areas at a disadvantage in their efforts to lose weight. Even when there is access to healthy foods, calorie-for-calorie, healthy foods are costlier than unhealthy ones, which create additional barriers to healthy eating for underprivileged individuals [108]. Research in this area has great potential for contributing to improving diet and related outcomes, but many associations remain to be clarified [105]. Given these barriers, clinicians should offer low-cost recipe ideas, resources for SNAP-benefit eligible farmers' markets, and shopping tips for low-income patients.

Similarly, the built environment in low-SES areas can impact physical activity opportunities and habits. Research has shown that aspects of the built environment such as destinations (i.e., shops, restaurants, parks), land use, streetscape features, and street and intersection amenities are related to walking for transportation, while esthetic neighborhood variables are related to leisure physical activity and walking [109]. However, in low SES or predominantly minority neighborhoods, there are often fewer facilities for physical activity and poorer features of the built environment. This has been associated with lower physical activity and more overweight among individuals living in these neighborhoods [110]. Interventions to address environmental disparities and promote safe and accessible physical activity require change at multiple levels. Changing environments and policies can affect whole communities on a relatively permanent basis [111]. Patients should be educated on ways to interact with their built environment and advocate for neighborhood-level changes such as organizing a park cleanup or contacting city officials to help improve sidewalk quality [112].

3.5 Comorbid Medical Conditions and Weight Management

Patients with obesity frequently suffer from one or more of a number of medical comorbidities. Often behavioral specialists are tasked with not only evaluating and treating obesity, but also with addressing various issues related to the medical consequences of obesity. Following we briefly discuss the management of pain, diabetes, and obstructive sleep apnea, common conditions comorbid to obesity.

3.5.1 Pain Management

Chronic pain and obesity frequently co-occur. Among those with chronic pain, a higher BMI has been associated with reduced activity and disability [113]. Obesity may contribute to musculoskeletal or neuropathic pain by placing extra stress on joints or through its association with fibromyalgia and/or type 2 diabetes [113, 114]. In turn, pain often limits physical activity, further exacerbating weight gain and obesity. Pain and obesity can both independently reduce quality of life, and when they co-occur, patients experience significant distress and disability. Though pain medications may offer some degree of relief for some individuals, there are risks and side effects associated with their chronic use.

Weight reduction can improve pain and reduce disability among obese patients [115]. This is particularly true when weight loss is significant, for instance, in the context of weight loss surgery (WLS). Research has shown that patients experience significant relief from joint pain, low back pain, and disability following WLS [116, 117]. However, even in the absence of significant weight loss, behavioral pain management techniques can be beneficial for patients with obesity. Pain treatment involves changing patients' relationship to pain: decatastrophizing and increasing adaptive coping behaviors including relaxation practice and pleasant activity scheduling. Interventions also include education regarding the relationship between chronic pain and obesity. Physical activity is a primary target of intervention, given its beneficial effects for weight loss and chronic pain. Activity pacing is a critical component of treatment, such that patients are instructed to take rest breaks before their pain spikes, in order to gradually prolong activity. Treatment also focuses on identifying triggers for overeating, sedentary behavior, and pain; planning strategies to overcome barriers; and identifying and challenging automatic thoughts about weight and pain content [118].

3.5.2 Diabetes Management

Obesity is linked to insulin resistance, the precursor to type 2 diabetes. Weight loss may postpone or prevent the onset of diabetes; however, once diabetes has developed, many of the treatments available (e.g., insulin or certain oral hypoglycemic agents) can induce weight gain [119]. In addition, research suggests that among patients with diabetes, those with severe obesity (BMI $\geq$ 35 kg/m^2) may be less likely to prioritize changing diet and physical activity as part of their goals, or to achieve those goals, and more likely to find weight control to be a greater burden. Further, these issues seem to worsen with increasing severity of obesity [120]. Therefore, enhancing self-care may need to be a primary focus of diabetes care [121] and one for which behavioral specialists may be particularly well suited. Areas for intervention by a behavioral specialist may include behavioral problem-solving to enhance adherence to self-monitoring of blood glucose, following a diabetic diet, and taking medications, or even to help patients overcome needle phobia if this is a significant barrier to appropriate diabetes self-care.

3.5.3 Obstructive Sleep Apnea

The prevalence of obstructive sleep apnea (OSA) in US adults is estimated to be approximately 5 %, with a higher prevalence in men than women. However, among individuals with obesity, OSA prevalence is higher, reaching approximately 11 % [122]. Obesity significantly increases the risk for OSA, and at least 70 % of patients with OSA have obesity [123]. Weight loss (achieved through either surgical or nonsurgical means) is likely to effect improvements in OSA among individuals with obesity.

Conversely, OSA may also contribute to weight gain and obesity, and it is a known contributor to cardiometabolic risk [124]. Effective treatment of OSA may in fact lead to weight loss, and it has been found that patients who are adherent to continuous positive airway pressure (CPAP) treatment have larger decreases in BMI than those who do not adhere to treatment [125]. However, patients often find it difficult to tolerate CPAP use, and this is one arena in which a behavioral specialist can be helpful, through CPAP desensitization and relaxation training.

3.6 Case Example

Monica is a 55-year-old African American female, who was referred by her primary care doctor for a comprehensive evaluation and treatment of Class I Obesity. At the time of referral, her BMI was 34 and she had just been diagnosed with "prediabetes" based on elevated blood glucose findings. This recent diagnosis had heightened Monica's concerns about her weight and overall health, and she was motivated to explore cognitive-behavioral treatment for her obesity.

During her initial evaluation, Monica shared that her weight had been a lifelong struggle and that there was a strong family history of obesity. As a child, she was exposed to both physical and emotional abuse. Although she did not meet full criteria for PTSD at the time of the evaluation, it became clear that many of her early experiences were continuing to affect her eating behaviors. Her mother suffered from schizophrenia, her father left the family when she was 6 years old, and she had three younger siblings. Financial resources were limited and her mother often used food as a source of reward or punishment. The availability of food in her childhood household was unpredictable and she associated a "full belly" with security and comfort. Monica was a hardworking and resilient child and she eventually earned a scholarship to attend a private high school and a junior college. She married, pursued a government job, and had three children. However, she cited numerous life stressors, including her recent divorce and the sale of her home, as contributions to her increased weight gain in the past 5 years. She also noted that menopause may have been a factor in her more recent weight gain. In terms of physical activity, she described a fairly sedentary lifestyle, with her 20 min walk from the train as her only form of regular exercise. She did not describe any physical injuries or limitations to her mobility. Since her divorce, she also noted increased financial concerns, difficulties affording healthier foods, and less cooking at home. While her symptoms did not meet full diagnostic criteria for depression, she noted intermittent feelings of sadness and loneliness and endorsed increased occasional emotional eating of comfort foods in response to these feelings. When asked about the structure of her eating, she admitted to skipping breakfast and drinking a highly sweetened coffee on her daily commute to work, and often relying on takeout or fast foods for lunch and dinner. She denied binge eating, but noted large portion sizes at both lunch and dinner. Additionally, she noted snacking on sweets in the evenings, particularly when feeling lonely. While her reported intake of alcoholic beverages did not place her at high risk of being harmed by alcohol, she did note a pattern of 1–2 glasses of wine several nights per week in order to wind down after work, which was contributing excess calories to her overall intake. Upon reflection, she did admit that her sleep was fitful and disturbed, often falling asleep with the television on. She appeared quite motivated to pursue a healthier lifestyle and noted her health as a primary source of motivation. Following the initial evaluation, she agreed to pursue a course of cognitive-behavioral therapy, with the goal of weight loss, but more importantly a stronger, healthier lifestyle.

Initial sessions contained a blend of psychoeducation modules and behavioral problem-solving modules to improve eating structure, nutritional knowledge, and physical activity. The rationale of structured, planned meals and snacks was introduced as a method to maintain a healthy metabolism, stabilize blood sugars, and avoid excessive hunger, which drove consumption of large portions. Education about appropriate portion sizes and reading food labels was also provided. Initially, Monica was concerned about eating breakfast, as she had never been a "breakfast person" and doubted that she could "force" herself to eat in the morning. The importance of protein as a source of energy was a novel concept for Monica and she eventually developed a list of acceptable and convenient breakfast choices, including a hard boiled egg; whole wheat toast with peanut butter; and plain, unsweetened oatmeal with milk and sliced almonds. She also agreed to gradually decrease her use of sugar in her morning coffee. The idea of "planned snacks" was also introduced as an important component of dietary structure and she agreed on several items such as almonds, cheese sticks, and veggie sticks that could easily be transported to work and would promote lasting satiety. She also began to plan ahead and pack lunches, rather than relying on takeout foods at work. Given her recent financial pressures, she also realized that bringing her own lunch/snacks to work led to tremendous monetary savings. While Monica had resisted cooking since her divorce, she agreed to explore recipes and gradually began preparing dinner for herself at home, with the goal of preparing foods ahead of time on weekends whenever possible. She noted the benefits of this strategy, as she had often felt too tired to cook after her long commute and had gravitated toward quick, unhealthy takeout choices in the past. Along with all of these suggested changes, she agreed to keep detailed daily food records and brought those to treatment sessions, leading to collaborative problem-solving when less desirable options were reported.

In addition to monitoring of food intake, the importance of physical activity as a component of weight loss was discussed in early sessions. Initial problem-solving focused on identifying feasible forms of exercise and committing to regular weekly exercise sessions, in addition to increasing daily steps (e.g., taking stairs, parking further away). She noted that walking was her preferred form of activity and agreed to contact a local friend who had also expressed an interest in getting healthier. Together, they agreed to meet three times per week in the mornings before work and to walk for 30–45 min. Monica found that walking with her friend increased her accountability and also led to decreased feelings of isolation/loneliness, as they enjoyed their morning chats. As the weather became colder, Monica and her friend agreed to join a reasonably priced local gym and began to expand their repertoire of exercises to dance classes and light weight training.

As sessions progressed, Monica made reasonable progress with structure and exercise, along with modest decreases in weight loss. The focus shifted to further addressing beliefs about food and emotional/physical security, which had developed in response to her early childhood experiences. Given the limited availability of food in her childhood household, maladaptive beliefs about "cleaning her plate" and wasting food were addressed. Thought records and cognitive restructuring were also helpful in identifying and addressing other maladaptive thoughts around food, such as "I must have a full belly in order to feel safe and loved." Monica focused on new ways to make herself feel safe and secure and reframed many of her underlying beliefs about food. Nonfood rewards were discussed, such as buying herself a magazine or a small bouquet of flowers at the checkout counter, rather than candies, as she had done in the past. She also focused on initiating more social activities in the evenings (e.g., registering for an adult education course, volunteering in a community group), as triggers for her emotional eating were often related to feelings of loneliness. In addition, distress tolerance skills and relaxation exercises (e.g., diaphragmatic breathing) were used to cope with stress and painful emotions. Thought records were also useful in addressing "All or Nothing" cognitive distortions, such as "I made the mistake of eating some candy, so I may as well throw in the towel and eat whatever I want." In order to further address "Black and White" thinking, the "80/20 rule" was introduced to reinforce that perfection is not realistic, but that the goal is to try to make the right choice about 80 % of the time.

Given the important connection between sleep hygiene and weight loss, nightly sleep patterns were also addressed through a sleep hygiene module. Monika worked to adopt a healthier routine in preparing for sleep, by developing a relaxing nightly ritual and minimizing exposure to electronics (including TV, Facebook, and phone) for 1 h before bedtime. She also agreed to significantly decrease her intake of wine, as she noted a connection between even modest alcohol intake and restless, disturbed sleep. This decision was further reinforced by noting the benefits of decreased caloric intake.

By the conclusion of 6 months of treatment, Monica had lost approximately 10 % of her initial body weight and her blood work no longer showed a propensity toward diabetes. She also felt stronger and more connected to her body, through a routine of regular exercise. She was encouraged to maintain contact through booster visits and to continue to strive for small stepwise goals, comparing herself to where she was yesterday, not 10 years ago.

References

1. Flegal KM, Carroll MD, Kit BK, Ogden CL. Prevalence of obesity and trends in the distribution of body mass index among US adults, 1999–2010. JAMA. 2012;307(5):491–7.
2. Swinburn BA, Sacks G, Hall KD, McPherson K, Finegood DT, Moodie ML, et al. The global obesity pandemic: shaped by global drivers and local environments. Lancet. 2011;378(9793):804–14.
3. Farooqi IS, O'Rahilly S. Genetic factors in human obesity. Obes Rev. 2007;8(s1):37–40.
4. Kral TV, Allison DB, Birch LL, Stallings VA, Moore RH, Faith MS. Caloric compensation and eating in the absence of hunger in 5- to 12-year-old weight-discordant siblings. Am J Clin Nutr. 2012;96(3):574–83.
5. Llewellyn CH, Trzaskowski M, van Jaarsveld CH, Plomin R, Wardle J. Satiety mechanisms in genetic risk of obesity. JAMA Pediatr. 2014;168(4):338–44.
6. Shea JL, Randell EW, Sun G. The prevalence of metabolically healthy obese subjects defined by BMI and dual-energy X-ray absorptiometry. Obesity. 2011;19(3):624–30.
7. Mitchell NS, Catenacci VA, Wyatt HR, Hill JO. Obesity: overview of an epidemic. Psychiatr Clin North Am. 2011;34(4):717–32.
8. Padwal RS, Pajewski NM, Allison DB, Sharma AM. Using the Edmonton obesity staging system to predict mortality in a population-representative cohort of people with overweight and obesity. CMAJ. 2011;183(14):E1059–66.
9. Schneider HJ, Friedrich N, Klotsche J, Pieper L, Nauck M, John U, et al. The predictive value of different measures of obesity for incident cardiovascular events and mortality. J Clin Endocrinol Metab. 2010;95(4):1777–85.
10. Berkowitz RI, Fabricatore AN. Obesity, psychiatric status, and psychiatric medications. Psychiatr Clin North Am. 2011;34(4):747–64.
11. Gariepy G, Nitka D, Schmitz N. The association between obesity and anxiety disorders in the population: a systematic review and meta-analysis. Int J Obes (Lond). 2010;34(3):407–19.
12. Wadden TA, Butryn ML, Sarwer DB, Fabricatore AN, Crerand CE, Lipschutz PE, et al. Comparison of psychosocial status in treatment-seeking women with class III vs. class I–II obesity. Obesity. 2006;14 Suppl 2:90S–8.
13. Malik S, Mitchell JE, Engel S, Crosby R, Wonderlich S. Psychopathology in bariatric surgery candidates: a review of studies using structured diagnostic interviews. Compr Psychiatry. 2014;55(2):248–59.
14. Simon GE, Von Korff M, Saunders K, Miglioretti DL, Crane PK, van Belle G, et al. Association between obesity and psychiatric disorders in the US adult population. Arch Gen Psychiatry. 2006;63(7):824–30.
15. Sharma S, Fulton S. Diet-induced obesity promotes depressive-like behaviour that is associated with neural adaptations in brain reward circuitry. Int J Obes (Lond). 2013;37(3):382–9.
16. Atlantis E, Baker M. Obesity effects on depression: systematic review of epidemiological studies. Int J Obes (Lond). 2008;32(6):881–91.
17. Sobal J, Stunkard AJ. Socioeconomic status and obesity: a review of the literature. Psychol Bull. 1989;105(2):260–75.
18. Tussing-Humphreys LM, Fitzgibbon ML, Kong A, Odoms-Young A. Weight loss maintenance in African American women: a systematic review of the behavioral lifestyle intervention literature. J Obes. 2013;2013:437369.
19. Kirk SF, Penney TL, McHugh TL, Sharma AM. Effective weight management practice: a review of the lifestyle intervention evidence. Int J Obes (Lond). 2012;36(2):178–85.
20. Wing RR. Behavioral weight control. In: Wadden TA, Stunkard AJ, editors. Handbook of obesity treatment. New York: Guilford; 2002. p. 301–16.
21. Douketis JD, Macie C, Thabane L, Williamson DF. Systematic review of long-term weight loss studies in obese adults: clinical significance and applicability to clinical practice. Int J Obes (Lond). 2005;29(10):1153–67.

22. Armstrong MJ, Mottershead TA, Ronksley PE, Sigal RJ, Campbell TS, Hemmelgarn BR. Motivational interviewing to improve weight loss in overweight and/or obese patients: a systematic review and meta-analysis of randomized controlled trials. Obes Rev. 2011;12(9):709–23.

23. Sheehan DV, Lecrubier Y, Sheehan KH, Amorim P, Janavs J, Weiller E, et al. The Mini-International Neuropsychiatric Interview (MINI): the development and validation of a structured diagnostic psychiatric interview for DSM-IV and ICD-10. J Clin Psychiatry. 1998;59:22–33.

24. Kroenke K, Spitzer RL. The PHQ-9: a new depression diagnostic and severity measure. Psychiatr Ann. 2002;32(9):1–7.

25. Beck AT, Steer RA, Brown GK. Beck depression inventory-II. San Antonio: Psychological Corporation; 1996.

26. Beck AT, Epstein N, Brown G, Steer RA. An inventory for measuring clinical anxiety: psychometric properties. J Consult Clin Psychol. 1988;56(6):893.

27. Henry JD, Crawford JR. The short-form version of the Depression Anxiety Stress Scales (DASS-21): construct validity and normative data in a large non-clinical sample. Br J Clin Psychol. 2005;44(2):227–39.

28. Cohen S, Kamarck T, Mermelstein R. A global measure of perceived stress. J Health Soc Behav. 1983;24(4):385–96.

29. Weathers F, Litz B, Keane T, Palmieri P, Marx B, Schnurr P. The PTSD checklist for DSM-5 (PCL-5). Scale available from the National Center for PTSD. 2013.

30. Cash TF. Body-image attitudes: evaluation, investment, and affect. Percept Mot Skills. 1994;78(3c):1168–70.

31. Garner DM, Garfinkel PE. The eating attitudes test: an index of the symptoms of anorexia nervosa. Psychol Med. 1979;9(2):273–9.

32. Garner DM. EDI 3: Eating disorder inventory-3: professional manual. Lutz: Psychological Assessment Resources; 2004.

33. Thomas S, Reading J, Shephard RJ. Revision of the Physical Activity Readiness Questionnaire (PAR-Q). Can J Sport Sci. 1992;17(4):338–45.

34. Craig CL, Marshall AL, Sjostrom M, Bauman AE, Booth ML, Ainsworth BE, et al. International physical activity questionnaire: 12-country reliability and validity. Med Sci Sports Exerc. 2003;35(8):1381–95.

35. Brownell KD, Hager DL, Leermakers E. The weight loss readiness test II, version 4.1. Dallas: American Health Publishing Company; 2004.

36. Amtmann D, Cook KF, Jensen MP, Chen WH, Choi S, Revicki D, et al. Development of a PROMIS item bank to measure pain interference. Pain. 2010;150(1):173–82.

37. Cleeland CS, Ryan KM. Pain assessment: global use of the Brief Pain Inventory. Ann Acad Med Singapore. 1994;23(2):129–38.

38. Vaglio J, Conard M, Poston WS, O'Keefe J, Haddock CK, House J, et al. Testing the performance of the ENRICHD social support instrument in cardiac patients. Health Qual Life Outcomes. 2004;2(1):1–5.

39. Sallis JF, Grossman RM, Pinski RB, Patterson TL, Nader PR. The development of scales to measure social support for diet and exercise behaviors. Prev Med. 1987;16(6):825–36.

40. Laska MN, Borradaile KE, Tester J, Foster GD, Gittelsohn J. Healthy food availability in small urban food stores: a comparison of four US cities. Public Health Nutr. 2010;13(7):1031–5.

41. Glanz K, Sallis JF, Saelens BE, Frank LD. Nutrition Environment Measures Survey in stores (NEMS-S): development and evaluation. Am J Prev Med. 2007;32(4):282–9.

42. Saelens BE, Sallis JF, Black JB, Chen D. Neighborhood-based differences in physical activity: an environment scale evaluation. Am J Public Health. 2003;93(9):1552–8.

43. Allison KC, Wadden TA, Sarwer DB, Fabricatore AN, Crerand CE, Gibbons LM, et al. Night eating syndrome and binge eating disorder among persons seeking bariatric surgery: prevalence and related features. Obesity (Silver Spring). 2006;14 Suppl 2:77S–82.

44. Jakicic JM. Exercise in the treatment of obesity. Endocrinol Metab Clin North Am. 2003;32(4):967–80.

45. Wadden TA, Butryn ML, Wilson C. Lifestyle modification for the management of obesity. Gastroenterology. 2007;132(6):2226–38.

46. Prevention CfDCa. How much physical activity do adults need? 2015 [updated June 4, 2015; cited 2015 November 4].

47. Foster GD, Makris AP, Bailer BA. Behavioral treatment of obesity. Am J Clin Nutr. 2005;82 (1 Suppl):230S–5.

48. Renjilian DA, Perri MG, Nezu AM, McKelvey WF, Shermer RL, Anton SD. Individual versus group therapy for obesity: effects of matching participants to their treatment preferences. J Consult Clin Psychol. 2001;69(4):717–21.

49. Diabetes Prevention Program Research Group. The Diabetes Prevention Program (DPP): description of lifestyle intervention. Diabetes Care. 2002;25(12):2165–71.

50. Brownell KD. The LEARN program for weight management. Dallas: American Health Publishing; 2000.

51. Linde JA, Jeffery RW, French SA, Pronk NP, Boyle RG. Self-weighing in weight gain prevention and weight loss trials. Ann Behav Med. 2005;30(3):210–6.

52. Madigan CD, Aveyard P, Jolly K, Denley J, Lewis A, Daley AJ. Regular self-weighing to promote weight maintenance after intentional weight loss: a quasi-randomized controlled trial. J Public Health (Oxf). 2014;36(2):259–67.

53. Wing RR, Tate DF, Gorin AA, Raynor HA, Fava JL, Machan J. STOP regain: are there negative effects of daily weighing? J Consult Clin Psychol. 2007;75(4):652–6.

54. Sarwer DB, von Sydow GA, Vetter ML, Wadden TA. Behavior therapy for obesity: where are we now? Curr Opin Endocrinol Diabetes Obes. 2009;16(5):347–52.

55. Donnelly JE, Blair SN, Jakicic JM, Manore MM, Rankin JW, Smith BK. American college of sports medicine position stand. Appropriate physical activity intervention strategies for weight loss and prevention of weight regain for adults. Med Sci Sports Exerc. 2009;41(2):459–71.

56. Wadden TA, Crerand CE, Brock J. Behavioral treatment of obesity. Psychiatr Clin North Am. 2005;28(1):151–70. ix.

57. Pearson ES. Goal setting as a health behavior change strategy in overweight and obese adults: a systematic literature review examining intervention components. Patient Educ Couns. 2012;87(1):32–42.

58. Rollnick S, Miller WR, Butler C. Motivational interviewing in health care: helping patients change behavior. New York: Guilford; 2008.

59. DiLillo V, Siegfried NJ, West DS. Incorporating motivational interviewing into behavioral obesity treatment. Cogn Behav Pract. 2003;10(2):120–30.

60. Yale Rudd Center. Motivational interviewing for diet/exercise and obesity. 2007. http://www.yaleruddcenter.org/resources/bias_toolkit/toolkit/Module-2/2-07-MotivationalStrategies.pdf. Accessed 25 Jan 2015.

61. Cortese S, Angriman M, Maffeis C, Isnard P, Konofal E, Lecendreux M, et al. Attention-Deficit/Hyperactivity Disorder (ADHD) and obesity: a systematic review of the literature. Crit Rev Food Sci Nutr. 2008;48(6):524–37.

62. Altfas JR. Prevalence of attention deficit/hyperactivity disorder among adults in obesity treatment. BMC Psychiatry. 2002;2:9.

63. Vocks S, Tuschen-Caffier B, Pietrowsky R, Rustenbach S, Kersting A, Herpertz S. Meta-analysis of the effectiveness of psychological and pharmacological treatments for binge eating disorder. Int J Eat Disord. 2010;43(3):205–17.

64. Grilo CM, Masheb RM, Wilson GT. Subtyping binge eating disorder. J Consult Clin Psychol. 2001;69(6):1066–72.

65. Gladis MM, Wadden TA, Vogt R, Foster G, Kuehnel RH, Bartlett SJ. Behavioral treatment of obese binge eaters: do they need different care? J Psychosom Res. 1998;44(3–4):375–84.

66. Wilson G, Wilfley D, Agras W, Bryson S. Psychological treatments of binge eating disorder. Arch Gen Psychiatry. 2010;67(1):94–101.

67. Fairburn C. Overcoming binge eating. 2nd ed. New York: Guilford; 2013.

68. Sairanen E, Lappalainen R, Lapveteläinen A, Tolvanen A, Karhunen L. Flexibility in weight management. Eat Behav. 2014;15(2):218–24.
69. Adams CE, Leary MR. Promoting self-compassionate attitudes toward eating among restrictive and guilty eaters. J Soc Clin Psych. 2007;26(10):1120–44.
70. Fontaine KR, Barofsky I. Obesity and health-related quality of life. Obes Rev. 2001;2(3):173–82.
71. Cash TF, Pruzinsky TE. Body images: development, deviance, and change. New York: Guilford; 1990.
72. Friedman KE, Reichmann SK, Costanzo PR, Musante GJ. Body image partially mediates the relationship between obesity and psychological distress. Obes Res. 2002;10(1):33–41.
73. Grogan S. Body image and health: contemporary perspectives. J Health Psychol. 2006;11(4):523–30.
74. Chang VW, Christakis NA. Self-perception of weight appropriateness in the United States. Am J Prev Med. 2003;24(4):332–9.
75. Mack KA, Anderson L, Galuska D, Zablotsky D, Holtzman D, Ahluwalia I. Health and sociodemographic factors associated with body weight and weight objectives for women: 2000 behavioral risk factor surveillance system. J Womens Health. 2004;13(9):1019–32.
76. Snooks MK, Hall SK. Relationship of body size, body image, and self-esteem in African American, European American, and Mexican American middle-class women. Health Care Women Int. 2002;23(5):460–6.
77. McCabe MP, Ricciardelli LA. Body image dissatisfaction among males across the lifespan: a review of past literature. J Psychosom Res. 2004;56(6):675–85.
78. Phillips KA, Kim JM, Hudson JI. Body image disturbance in body dysmorphic disorder and eating disorders. Obsessions or delusions? Psychiatr Clin North Am. 1995;18(2):317–34.
79. Espeset EM, Nordbo RH, Gulliksen KS, Skarderud F, Geller J, Holte A. The concept of body image disturbance in anorexia nervosa: an empirical inquiry utilizing patients' subjective experiences. Eat Disord. 2011;19(2):175–93.
80. Grant JR, Cash TF. Cognitive-behavioral body image therapy: comparative efficacy of group and modest-contact treatments. Behav Ther. 1996;26(1):69–84.
81. Cash T. The body image workbook: an eight-step program for learning to like your looks. Oakland: New Harbinger Publications; 2008.
82. Callaghan GM, Sandoz EK, Darrow SM, Feeney TK. The body image psychological inflexibility scale: development and psychometric properties. Psychiatry Res. 2015;226(1):45–52.
83. Buchwald H, Avidor Y, Braunwald E, Jensen MD, Pories W, Fahrbach K, et al. Bariatric surgery: a systematic review and meta-analysis. JAMA. 2004;292(14):1724–37.
84. Sarwer DB, Wadden TA, Moore RH, Baker AW, Gibbons LM, Raper SE, et al. Preoperative eating behavior, postoperative dietary adherence, and weight loss after gastric bypass surgery. Surg Obes Relat Dis. 2008;4(5):640–6.
85. de Zwaan M, Hilbert A, Swan-Kremeier L, Simonich H, Lancaster K, Howell L, et al. Comprehensive interview assessment of eating behavior 18–35 months after gastric bypass surgery for morbid obesity. Surg Obes Relat Dis. 2010;6(1):79–85.
86. de Zwaan M, Enderle J, Wagner S, Muhlhans B, Ditzen B, Gefeller O, et al. Anxiety and depression in bariatric surgery patients: a prospective, follow-up study using structured clinical interviews. J Affect Disord. 2011;133(1–2):61–8.
87. Scholtz S, Bidlake L, Morgan J, Fiennes A, El-Etar A, Lacey J, et al. Long-term outcomes following laparoscopic adjustable gastric banding: postoperative psychological sequelae predict outcome at 5-year follow-up. Obes Surg. 2007;17(9):1220–5.
88. Beck N, Johannsen M, Støving R, Mehlsen M, Zachariae R. Do postoperative psychotherapeutic interventions and support groups influence weight loss following bariatric surgery? A systematic review and meta-analysis of randomized and nonrandomized trials. Obes Surg. 2012;22(11):1790–7.
89. Elakkary E, Gazayerli MM. Laparoscopic adjustable gastric band: do support groups add to the weight loss? Obes Surg. 2004;14(8):1139–40.

90. Kaiser KA, Franks SF, Smith AB. Positive relationship between support group attendance and one-year postoperative weight loss in gastric banding patients. Surg Obes Relat Dis. 2011;7(1):89–93.
91. Song Z, Reinhardt K, Buzdon M, Liao P. Association between support group attendance and weight loss after Roux-en-Y gastric bypass. Surg Obes Relat Dis. 2008;4(2):100–3.
92. Rudolph A, Hilbert A. Post-operative behavioural management in bariatric surgery: a systematic review and meta-analysis of randomized controlled trials. Obes Rev. 2013;14(4):292–302.
93. Vidot DC, Prado G, Cruz-Munoz N, Cuesta M, Spadola C, Messiah SE. Review of family-based approaches to improve postoperative outcomes among bariatric surgery patients. Surg Obes Relat Dis. 2015;11(2):451–8.
94. Xi B, Mi J, Zhao M, Zhang T, Jia C, Li J, et al. Trends in abdominal obesity among U.S. children and adolescents. Pediatrics. 2014;134(2):e334–9.
95. Moore LM, Fals AM, Jennelle PJ, Green JF, Pepe J, Richard T. Analysis of pediatric waist to hip ratio relationship to metabolic syndrome markers. J Pediatr Health Care. 2015;29(4):319–24.
96. Zeller MH, Inge TH, Modi AC, Jenkins TM, Michalsky MP, Helmrath M, et al. Severe obesity and comorbid condition impact on the weight-related quality of life of the adolescent patient. J Pediatr. 2015;166(3):651–9.e4.
97. Black WR, Davis AM, Gillette ML, Short MB, Wetterneck CT, He J. Health-related quality of life in obese and overweight, treatment-seeking youth. Ethn Dis. 2014;24(3):321–7.
98. Riverin M, Tremblay A. Obesity and ADHD. Int J Obes. 2009;33(8):945.
99. Murphy RA, Reinders I, Garcia ME, Eiriksdottir G, Launer LJ, Benediktsson R, et al. Adipose tissue, muscle, and function: potential mediators of associations between body weight and mortality in older adults with type 2 diabetes. Diabetes Care. 2014;37(12):3213–9.
100. Avena NM, Murray S, Gold MS. Comparing the effects of food restriction and overeating on brain reward systems. Exp Gerontol. 2013;48(10):1062–7.
101. Ogden CL, Carroll MD, Kit BK, Flegal KM. Prevalence of obesity among adults: United States, 2011–2012. NCHS Data Brief. 2013;131:1–8.
102. Ogden CL, Lamb MM, Carroll MD, Flegal KM. Obesity and socioeconomic status in adults: United States, 2005–2008. NCHS Data Brief. 2010;50:1–8.
103. Morland KB, Evenson KR. Obesity prevalence and the local food environment. Health Place. 2009;15(2):491–5.
104. Sallis JF, Glanz K. Physical activity and food environments: solutions to the obesity epidemic. Milbank Q. 2009;87(1):123–54.
105. Gordon-Larsen P. Food availability/convenience and obesity. Adv Nutr. 2014;5(6):809–17.
106. Morland K, Diez Roux AV, Wing S. Supermarkets, other food stores, and obesity: the atherosclerosis risk in communities study. Am J Prev Med. 2006;30(4):333–9.
107. Zenk SN, Schulz AJ, Israel BA, James SA, Bao S, Wilson ML. Fruit and vegetable access differs by community racial composition and socioeconomic position in Detroit, Michigan. Ethn Dis. 2006;16(1):275–80.
108. Beaulac J, Kristjansson E, Cummins S. A systematic review of food deserts, 1966–2007. Prev Chronic Dis. 2009;6(3):A105.
109. Cain KL, Millstein RA, Sallis JF, Conway TL, Gavand KA, Frank LD, et al. Contribution of streetscape audits to explanation of physical activity in four age groups based on the Microscale Audit of Pedestrian Streetscapes (MAPS). Soc Sci Med. 2014;116:82–92.
110. Gordon-Larsen P, Nelson MC, Page P, Popkin BM. Inequality in the built environment underlies key health disparities in physical activity and obesity. Pediatrics. 2006;117(2):417–24.
111. Sallis JF, Cervero RB, Ascher W, Henderson KA, Kraft MK, Kerr J. An ecological approach to creating active living communities. Annu Rev Public Health. 2006;27:297–322.
112. Linton LS, Edwards CC, Woodruff SI, Millstein RA, Moder C. Youth advocacy as a tool for environmental and policy changes that support physical activity and nutrition: an evaluation study in San Diego County. Prev Chronic Dis. 2014;11:E46.

113. Marcus DA. Obesity and the impact of chronic pain. Clin J Pain. 2004;20(3):186–91.

114. Ursini F, Naty S, Grembiale RD. Fibromyalgia and obesity: the hidden link. Rheumatol Int. 2011;31(11):1403–8.

115. Christensen R, Bartels EM, Astrup A, Bliddal H. Effect of weight reduction in obese patients diagnosed with knee osteoarthritis: a systematic review and meta-analysis. Ann Rheum Dis. 2007;66(4):433–9.

116. Melissas J, Kontakis G, Volakakis E, Tsepetis T, Alegakis A, Hadjipavlou A. The effect of surgical weight reduction on functional status in morbidly obese patients with low back pain. Obes Surg. 2005;15(3):378–81.

117. Peltonen M, Lindroos AK, Torgerson JS. Musculoskeletal pain in the obese: a comparison with a general population and long-term changes after conventional and surgical obesity treatment. Pain. 2003;104(3):549–57.

118. Janke EA, Fritz M, Hopkins C, Haltzman B, Sautter JM, Ramirez ML. A randomized clinical trial of an integrated behavioral self-management intervention Simultaneously Targeting Obesity and Pain: the STOP trial. BMC Public Health. 2014;14:621.

119. Jeon WS, Park CY. Antiobesity pharmacotherapy for patients with type 2 diabetes: focus on long-term management. Endocrinol Metab (Seoul). 2014;29(4):410–7.

120. Dixon JB, Browne JL, Mosely KG, Rice TL, Jones KM, Pouwer F, et al. Severe obesity and diabetes self-care attitudes, behaviours and burden: implications for weight management from a matched case-controlled study. Results from Diabetes MILES—Australia. Diabet Med. 2014;31(2):232–40.

121. Wermeling M, Thiele-Manjali U, Koschack J, Lucius-Hoene G, Himmel W. Type 2 diabetes patients' perspectives on lifestyle counselling and weight management in general practice: a qualitative study. BMC Fam Pract. 2014;15:97.

122. Li C, Ford ES, Zhao G, Croft JB, Balluz LS, Mokdad AH. Prevalence of self-reported clinically diagnosed sleep apnea according to obesity status in men and women: National Health and Nutrition Examination Survey, 2005–2006. Prev Med. 2010;51(1):18–23.

123. Tuomilehto H, Seppa J, Uusitupa M. Obesity and obstructive sleep apnea—clinical significance of weight loss. Sleep Med Rev. 2013;17(5):321–9.

124. Drager LF, Togeiro SM, Polotsky VY, Lorenzi-Filho G. Obstructive sleep apnea: a cardiometabolic risk in obesity and the metabolic syndrome. J Am Coll Cardiol. 2013;62(7):569–76.

125. Rishi MA, Copur AS, Nadeem R, Fulambarker A. Effect of positive airway pressure therapy on body mass index in obese patients with obstructive sleep apnea syndrome: a prospective study. Am J Ther. 2016;23(2):e422–8.

Additional Resources

Books

Brownell KD. The LEARN program for weight management 2000. Dallas: American Health Publishers; 2000.

Burns DD. Feeling good: The new mood therapy. New York, NY: Avon Books, 1980.

Cash T. The body image workbook. Oakland, CA: New Harbinger Publications, Inc., 1997; 2nd Edition, 2008.

Davis M, Robbins Eshelman, E, McKay, M. The relaxation & stress reduction workbook. Oakland, CA: New Harbinger Publications, Inc., 2008.

Fairburn C. Overcoming binge eating, 2nd Ed. New York, NY: Guilford Press; 2013.

Furtado MM, Schultz L, Ewing J. Recipes for life after weight-loss surgery. Beverly, MA: Fairwinds Press, 2011.

Greenberger D, Padesky C. Mind over mood, second edition: Change how you feel by changing the way you think. New York, NY: Guilford Press, 2016.

Johnson C. Self-esteem comes in all sizes. Carlsbad, CA: Gurze Books, 2001.

Roth G. Breaking free from emotional eating. New York, NY. Plume/Penquin Books, 1984.

Satter E. How to get your kid to eat... But not too much. Boulder, CO: Bull Publishing Company, 1987.

Satter E. Your child's weight: Helping without harming. Madison, WI: Kelcy Press, 2005.

Satter E. Secrets of feeding a healthy family: How to eat, raise good eaters, how to cook. Madison, WI: Kelcy Press, 2008.

Websites

Mindless Eating—Brian Wansink. http://mindlesseating.org/.

Motivational Interviewing. http://www.yaleruddcenter.org/resources/bias_toolkit/toolkit/Module-2/2-07-MotivationalStrategies.pdf.

National Institute of Diabetes and Digestive and Kidney Diseases. http://www.niddk.nih.gov/health-information/health-statistics/Pages/overweight-obesity-statistics.aspx.

The Center for Mindful Eating. http://www.thecenterformindfuleating.org/.

Chapter 4
Cognitive and Behavioral Approaches for Treating Substance Use Disorders Among Behavioral Medicine Patients

Allison K. Labbe, Julie Yeterian, Julianne G. Wilner, and John F. Kelly

4.1 Introduction

Substance use and substance use disorders (SUD), including alcohol, are a serious public health concern. For example, from 2010 to 2012 the rate of heroin overdose doubled [1], and from 1999 to 2010 the overdose rate from prescription opioid medications has quadrupled [1]. In fact, in 2012 drug overdose was the leading cause of injury death among people aged 18–64 years, and overdose caused more deaths than motor vehicle accidents [1]. And, in 2011 drug misuse was related to 2.5 million emergency department visits [2]. Especially among individuals with a co-occurring medical condition, substance use can negatively affect treatment adherence (e.g., [3–16]) as well as disease progression and outcome (e.g., [17–21]), and it is significantly related to increased mortality, particularly among medically ill people (e.g., [5, 9, 10, 22]).

A.K. Labbe, Ph.D. (✉) • J.G. Wilner, M.A.
Behavioral Medicine Service, Department of Psychiatry, Massachusetts General Hospital, Harvard Medical School, Boston, MA, USA
e-mail: aklabbe@mgh.harvard.edu; jgwilner@mgh.harvard.edu

J. Yeterian, M.A.
Department of Psychiatry, Center for Addiction Medicine, Massachusetts General Hospital, Boston, MA, USA
e-mail: jyeterian@mgh.harvard.edu

J.F. Kelly, Ph.D.
Department of Psychiatry, Harvard Medical School, Massachusetts General Hospital, 60 Staniford Street, Boston, MA 02114, USA

Department of Psychiatry, Center for Addiction Medicine, Massachusetts General Hospital, Boston, MA, USA
e-mail: jkelly11@mgh.harvard.edu

© Springer Science+Business Media New York 2017
A.-M. Vranceanu et al. (eds.), *The Massachusetts General Hospital Handbook of Behavioral Medicine*, Current Clinical Psychiatry, DOI 10.1007/978-3-319-29294-6_4

Substance use disorders are caused by the interaction of multiple variables. These include genetic, biological, and environmental factors, as well as exposure to the specific drug. Addiction has a strong genetic component, accounting for approximately 50 % of the risk [23, 24]. When this predisposition is combined with stress-inducing environmental factors, such as developmental trauma, poverty, unemployment, and psychiatric illness, along with exposure to substances (especially during teenage years), risk for developing SUD increases [25]. Drug-specific pharmacological effects, as well as the potency, concentration, and speed at which the drug reaches the brain following administration, also independently influence perceived reward and SUD risk. The fastest routes to the brain are via the lungs (smoking), followed by injection (intravenous), nasal (snorting), and oral (drinking/eating).

SUD presentation in clinical practice is highly heterogeneous and will differ within and across settings. In fact, the DSM-5 [26] diagnosis of SUD encompasses a broad range of severity. Individuals are diagnosed with mild (2–3 symptoms), moderate (4–5 symptoms), or severe (6 or more symptoms) SUD, depending on how many of the 11 symptoms they endorse. Individuals who use substances, but do not endorse at least two symptoms of SUD would not be classified as having the disorder.

The rates of alcohol and other substance use disorders in the United States are high. In 2013, 21.6 million people were classified with DSM-IV dependence or abuse [25]. Among this group, 14.7 million people were classified with alcohol abuse or dependence, 4.2 million met criteria for marijuana abuse or dependence, and 1.9 million met for prescription opioid abuse or dependence [25]. What is noteworthy is that 20.2 million people in the United States ages 12 and older who were classified as needing treatment for a substance use disorder did not receive specialty treatment, and that only 4.5 % of these people classified as needing treatment believed they actually needed treatment [25]. Overall, the data indicate that people with a substance use disorder are especially undertreated.

4.1.1 Chapter Overview

Treating a substance use disorder can be challenging. Potentially complicating the treatment of an SUD is the presence of a comorbid chronic medical condition. Not only can problematic alcohol or substance use cause the onset or acquisition of some medical conditions, active alcohol and other substance use can exacerbate medical problems, complicate the treatment of medical problems, and have adverse effects on disease course and prognosis. To illustrate these complications and how to effectively address them using cognitive–behavioral interventions, we have organized this chapter into six sections: (1) the prevalence, clinical presentations, and complications of having a comorbid alcohol or other substance use disorder across five significant medical conditions; (2) description of cognitive and behavioral approaches to addressing alcohol and other drug use disorders in medical settings;

(3) a brief overview of the empirical support for CBT approaches for alcohol and other substance use disorders; (4) implementation of CBT in addressing these clinical challenges; (5) implementation of harm reduction approaches to reduce harm caused by substances when abstinence is clinically unfeasible; and (6) a case example that highlights CBT principles and techniques in practice.

4.1.2 Prevalence, Clinical Presentations, and Implications of a Comorbid Substance Use Disorder Among Behavioral Medicine Patient Populations

In this section, we describe the epidemiology and practice implications of addressing alcohol and other substance use disorders across five high volume and/or high burden medical conditions: cancer, HIV/AIDs, hepatitis C, diabetes, and chronic pain.

Cancer. Alcohol use has been linked to an increased risk for developing various types of cancer. Meta-analyses have found that alcohol consumption has been linked to cancer of the mouth, pharynx, larynx, esophagus, liver, female breast, stomach, colon, rectum, and ovaries [27–29]. Further, studies show that the relative risk for developing cancer due to alcohol consumption is associated with quantity of alcohol consumed. For example, Bagnardi and colleagues [27] found that the greatest relative risk of developing cancer occurred for cancers of the oral cavity (i.e., mouth, larynx, pharynx) and esophagus and that the relative risk substantially increased as the quantity of alcohol consumed increased. Specifically, the relative risk of developing cancer of the oral cavity associated with consuming 2, 4, and 8 standard drinks per day was 1.73, 2.77, and 5.75, respectively. In other words, among people who consumed eight standard drinks per day, their relative risk of developing mouth, larynx, or pharynx cancer was nearly six times greater than for abstainers. Similar rates were found by Bagnardi et al. [28] and Rehm et al. [29]. These findings are important given that the rates of an alcohol use disorder among cancer patients is up to five times higher than the general population [30–33].

Alcohol consumption has shown to have a substantial effect on disease progress and mortality for some cancers. Araújo and colleagues [22] found that, among colorectal cancer (CRC) patients, the odds of developing stage III and IV tumors was 2.22 times greater, and the odds of dying were 1.71 times greater, among the patients who consumed alcohol compared to the patients who did not. Maeda et al. [17] found that alcohol consumption was an independent predictor of liver metastases among CRC patients. Findings are similar among patients with lung cancer in that alcohol abuse is associated with increased surgical resection complications, increased risk of postoperative mortality, faster disease progression and worse prognosis [34–36]. The effects of alcohol on breast cancer are mixed. Some studies have found that drinking more than one alcoholic drink per day (i.e., ≥10 g of alcohol) was associated with a 1 % increased risk of death from breast cancer [37–39]. However, one of the largest pooled investigations examining data from over 9300 breast cancer survivors found no significant associations between post-diagnosis alcohol consumption and breast cancer recurrence or mortality [40].

Last, among patients with cancer, problematic alcohol and/or other substance use has been shown to be associated with increased pain sensitivity [33], difficulties in adequately treating one's pain [30], limited social supports, and dysfunctional family structures [41] which can negatively affect quality of life and survival [42, 43] and poor treatment adherence [3].

HIV/AIDS. By the end of 2010, the prevalence of HIV in the United States was approximately 1.1 million people. The incidence of HIV in 2010 was approximately 47,745 and injection drug use (IDU) or male-to-male sexual contact in the setting of IDU accounted for 9.7 % of these new infections [44]. Not only are rates of alcohol and drug use, and alcohol and substance use disorders, high among individuals with HIV (at least twice that of the general population; [4, 45, 46]), use of alcohol and other drugs are also associated with an increased risk for HIV infection. Buchacz and colleagues [47] found that HIV incidence among amphetamine users was 6.3 % per year, compared to 2.1 % per year among non-users. Other studies have found that use of "poppers" was associated with increased hazard rates of HIV seroconversion (HR 2.10–3.89; [48, 49]). A recent meta-analysis examining the effects of alcohol consumption on HIV incidence found that alcohol consumers were at a 77 % increased risk of HIV infection, those consuming alcohol at the time of or prior to sexual relations were at an 87 % increased risk of HIV, and binge drinkers were twice as likely to become infected with HIV compared to non-binge drinkers [50].

One of the primary reasons for the higher HIV incidence among people who engage in alcohol and substance use is engaging in risky sexual practices due to the disinhibitory effect that alcohol and drugs cause. Mimiaga and colleagues found, for example, that those HIV+ individuals who reported engaging in unprotected anal sex had higher odds of polydrug, marijuana, amphetamine, opiate, and injection drug use. Similarly, they found that unprotected vaginal sex was associated with polydrug and crack-cocaine use [4]. Further, research has found that any alcohol consumption, problematic drinking, and alcohol use in sexual contexts were associated with a 63 % increase, 69 % increase, and a 95 % increase, respectively, in engaging in unprotected sex among people living with HIV/AIDS [51].

Finally, there is substantial evidence demonstrating the various adverse consequences that alcohol and substance use can have on HIV treatment adherence, disease progression, and mortality. Specifically, studies show that alcohol and substance use negatively affects CD4 cell counts, viral load, highly active antiretroviral therapy (HAART) uptake and adherence, healthcare utilization, and liver function [4–12, 14, 52].

Hepatitis C (HCV). Hepatitis C virus (HCV) is the most common chronic bloodborne infection in the United States with 3.2 million people chronically infected [105, 106]. Chronic HCV infection is the leading cause of cirrhosis and hepatocellular carcinoma, as well as a primary reason for liver transplantation [53]. Injection drug use (IDU) is the most common route of transmission of HCV in the United States and accounts for at least 70 % of all new HCV infections [54] A recent report demonstrated that each HCV+ person who engages in IDU will infect another 20 people with HCV and that this rapid transmission occurs within the first 3 years of infection [55]. Though injection drug use is most highly related to incidence of HCV infection, non-injection use of other substances (i.e., heroin, crack, cocaine) is also associated with HCV incidence rates of 5–29 %, depending on the substance used, gender, and age [56]. Alcohol use is very common among people with HCV, with rates of heavy alcohol use among HCV patients is nearly eight times higher than the general population (41 % vs. 5 %, respectively; [57]).

Few studies have been conducted to examine the effects of ongoing substance use on the course of HCV disease progression, primarily due to the fact that people who engage in injection drug use do not regularly undergo liver biopsy and are difficult to monitor over time [18]. However, one study examining the natural history of disease progression among people who acquired HCV from IDU found that the relative incidence of developing end-stage liver disease (ESLD) significantly increased as frequency of IDU increased [18]. Moreover, injection drug use is associated with low rates of HCV treatment uptake, with approximately only 1–6 % initiating treatment [15, 16]. Alcohol use in HCV has been shown to increase severity and progression of liver disease, increase incidence and prevalence of cirrhosis, decrease effectiveness of interferon treatment, decrease immune response, increase viral load, increase liver fibrosis, and increase treatment discontinuation [58–60]. Generally, given that heavy alcohol use and HCV infection independently are known to potentially cause cirrhosis, when combined together they produce a synergistic effect that hastens liver fibrosis and cirrhosis [18–21]. In fact, Corrao and Arico [19] found that, among HCV-infected heavy drinkers (i.e., consuming between 9 and 12 alcoholic drinkers per day), the risk for developing cirrhosis was 100 times greater than for HCV-infected individuals who did not consume alcohol.

Diabetes. The prevalence of diabetes has increased substantially in recent years [61]. In 2013, an estimated 382 million individuals globally were living with diabetes, and that number is expected to rise to 592 million by 2035 [62]. Substance use, specifically heavy alcohol use, is associated with an increased risk for type 2 diabetes [63]. Although some evidence suggests that mild to moderate alcohol use is associated with a decreased risk for type 2 diabetes [63–65], more rigorous recent research suggests this research was confounded by lack of control of important explanatory variables. Recent studies suggest there is likely no alcohol-related health benefit even from mild-moderate amounts of alcohol consumption [66, 67].

Despite these facts, for patients with diabetes, rates of co-occurring alcohol and other substance disorders are higher among patients with diabetes than the general population. A study by the National Institute on Alcohol Abuse and Alcoholism (NIAAA) reported that, among primary care patients diagnosed with diabetes, 13.4 % met criteria for at-risk drinking, and 11.1 % of these risky drinkers met criteria for current alcohol dependence [68], compared to estimated prevalence rates of heavy alcohol use of 6.3 % in the general population [25]. A review of diabetic young people (age 17–24, mean age 21) using substances found that more than 50 % of participants reported using cannabis (80 %), ecstasy (60 %), and heroin (30 %); 70 % were poly-drug users [69].

Elevated rates of substance and alcohol use within diabetic patients are of particular concern as they are associated with poorer medication adherence, which is essential for maximizing one's prognosis in diabetes [70]. Consequently, alcohol abuse and dependence is likely associated with increased morbidity and mortality in diabetes, especially given the complications of non-adherence [71].

Non-cancer Chronic Pain. Chronic pain is a widely prevalent and interfering disease and co-occurs with substance use at a high rate [72]. As many as five to seven million patients with a substance use disorder also report pain [73] although this number may not be fully representative of the full population [72].

A significant issue with regard to treating chronic pain, especially among patients with a substance use disorder, is that the opioids used to treat the pain (e.g., morphine, codeine, oxycodone) may be posited as "the problem," "the solution," or a combination of both [73]. Patients tend to misuse opioids for a number of reasons that are linked to various implications and consequences. Individuals may misunderstand the correct use of opioids, including using opioids to obtain relief from depressive or anxious symptoms, insomnia, or a host of other symptoms. Additionally, patients dependent on opioids may overuse opioids even once the pain has subsided to reduce withdrawal symptoms [74]. Regardless, if a substance use disorder predominates within a clinical setting, aggressive management of an underlying pain problem is likely to be ineffective if not coordinated appropriately with treatment for the concurrent SUD [73].

Substance use proves to be problematic to individuals living with chronic pain as it has been shown that persons with substance use disorders are less likely to receive effective pain treatment [75]. The stress of a lack of adequate treatment of pain may itself serve as a trigger to relapse to substance use [73]. Along these lines, research has shown that a large proportion of patients with chronic pain underuse their opioid prescription medications [76, 77], often citing concerns about adverse effects, particularly addiction [78, 79]. Though little research exists that specifically examines reasons for underuse among chronic pain patients with a history of a substance use disorder, one study found that half of the "under-users" were concerned about addiction which was reflective of their history with substance use disorders [79]. Underuse of medication can leave pain untreated, which, as stated previously, is a potential trigger for relapse. It is therefore important for clinicians treating patients with chronic pain to be aware of whether a patient is in recovery from a substance use disorder in order to anticipate and prevent potential relapse. It is also imperative to discuss the possibility of relapse and associated consequences with patients over the course of therapy, especially when the use of prescription opioids are incorporated within the treatment regimen as they may lead to physical dependency and possible misuse (either overuse or underuse). However, the clinician should also be sensitive not to inadvertently minimalize the patient's complaints of pain, and see the patient's willingness to discuss past (or current) substance problems as an opportunity for readiness for change. This will also aid in stigma reduction, harm reduction, and overall patient care [73].

It is important to note that opioid medications tend to be the first-line approach to treating pain. However, research has shown that, patients who continue to take opioid medications at least 2 months post-trauma tend to have higher rates of psychological distress, less effective coping strategies, and higher scores on disability compared to patients who do not take opioids [80].

Given that long-term use of an opioid increases one's risk of developing physical dependency and misuse/abuse, it is important for a clinician working with patients with chronic pain and a history of a substance use disorder to also consider prescribing psychosocial treatments for pain management, such as CBT or other efficacious skills-based interventions.

In summary, problematic alcohol and substance use is related to a wide variety of negative outcomes, including mortality. However, particularly among medically ill individuals, alcohol and substance use are related to disease acquisition, hastening of disease progression, increased mortality, and poor medical treatment adherence. Consequently, if the underlying substance use disorder can be effectively treated, this would translate to improved disease outcomes. Accordingly, we will now describe a cognitive behavioral approach for the treatment of substance use disorders, with particular attention paid to individuals with a co-occurring medical condition.

4.1.3 Cognitive Behavioral Approaches for Treating Substance Use Disorders

From the standpoint of social-cognitive learning theory [81], onset and maintenance of SUD is related to observing social modeling of substance use, receiving social encouragement and support for drug use, and possessing positive beliefs about drugs' effects (also known as "expectancies"). In addition, SUD onset risk and relapse following periods of abstinence are believed to be increased by inadequate skills to cope with life-stressors and a lack of alternative rewarding activity options. Substance use is believed to act as the predominant coping response to aversive stimuli among individuals with SUD. Consequently, cognitive behavioral therapy (CBT) is often based around addressing these presumed cognitive and behavioral deficits.

Cognitive behavioral approaches teach skills for managing threats to sobriety on an ongoing basis, in order to reduce one's risk for relapse. "Relapse Prevention" is a general term that encompasses cognitive behavioral, skills-based approaches. Based on the cognitive behavioral model, Relapse Prevention focuses on identifying personal predictors of relapse, including contextual factors (e.g., high-risk situations) and tonic (stable) processes (e.g., thought patterns, distal risk factors), and implementing skills to cope with these in order to prevent relapse [82].

At least some client motivation for change is a prerequisite for the successful implementation of CBT/Relapse Prevention skills. If the client is not motivated to learn and implement skills, CBT is unlikely to be effective. Clients are often ambivalent about changing their substance use and may present with varying levels of motivation. As such, therapists may wish to incorporate motivational enhancement strategies (e.g., Motivational Interviewing; [83]; www.motivationalinterviewing.org) into CBT/Relapse Prevention approaches, as client motivation typically waxes and wanes. It is also important to note that, while some clients may be able to stop using drugs/alcohol safely on an outpatient basis while participating in CBT/Relapse Prevention, others, who are more severely addicted or who have medical issues that could be complicated by withdrawal (e.g., acute coronary syndrome, sepsis, pregnancy), will need to undergo detoxification and stabilization under medical supervision before beginning CBT/Relapse Prevention.

Assessment Measures. Before beginning treatment therapists may wish to conduct a comprehensive assessment of patients' substance use and treatment history, mental and physical health, risk behaviors, and social, legal, and vocational needs. The Global Appraisal of Individual Needs (GAIN; [84]) and Addiction Severity Index (ASI; [85]) are excellent examples of such comprehensive, multidimensional assessments. Both require training to administer. Upon intake and throughout treatment, therapists may wish to use additional assessment tools to monitor patients' degree of craving for alcohol and/or other drugs (Craving Questionnaire; [86]), motivation/commitment to sobriety (Commitment to Sobriety Scale [CSS]; [87]), and the intrinsic and environmental resources that can support patients' recovery (i.e., recovery capital; Assessment of Recovery Capital [ARC]; [88]). Ongoing measurement of anxiety (Generalized Anxiety Disorder 7-item scale [GAD-7]; [89]), and depression (Patient Health Questionnaire [PHQ-9]; [90]) symptoms is also important, as these are often related to substance use and withdrawal.

4.1.4   Empirical Support for CBT in the Treatment of SUD

Numerous quantitative reviews of CBT and Relapse Prevention for SUD have demonstrated the efficacy of these treatment approaches. One meta-analytic review that included 53 randomized controlled trials of CBT for adults with SUD found a positive treatment effect (e.g., improved abstinence rates, fewer drinking/using days) of a small magnitude (Hedges's $g = 0.14$), which diminished by 12 months post-treatment ($g = 0.096$). However, a majority (58%) of these patients still fared better than patients in active comparison conditions, which included such treatments as discussion groups, interpersonal therapy, 12-step facilitation, communication skills training, support counseling, and medication [91]. The magnitude of the effect of treatment increased when CBT was combined with another psychosocial treatment (e.g., motivational interviewing, contingency management, social support, behavioral therapy) ($g = 0.305$) and, when compared to no-treatment controls, CBT demonstrated a large effect on substance use outcomes ($g = 0.796$). Another meta-analysis comprises 34 studies found a similar small treatment effect for CBT alone (Cohen's $d = 0.28$) and found post-treatment abstinence rates to be 27.1% [92].

Though Relapse Prevention is an influential cognitive behavioral approach to the treatment of SUD, a primary distinction between CBT and Relapse Prevention is that CBT is more often used to describe a primary, or stand-alone, treatment based on the cognitive behavioral model, whereas Relapse Prevention is more often utilized to describe a type of treatment that occurs after a patient obtain abstinence and is working to stay in recovery [82]. Meta-analytic reviews specifically examining the effects of Relapse Prevention have demonstrated similar results as general CBT. Irvin and colleagues [93] and Dutra and colleagues [92] both found small overall treatment effects for Relapse Prevention ($r = 0.14$ and $d = 0.32$, respectively).

Importantly, Irvin's review also showed that Relapse Prevention produced a large change in psychosocial adjustment ($r=0.48$). Dutra and colleagues [92] found that Relapse Prevention produced the largest post-treatment abstinence rates (39.0 %) compared to general CBT alone (27.1 %) and contingency management alone (31.0 %). Irvin and colleagues [93] suggested that one reason why the magnitude of the effect size of Relapse Prevention on substance use outcomes was not larger might have been due to the fact that most studies utilized Relapse Prevention immediately following another primary intervention, or as a supplement to another treatment, and so a true comparison between active treatment and no-treatment controls could not be adequately obtained.

4.1.4.1   Moderators of Treatment Outcomes

Type of Substance: Moderator analyses for CBT alone and for Relapse Prevention alone have demonstrated differential effects of treatment on outcome depending on the type of substance. Regarding CBT, stronger treatment effects were found with marijuana ($g=0.513$) than for alcohol or any other drug class [91]. Irvin et al. [93] discovered that Relapse Prevention was more effective for alcohol use and polysubstance use ($r=0.37$ and $r=0.27$, respectively) than for cocaine and cigarette smoking ($r=-0.03$ and $r=0.09$, respectively).

Treatment Format: Generally, meta-analyses of CBT/Relapse Prevention have found no differences in effectiveness for either CBT or Relapse Prevention by treatment format (group vs. individual; [91, 93]). As such, group CBT/Relapse Prevention may be the most cost-effective route for clinical delivery, but patient preference should be taken into consideration.

Despite the existence of methodological limitations in the randomized controlled trials that were utilized for the meta-analyses presented here, the most common being a limited number of studies examining the application of CBT/Relapse Prevention across several types of substances, the general findings are that CBT and Relapse Prevention are efficacious in the treatment of SUD. Continued research testing these treatment approaches with a more comprehensive range of substance use types will help elucidate the generalizability of CBT/Relapse Prevention.

4.1.5   Implementing CBT for SUD Among Patients with Medical Conditions

Setting the Stage. Treatment begins with a thorough exploration of the client's patterns of substance use, which can be accomplished using a *behavior chain analysis* (sometimes called a "functional analysis;" see Sect. 4.2). Here, the client and therapist collaboratively explore a recent, representative episode of substance use as a chronological sequence (chain) of events. The therapist asks the client to recall a recent, typical episode of substance use and to describe, in as much detail as possible, the situation (Where was he? Who was he with? What was he doing?) and related triggers (i.e., people, places, emotions, times of day, activities, or objects). These details provide information on what situational or contextual factors (i.e., "triggers" or "high-risk situations") put the client at risk for relapse. Then, the client is asked to report on what he was thinking at the time of use, as well as how he was feeling at the time of use (either emotionally or physically). Especially when working with patients with a comorbid medical condition, it is also important to identify the ways in which factors related to his or her medical condition are incorporated into the behavioral chain analysis. For example, is a client taking extra pain medication in response to experiencing distressing cancer-related pain? Or, is a client drinking alcohol as a way to cope with anxiety or stress related to managing his or her chronic illness? Additionally, collecting information about the method and quantity of alcohol/substance use and any other behaviors that are contemporaneous with using/drinking is important. This glimpse into the client's thought patterns provides valuable information about the nature and impact of his cognitive distortions, which informs the clinical approach to challenging these thoughts. Further, clients are often unaware of the emotional and affective drives that precipitate use, and these feelings can greatly impact the overall experience of getting high/intoxicated.

Finally, the therapist asks the client about the positive and negative results of using/drinking, both at the time and afterwards. It is crucial to gather information on the specific benefits the client receives from drinking or using drugs, as these are powerful reinforcers of substance use (e.g., immediate relief of physical pain that one may feel is intolerable, immediate reduction of anxiety and panicky feelings that one may feel consumed by when thinking about having a terminal illness; immediate escape from feelings of shame). Further, it is important to provide information about the needs that the client has that must be met in other ways if sobriety is to be maintained, such as learning to cope with triggers/high-risk situations (e.g., certain emotions, physical symptoms, attending medical appointments) and having fun or socializing without being intoxicated. In terms of negative results, clients are likely to talk about a variety of consequences, including hangovers, breaking a period of abstinence and having to "start all over," feeling bad about themselves, missing important medical appointments or not adhering to medical treatment appropriately, or noticing "flare ups" or worsening of their medical condition. While there are often short-term positive consequences of using, most clients who have a co-occurring medical condition present for SUD treatment after noticing that their alcohol or drug use is exacerbating their medical condition or hastening disease progression.

The behavior chain analysis sets the stage for further intervention, as it reveals the *function* of the substance use and highlights the difficulties that the client will encounter as he enters sobriety and the substance no longer serves those functions (see Table 4.1). It is also important in CBT to have a *written treatment goal* that is determined largely by the client and mutually agreed upon, so that the therapist and client will know whether the client is meeting or progressing towards his treatment goal from week to week. It can also be useful to collaborate with a client's medical providers to incorporate specific goals related to managing effectively his or her medical illness, especially as it relates to substance use. The combination of the treatment goal and the functional analysis helps the therapist and client to identify the steps that must be taken in order for the client to succeed.

Learning and Implementing Skills. CBT/Relapse Prevention skills generally fall into two related categories: (1) skills that are implemented in the moment when relapse risk is high (e.g., leaving a high-risk situation, urge surfing) and (2) lifestyle changes that reduce overall risk for relapse (e.g., changing social networks, self-care). It is necessary to attend to both sets of skills when treating SUD. CBT/Relapse Prevention skills can be mapped onto the behavior chain model of SUD (see Table 4.1).

Triggers and High-Risk Situations (HRS): Triggers can be external (e.g., certain people, certain places, time of day, seeing medication bottles) or internal (e.g., positive or negative emotions; feeling ill from medication side effects). Many external triggers can be avoided, which is a basic skill for managing them, but this is another area which clients are likely to be ambivalent about changing. Avoiding triggers usually entails making changes to one's social network in order to lessen exposure to people who use/drink and increase exposure to sober or recovering people. Particularly for young adult and adolescent clients, changing the social network is a major treatment challenge, as drug and alcohol use frequently occurs in a social context [94, 95] and the social network is funneled over time to mainly include fellow drug and alcohol users. Though many external triggers can be avoided, for behavioral medicine patients there are also several external triggers that cannot (or should not) be avoided. In this manner, it is important to work with the client to identify what thoughts and feelings come up when these external triggers (e.g., seeing medication bottles, taking medications, attending medical appointments, receiving lab results) present themselves, and problem-solving ways to approach (rather than avoid) these triggers without using alcohol or drugs. Additional strategies include identifying and challenging inaccurate thoughts about one's ability to approach these particular triggers without using and finding alternative behaviors to substance use to cope.

Internal triggers (i.e., certain emotional states, physical symptoms) cannot be avoided and must be tolerated without the use of drugs and alcohol (often called "distress tolerance"). Ongoing self-care efforts such as getting adequate sleep, eating healthfully, exercising regularly, and managing stress can lessen emotionality and thus decrease the intensity of these internal triggers. Self-care can be a major treatment target, as many clients with SUD experience at least some deficiencies in their self-care during periods of active use. Some clients with more severe addictions will have completely neglected their self-care and can have a variety of nutritional and medical problems as a result. Further, self-care can decline when a patient is also struggling with intense or incapacitating physical symptoms associated with his or her medical condition, or side effects from its treatment, such as experiencing nausea and fatigue from chemotherapy treatments, HIV medications, and/or HCV treatment. Therefore, it is of particular significance to problem-solve ways to increase one's self-care as a way to reduce triggers to use substances, as well as to improve one's overall sense of well-being.

Thoughts: When examining cognitions, it is important to examine any thought pattern that predisposes the client to substance use. This can include thoughts that

Table 4.1 Cognitive–behavioral model of SUD and related interventions

Behavior chain model element	Theoretical deficits/clinical targets	Interventions
Triggers and high-risk situations (HRS)	• Limited awareness of the maintaining conditions of substance use	• Identifying triggers and HRS
	• Limited awareness of high-risk situations that precipitate relapse	• Avoiding HRS when possible
		• Changing social networks to lessen exposure to HRS
		• Increase skills to cope effectively with HRS that cannot be avoided
Thoughts	• Cognitive errors in risk appraisal (e.g., underestimation of risk)	• Identifying patterns of problematic thinking
	• Positive outcome expectancies for substance use	• Challenging problematic thinking, alone or with another person
	• Abstinence violation effect	• Use of cognitive distraction
Feelings	• Limited ability to identify and understand feelings	• Grounding
	• Reluctance or inability to tolerate negative emotions	• Breathing exercises
		• Distress tolerance (e.g., distraction, acceptance)
		• Urge surfing
		• Indirect mechanisms (changing thoughts and behaviors, e.g., assertiveness training)
Behaviors	• Insufficient knowledge of effective alternative coping skills	• Making a decision to delay use
	• Lack of confidence in the ability to deploy coping skills	• Escaping/leaving HRS
		• Substitute behaviors that are incompatible with using (e.g., exercise)
		• Drink/drug refusal skills
		• Assertiveness training
Positive consequences (of substance use)	• Limited awareness of the short-term benefits of substance use that increase the probability of use	• Increasing pleasant activities
	• Lack of non-drug rewards	• Relearning how to have fun without being drunk/high
		• Finding alternative ways to relax or feel good
		• Awareness of the benefits of sobriety
Negative consequences (of substance use)	• Inadequate appraisal of the negative impacts of substance use	• Increase awareness of the nature and impact of drug-related consequences
	• Limited understanding of how these can create a feedback loop for further substance use	• Problem-solving
		• Goal-setting

are directly about using/drinking (e.g., "I deserve a drink because I am in so much pain." "I can take just one hit." "I've got a terminal illness, so why not?"), as well as thoughts that are indirectly related (e.g., "I can't stand to feel sick anymore." "I want to relax."). Clients may also have distorted viewpoints about sobriety or recovery ("These urges will last forever."), which can decrease their self-efficacy for abstinence and predispose them to relapse. The first step towards addressing these problematic thought patterns is to identify what they are and how much the client believes them. The therapist can use Socratic questioning to gently challenge the client to come up with other interpretations (e.g., "What evidence do you have that that might not be true?" "Have you ever had an urge that didn't go away?"). It is also helpful for the therapist to familiarize the clients with common "thinking traps" (e.g., "jumping to conclusions," "emotional reasoning," "black and white thinking") and ask them to identify these as they arise in their thinking. For example, many individuals with SUD jump to conclusions about their inability to remain sober over the long-term, romanticize/glorify their substance use, or catastrophize their emotional experience ("This feeling will *never* go away!"). Teaching the client to identify these kinds of cognitive distortions and develop a more realistic view of substance use and sobriety can help sustain motivation, build self-efficacy, and decrease the risk for relapse.

Feelings: Many types of feelings, including urges, cravings, and physical sensations related to medical illness or treatment side-effects, can put clients at risk for drinking/using. As with high-risk situations and thoughts, the therapist should help the client identify which feelings put him at greatest risk for using/drinking. It should also be emphasized that urges and cravings are a normal part of stopping substance use and do not have to cause the client to drink/use. For example, having an urge to drink and actually drinking are two very different things. The therapist and client can then explore the function of substance use in relation to feelings, for example to "numb" negative emotions or enhance positive emotions. Often, clients must relearn how to feel their feelings without attempting to numb, avoid, enhance, or otherwise interfere with them. Distress tolerance techniques [96] such as acceptance of feelings or temporary distraction can be very helpful, as can grounding [97] and breathing exercises, which help clients bring their focus back to the present. Similarly, clients may be taught "urge surfing," a mindfulness-based technique where clients visualize their urges as waves and "ride the wave" as it peaks in intensity and then subsides [98]. Over time, this can help to break the association between having an urge and using a drug or taking a drink. Further, distress tolerance strategies can be beneficial in teaching clients ways to more effectively cope with painful and/or uncomfortable medical symptoms that will be more helpful and healthful in the long term.

Behaviors: CBT/Relapse Prevention for SUD ultimately seeks to eliminate drinking/drug use behavior, which involves using "in the moment" skills that prevent or take the place of drinking or using drugs. As such, it is important to brainstorm feasible, alternative behaviors to drinking or using substances in which the client can engage when faced with a high-risk situation and/or is experiencing strong urges to use. These may include leaving the situation, delaying the decision to use (coupled with urge surfing), or doing something that is incompatible with using (e.g., exercise, reading literature that reminds the client of the significant negative health consequences of one's use with relation to his or her chronic medical condition, calling a sober support person). Assertive communication skills are also important, as it is common for people to use/drink in response to a direct offer of drugs or alcohol. The therapist and client can identify alternative behaviors and can role-play drink/drug refusal skills in session in order to prepare the client for real-world encounters.

Positive Results: When a substance is given up, individuals with SUD and a comorbid medical illness need to find new ways to achieve the positive results that drinking/using achieved or they may soon find themselves seeking the drug again. This often involves relearning how to have fun while doing things sober, increasing pleasant activities in general in order to build a sense of fulfillment, and finding and learning effective and healthful ways to manage stress, especially as it relates to medical issues. Clients may also want to consider attending support groups for people managing medical illness as a way to broaden their support network, as well as hear similar patients' suggestions or methods for coping. It is important for the therapist and client to brainstorm and identify activities that are rewarding and achievable, in order to help the client to rebuild a meaningful, fulfilling life. At its core, this therapeutic area is about identifying the benefits of sobriety (vs. the benefits of using/drinking) and finding ways to experience those benefits in daily life.

Negative Results: Identifying and reminding the client of the numerous negative consequences, especially those potentially affecting their health, resulting from their substance use can be an important source of continued motivation for sobriety, particularly when coupled with the identified benefits of sobriety. Some of these problems will resolve on their own once the client stops drinking/using; however, others will need to be actively addressed through goal-setting and problem-solving. Overall, it is important to routinely review the progress that the client has made, as this can be very rewarding for the client and helps sustain motivation over time.

Ongoing Monitoring and Between-Session Practice: CBT emphasizes between-session monitoring and practice of skills learned in session. Particularly when treating SUD, the time between sessions is extremely important because the client uses this time to figure out how to effectively implement skills on his own. It is helpful to do more monitoring in earlier sessions (e.g., with the behavior chain), as the therapist and client are gathering information about substance use patterns and related relapse risks. In particular for SUD clients with a co-occurring medical illness, continual monitoring of substance use patterns may be necessary since a client's health-related triggers/high-risk situations may wax and wane as a function of medical treatment regimens begin and end. Gradually, the focus shifts towards practicing specific skills between sessions that are mutually agreed upon by therapist and client. As the client learns skills and becomes adept at using them, he can begin to monitor the impact of using the skills in everyday life. Further, it is helpful to communicate with a client's medical provider to obtain medical lab results that can reflect improvements in a client's medical condition as a result of quitting substance use, such as viral load count, liver enzyme levels, blood glucose levels, and tumor progression. This biofeedback can serve to maintain or even bolster one's motivation to stay abstinent.

4.1.6   Harm Reduction

Harm reduction refers to practicing a set of strategies designed to reduce the harmful consequences associated with engaging in particular behaviors, such as substance use. Harm reduction strategies acknowledge that individuals who use substances initially may be unwilling or unable to reduce or stop their use. As such, harm reduction strategies place greater priority on reducing harm to the health of the individual using substances, as well as the general public, than on abstinence [99]. Among other assumptions of the harm reduction perspective is the assumption that many of the harmful consequences of substance use (e.g., overdose, acquisition and transmission of HIV and/or HCV, motor vehicle accidents) can be eliminated without achieving abstinence [100].

Harm reduction policies and practices have been utilized with success in several Western European countries since the 1920s. However, it more recently became adopted in the United States among HIV/AIDS service providers in response to the association of HIV/AIDS risk and injection drug use [100]. In this regard, HIV/AIDS prevention took priority over substance use prevention because of the idea that the preventable harm of HIV/AIDS was more important than the need to adhere to an abstinence-based approach to substance use [100]. The most notable harm reduction strategy associated with substance use includes needle and syringe programs (also referred to as needle exchange programs), with strong evidence that this approach is effective in reducing HIV and HCV-risk behaviors [101]. However, other harm reduction interventions include methadone and other opioid replacement therapies for individuals with opiate dependence, heroin prescribing (though this is not currently legal in the United States), information/education, "drug consumption rooms" which is a term describing rooms that are provided for substance use to avoid associated harms, and early warning systems which can act at sentinel systems within communities that alert substance users to hazards to contaminated or adulterated drugs (see [101] for full review).

However, with respect to harm reduction among behavioral medicine patients who also have a comorbid substance use disorder, an additional goal will likely be developing strategies to reduce the harm associated with not engaging in medical treatment due to one's alcohol or substance use (e.g., non-adherence to medication, checking blood-glucose levels, attending clinic appointments). Here, motivational interviewing can be practiced to help the patient recognize and acknowledge the pros of properly engaging in care and the cons of not properly engaging in care. Additionally, education can be provided regarding the ways in which alcohol and substance use can interfere with effective management of one's medical condition, as well as disease course. Last, problem-solving strategies can be utilized to identify common times when the patient is non-adherent with treatment, especially due to alcohol and substance use, and brainstorm strategies for overcoming these obstacles.

4.1.7 Case Example

Mr. J. is a 44-year-old Caucasian, heterosexual, widowed male who presented for individual treatment for opioid dependence and severe depression and anxiety following a relapse to IV heroin (1 g/day) use after being abstinent from heroin for 12 years. In addition, Mr. J. has untreated chronic Hepatitis C. He reported that he is unsure when he acquired the virus, however acknowledged that it was most likely due to his frequent injection drug use. He has not had permanent employment in over 10 years, lives in an apartment that he shares with two other men who also struggle with substance use, and receives government assistance for housing and food. After having relapsed for approximately 6 months, Mr. J. presented to a detoxification program because he was "tired of always feeling sick from withdrawal symptoms and worrying about how I was going to get more heroin." He left treatment early and returned to IV heroin use for another month before he reengaged in treatment using the opioid partial agonist, buprenorphine/naloxone ("Suboxone") with a former provider; he had been taking Suboxone for nearly 6 years prior to this relapse. During the 12 years that Mr. J. was abstinent from heroin, he occasionally misused benzodiazepines to "help manage my anxiety." Additionally, Mr. J. had a history significant of alcohol dependence and had been in sustained full remission at the time of his heroin relapse, and met DSM-IV-TR diagnostic criteria at the time of intake for Major Depressive Disorder, Recurrent, Severe without psychotic features, and Generalized Anxiety Disorder. Mr. J. received detoxification and residential treatment several times before and has some experience with Alcoholics Anonymous (AA).

Mr. J. grew up with his parents and four siblings (two older sisters, one older brother, one younger brother). He described his childhood as good and his family as caring and supportive. He denied any family history of substance use or mental health problems. Mr. J. explained that, when he was in third grade, his older brother sustained severe burns on over 80 % of his body and that this event was very traumatic for him resulting in nightmares, which he still has about three times a year. He also reported that he has significant social phobia, which began around age 12, and experiences intense anxiety when faced with public speaking. Mr. J. said he believed that the shock of seeing his brother severely burned and the intense social phobia starting at a young age contributed to him using substances to help manage his emotions. He reported that he started smoking marijuana and drinking alcohol on the weekends around age 18 to cope with symptoms of depression.

From his early 1920s onward, Mr. J.'s alcohol and other substance use varied depending on the types of stressors he was experiencing. The most recent significant stressor for Mr. J. was the death of his wife due to breast cancer and the removal of his stepsons from his care, both occurring about 4 years ago. This combination of events precipitated a relapse to heavy alcohol use for 6 months (i.e., 12-pack of beer nightly). Currently, Mr. J. reports that he faces constant stressors with regard to managing his chaotic household, significant financial struggles, complete lack of a social support network, and managing severe depression and anxiety.

Mr. J. presented to individual treatment after being abstinent from heroin for approximately 1 month (and being maintained on Suboxone). He demonstrated a moderate level of motivation, acknowledging that he needed to comply with individual treatment in order to continue to receive Suboxone. However, he also recognized that he needs assistance in managing his mood symptoms and focused work on relapse prevention. Mr. J. also presented with severe depression and anxiety symptomatology, as evidenced by scoring a 24 on the Personal Health Questionnaire-9 [102] and a 17 on the Generalized Anxiety Disorders-7 questionnaire [89]. Since Mr. J. had been engaged in psychiatric care prior to his relapse, some time was taken initially to identify factors that may have contributed to his previous therapy treatment to be less effective than he anticipated. Mr. J. was able to articulate that the major contributing factors were that he did not consistently attend appointments, did not consistently engage in skills practice (i.e., homework), and he did not have enough therapeutic supports in place. The therapist utilized this feedback to help develop appropriate treatment parameters and goals. In collaboration with Mr. J. the following treatment goals were established and agreed upon: (1) attend at least two 12-step meetings each week; (2) obtain a sponsor; (3) attend and complete a local intensive outpatient program (IOP); and (4) comply with homework/skills practice (as evidenced by completing handouts, etc.). Last, given's Mr. J.'s untreated HCV, some time was spent discussing his thoughts and feelings about initiating HCV treatment. He explained that he would like to get treatment for the HCV but was unsure if he would be eligible given his substance use history, particularly his injection drug use history. He stated that treatment had not been offered to him in the past but he would like to pursue treatment now in an effort towards working to improve his overall quality of life. Accordingly, referral to and engagement in HCV treatment were added as the fifth goal of his treatment plan.

Since Mr. J. was abstinent from all substances at the commencement of treatment, the beginning of treatment was spent introducing Relapse Prevention. First, the therapist introduced and explained high-risk situations, as well as their role in the relapse process. Mr. J. was able to quickly identify that intense negative moods, particularly depression and anxiety, were high-risk situations for him. Additional high-risk situations included: interpersonal conflict with one of this roommates and his neighbors, not having money to pay the rent at the beginning of the month, being lonely, and having chronic medical issues (i.e., HCV). Next, the therapist explained the concept of "apparently irrelevant decisions" [103]. Here, the idea is that seemingly innocuous decisions may actually set someone up for relapse. In the case of Mr. J., an "apparently irrelevant decision" included deciding to go talk with his neighbor (from whom he has previously gotten illicit benzodiazepines) when he is feeling very anxious. Though Mr. J. thought that talking with someone when he was feeling anxious would be helpful, he failed to recognize that the particular person he chose to talk to was putting him at risk of relapse due to the immediate availability of drugs.

Once high-risk situations were identified, the therapist and Mr. J. spent the next several sessions working to construct functional analyses of how he typically responded to these situations, specifically focusing on ascertaining any maladaptive ways of thinking (i.e., "thought traps") that would increase the likelihood of Mr. J. engaging in alcohol or substance use. For example, a common maladaptive thought that Mr. J. had was, "I can't tolerate this feeling. I'm going to lose it if I don't do something." His belief in this thought ultimately led to him misusing a substance (often a benzodiazepine). Cognitive restructuring was practiced for this and similar thoughts to help Mr. J. recognize that thoughts/beliefs are not facts and to gain evidence that there had been several occasions when he was able to tolerate intense negative emotions and *not* engage in substance use.

As skills practice/homework, Mr. J. engaged in mood monitoring and thought tracking as a way to help him pay closer attention to his emotions, as he recognized that he usually did not realize how badly he was feeling until "it was too late." By monitoring his mood and his associated thoughts throughout the day, this allowed Mr. J. the opportunity to practice skills to manage his mood earlier on the behavioral chain, thus improving the likelihood that he would remain abstinent.

Since Mr. J. identified that his primary high-risk situation related to intense negative mood, several sessions were dedicated to finding ways to both better manage and improve his mood. Activity monitoring was initially utilized to see how Mr. J. was typically spending his time. This was reviewed in session, gaps in time were identified, and brainstorming was practiced to develop a list of tasks and activities in which Mr. J. could engage to help add more structure to his days. Additionally, Mr. J identified specific AA meetings that he could attend to help increase his weekly activities, as well as potentially increase his sober social network. Mr. J. demonstrated significant ambivalence regarding attending and participating in 12-step meetings. In response, the therapist employed motivational interviewing strategies to assess the pros and cons of attending AA vs. not attending. In the end, Mr. J. recognized that attending the meetings would be beneficial for him in the long term. Finally, the therapist taught specific skills to help Mr. J. cope in the moment with intense negative moods. These included mindfulness and distress tolerance skills drawn from Dialectical Behavior Therapy [96], journaling, and practicing "playing the tape forward," (i.e., thinking about how the behavior he chooses to engage in now may negatively or positively affect him later and using that information to help guide his decision of what behavior to engage in currently).

The focus of the first 12–15 sessions was to help Mr. J. gain stability with regard to his recovery and mood. Once this was achieved, the focus of the sessions shifted to work on achieving the fifth goal of his treatment plan, which was to get a referral for, and engage in, HCV treatment. Motivational interviewing was practiced to address issues around ambivalence and to identify the pros and cons of starting treatment vs. not. Since Mr. J. was unaware of the newer, more effective medications available to treat HCV, the therapist provided education on this topic. Further, he was reluctant to pursue treatment because of his drug use history and current use of Suboxone. Similarly, the therapist provided psychoeducation around these concerns. Also, Mr. J. was concerned about being able to attend all the necessary clinic appointments in order to be evaluated and start treatment. The therapist assisted Mr. J. in identifying barriers to scheduling and attending appointments, and problem-solving was practiced around these barriers. Additionally, Mr. J. recognized that he was engaging in "jumping to conclusions" about the ability to be treatment adherent. Cognitive restructuring was practiced to address and modify these thoughts; more helpful thoughts were created (e.g., "I don't think I'll be able to stick to the medicine regimen very well" was challenged and the restructured thought was, "I've been able to stick to long-term treatment before so it's likely I can do it again."). After several sessions of continued motivational and CBT work, Mr. J. finally made an appointment to start the process of engaging in treatment for his chronic Hepatitis C infection. In fact, once he started taking the steps for treatment, Mr. J. reported that he felt hopeful about his health and sees it as a major move forward in working to improve his quality of life.

Currently, Mr. J. is still engaged in individual CBT/Relapse Prevention for depression, anxiety, and opioid dependence. Compared to when he first presented for treatment, Mr. J. demonstrates significantly improved mood management. Though his depression and anxiety symptoms are still high (17 on the PHQ-9, 13 on the GAD-7), he has observed noticeable improvement. More importantly, Mr. J. reports that he feels his mood is more stable, and he attributes this to skills practice. Though there have been a few incidents of illicit use of benzodiazepines to manage his anxiety throughout treatment, Mr. J. is better able to articulate the high-risk situations that led to the slips and identify strategies he can aim to implement the next time he faces this type of high-risk situation. Last, Mr. J. is scheduled to start HCV medication treatment within the next 3 weeks.

4.1.8 Summary

Substance use and related conditions present as a complex constellation of symptoms and associated problems that can be challenging to treat effectively. A co-occurring medical condition or illness can add another layer of complexity to treatment. However, it is possible to treat a substance use disorder among medically ill patients, thus improving one's quality of life, response to treatment, and overall disease course. This chapter has described the prevalence, highlighted the theoretical basis for cognitive and behavioral interventions for SUD, and provided a case illustration of how such approaches can be utilized with patients with a co-occurring medical issue. Given the potential for periods of relapse along the path to full remission and sustained recovery from SUD, especially in the setting significant medical conditions, continued behavioral management and monitoring using CBT/RP approaches is likely to be beneficial.

4.2   Additional Resources

Understanding the function of substance use: Behavior chain monitoring form

Triggers: What was going on? What put me at risk for drinking/using?	Thoughts: What was going through my mind?	Feelings: How did I feel physically and emotionally?	Behaviors: What did I do next? (Substance use or coping skills)	Positive results: What did I like about drinking/ using?	Negative results: What bad things happened after I used/ drank?

Adapted from [104]

Websites	National Registry of Evidence-Based Programs and Practices (NREPP); www.nrepp.samhsa.gov
	Recovery Research Institute; www.recoveryanswers.org
	Motivational Interviewing; www.motivationalinterviewing.org
	National Institute on Drug Abuse (NIDA); www.drugabuse.gov
	National Institute on Alcohol Abuse and Alcoholism (NIAAA); www.niaaa.nih.gov
	Center for Disease Control and Prevention (CDC); www.cdc.gov
Treatment Manuals	Kadden, R., Carroll, K.M., Donovan, D., Cooney, N., Monti, P., Abrams, D., Litt, M. & Hester, R. (1994). *Cognitive-behavioral coping skills therapy manual: A clinical research guide for therapists treating individuals with alcohol abuse and dependence*. Project MATCH Monograph Series, Vol. 3. DHHS Publication No. 94-3724. Rockville, MD: NIAAA
	Carroll, KM. (1998). *Therapy Manuals for Drug Addiction. Manual 1: A Cognitive-Behavioral Approach: Treating Cocaine Addiction*. NIH Publication No. 98-4308. Rockville, MD: NIDA. (http://archives.drugabuse.gov/pdf/CBT.pdf)
	Webb, C.; Scudder, M.; Kaminer; Y., & Kadden, R. (2002). *The Motivational Enhancement Therapy and Cognitive Behavioral Therapy Supplement: 7 Sessions of Cognitive Behavioral Therapy for Adolescent Cannabis Users*, Cannabis Youth Treatment (CYT) Series, Volume 2. DHHS Pub. No. (SMA) 07-3954. Rockville, MD: Center for Substance Abuse Treatment, Substance Abuse and Mental Health Services Administration

References

1. Rudd RA, Paulozzi LJ, Bauer MJ, et al. Increases in heroin overdose deaths—28 states, 2010 to 2012. MMWR Morb Mortal Wkly Rep. 2014;63:849–54.
2. Substance Abuse and Mental Health Services Administration, Center for Behavioral Health Statistics and Quality. The DAWN report: highlights of the 2011 Drug Abuse Warning Network (DAWN) findings on Drug-Related Emergency Department Visits, Rockville; 2013.

3. Passik SD, Portenoy RK, Ricketts PI. Substance abuse issues in cancer patients. Part 1: prevalence and diagnosis. Oncology (Williston Park). 1998;12:517–21, 524.
4. Mimiaga MJ, Reisner SL, Grasso C, et al. Substance use among HIV-infected patients engaged in primary care in the United States: findings from the Centers for AIDS Research Network of Integrated Clinical Systems cohort. Am J Public Health. 2013;103:1457–67.
5. Azar MM, Springer SA, Meyer JP, et al. A systematic review of the impact of alcohol use disorders on HIV treatment outcomes, adherence to antiretroviral therapy and health care utilization. Drug Alcohol Depend. 2010;112:178–93.
6. Barve S, Kapoor R, Moghe A, et al. Focus on the liver: alcohol use, highly active antiretroviral therapy, and liver disease in HIV-infected patients. Alcohol Res Health. 2010;33:229–36.
7. Baum MK, Rafie C, Lai S, et al. Crack-cocaine use accelerates HIV disease progression in a cohort of HIV-positive drug users. J Acquir Immune Defic Syndr. 2009;50:93–9.
8. Catz SL, Kelly JA, Bogart LM, et al. Patterns, correlates, and barriers to medication adherence among persons prescribed new treatments for HIV disease. Health Psychol. 2000;19:124–33.
9. Chander G, Lau B, Moore RD. Hazardous alcohol use: a risk factor for non-adherence and lack of suppression in HIV infection. J Acquir Immune Defic Syndr. 2006;43:411–7.
10. Lucas GM, Cheever LW, Chaisson RE, et al. Detrimental effects of continued illicit drug use on the treatment of HIV-1 infection. J Acquir Immune Defic Syndr. 2001;27:251–9.
11. Lucas GM, Gebo KA, Chaisson RE, et al. Longitudinal assessment of the effects of drug and alcohol abuse on HIV-1 treatment outcomes in an urban clinic. AIDS. 2002;16:767–74.
12. Miguez MJ, Shor-Posner G, Morales G, et al. HIV treatment in drug abusers: impact of alcohol use. Addict Biol. 2003;8:33–7.
13. Parker GB, Hegarty B, Paterson A, et al. Predictors of post-natal depression are shaped distinctly by the measure of "depression". J Affect Disord. 2015;173:239–44.
14. Petry NM. Alcohol use in HIV patients: what we don't know may hurt us. Int J STD AIDS. 1999;10:561–70.
15. Grebely J, Raffa JD, Lai C, et al. Low uptake of treatment for hepatitis C virus infection in a large community-based study of inner city residents. J Viral Hepat. 2009;16:352–8.
16. Mehta SH, Genberg BL, Astemborski J, et al. Limited uptake of hepatitis C treatment among injection drug users. J Community Health. 2008;33:126–33.
17. Maeda M, Nagawa H, Maeda T, et al. Alcohol consumption enhances liver metastasis in colorectal carcinoma patients. Cancer. 1998;83:1483–8.
18. Thomas DL, Astemborski J, Rai RM, et al. The natural history of hepatitis C virus infection: host, viral, and environmental factors. J Am Med Assoc. 2000;284:450–6.
19. Corrao G, Aricò S. Independent and combined action of hepatitis C virus infection and alcohol consumption on the risk of symptomatic liver cirrhosis. Hepatology. 1998;27:914–9.
20. Ostapowicz G, Watson KJ, Locarnini SA, et al. Role of alcohol in the progression of liver disease caused by hepatitis C virus infection. Hepatology. 1998;27:1730–5.
21. Schiff ER. Hepatitis C, and alcohol. Hepatology. 1997;26:39S–42S.
22. Araújo RF, Lira GA, Guedes HG, et al. Lifestyle and family history influence cancer prognosis in Brazilian individuals. Pathol Res Pract. 2013;209:753–7.
23. Schuckit MA. An overview of genetic influences in alcoholism. J Subst Abuse Treat. 2009;36:S5–14.
24. Urbanoski KA, Kelly JF. Understanding genetic risk for substance use and addiction: a guide for non-geneticists. Clin Psychol Rev. 2012;32:60–70.
25. Substance Abuse and Mental Health Services Administration. Results from the 2013 National Survey on Drug Use and Health: summary of national findings. Rockville: Substance Abuse and Mental Health Services Administration; 2014.
26. American Psychiatric Association. Diagnostic and statistical manual of mental disorders, vol. 5. Washington, DC: Author; 2013.
27. Bagnardi V, Blangiardo M, La Vecchia C, et al. Alcohol consumption and the risk of cancer: a meta-analysis. Alcohol Res Health. 2000;25:263–70.

28. Bagnardi V, Blangiardo M, Vecchia CL, et al. A meta-analysis of alcohol drinking and cancer risk. Br J Cancer. 2001;85:1700–5.
29. Rehm J, Room R, Graham K, et al. The relationship of average volume of alcohol consumption and patterns of drinking to burden of disease: an overview. Addiction. 2003;98:1209–28.
30. Bruera E, Moyano J, Seifert L, et al. The frequency of alcoholism among patients with pain due to terminal cancer. J Pain Symptom Manage. 1995;10:599–603.
31. Dev R, Parsons HA, Palla S, et al. Undocumented alcoholism and its correlation with tobacco and illegal drug use in advanced cancer patients. Cancer. 2011;117:4551–6.
32. Jenkins CA, Schulz M, Hanson J, et al. Demographic, symptom, and medication profiles of cancer patients seen by a palliative care consult team in a tertiary referral hospital. J Pain Symptom Manage. 2000;19:174–84.
33. Parsons HA, Delgado-Guay MO, El Osta B, et al. Alcoholism screening in patients with advanced cancer: impact on symptom burden and opioid use. J Palliat Med. 2008;11:964–8.
34. Neuenschwander AU, Pedersen JH, Krasnik M, et al. Impaired postoperative outcome in chronic alcohol abusers after curative resection for lung cancer. Eur J Cardiothorac Surg. 2002;22:287–91.
35. Paull DE, Updyke GM, Baumann MA, et al. Alcohol abuse predicts progression of disease and death in patients with lung cancer. Ann Thorac Surg. 2005;80:1033–9.
36. Paull DE, Updyke GM, Davis CA, et al. Complications and long-term survival for alcoholic patients with resectable lung cancer. Am J Surg. 2004;188:553–9.
37. Fuchs CS, Stampfer MJ, Colditz GA, et al. Alcohol consumption and mortality among women. N Engl J Med. 1995;332:1245–50.
38. Harris HR, Bergkvist L, Wolk A. Alcohol intake and mortality among women with invasive breast cancer. Br J Cancer. 2012;106:592–5.
39. Jain MG, Ferrenc RG, Rehm JT, et al. Alcohol and breast cancer mortality in a cohort study. Breast Cancer Res Treat. 2000;64:201–9.
40. Kwan ML, Chen WY, Flatt SW, et al. Postdiagnosis alcohol consumption and breast cancer prognosis in the after breast cancer pooling project. Cancer Epidemiol Biomark Prev. 2013;22:32–41.
41. Hurcom C, Copello A, Orford J. The family and alcohol: effects of excessive drinking and conceptualizations of spouses over recent decades. Subst Use Misuse. 2000;35:473–502.
42. Passik SD, Theobald DE. Managing addiction in advanced cancer patients: why bother? J Pain Symptom Manage. 2000;19:229–34.
43. Rodrigue JR, Park TL. General and illness-specific adjustment to cancer: relationship to marital status and marital quality. J Psychosom Res. 1996;40:29–36.
44. Centers for Disease Control and Prevention. CDC fact sheet: new HIV infections in the United States; 2012.
45. Bing EG, Burnam MA, Longshore D, et al. Psychiatric disorders and drug use among human immunodeficiency virus-infected adults in the United States. Arch Gen Psychiatry. 2001;58:721–8.
46. Galvan FH, Bing EG, Fleishman JA, et al. The prevalence of alcohol consumption and heavy drinking among people with HIV in the United States: results from the HIV Cost and Services Utilization Study. J Stud Alcohol Drugs. 2002;63:179.
47. Buchacz K, McFarland W, Kellogg TA, et al. Amphetamine use is associated with increased HIV incidence among men who have sex with men in San Francisco. AIDS. 2005;19:1423–4.
48. Ostrow DG, Plankey MW, Cox C, et al. Specific sex drug combinations contribute to the majority of recent HIV seroconversions among MSM in the MACS. J Acquir Immune Defic Syndr. 2009;51:349–55.
49. Plankey MW, Ostrow DG, Stall R, et al. The relationship between methamphetamine and popper use and risk of HIV seroconversion in the multicenter AIDS cohort study. J Acquir Immune Defic Syndr. 2007;45:85–92.

50. Baliunas D, Rehm J, Irving H, et al. Alcohol consumption and risk of incident human immunodeficiency virus infection: a meta-analysis. Int J Public Health. 2010;55:159–66.
51. Shuper PA, Joharchi N, Irving H, et al. Alcohol as a correlate of unprotected sexual behavior among people living with HIV/AIDS: review and meta-analysis. AIDS Behav. 2009;13:1021–36.
52. Paterson DL, Swindells S, Mohr J, et al. Adherence to protease inhibitor therapy and outcomes in patients with HIV infection. Ann Intern Med. 2000;133:21–30.
53. Sylvestre DL, Loftis JM, Hauser P, et al. Co-occurring Hepatitis C, substance use, and psychiatric illness: treatment issues and developing integrated models of care. J Urban Health. 2004;81:719–34.
54. AASLD/IDSA/IAS–USA. Recommendations for testing, managing, and treating hepatitis C. http://www.hcvguidelines.org. Accessed April 24, 2014.
55. Magiorkinis G, Sypsa V, Magiorkinis E, et al. Integrating phylodynamics and epidemiology to estimate transmission diversity in viral epidemics. PLoS Comput Biol. 2013;9:e1002876.
56. Tortu S, Neaigus A, McMahon J, et al. Hepatitis C among noninjecting drug users: a report. Subst Use Misuse. 2001;36:523–34.
57. Basseri B, Yamini D, Chee G, et al. Comorbidities associated with the increasing burden of hepatitis C infection. Liver Int. 2010;30:1012–8.
58. Bhattacharya R, Shuhart MC. Hepatitis C and alcohol: interactions, outcomes, and implications. J Clin Gastroenterol. 2003;36:242–52.
59. Pierson R. Update 2—Abbott hepatitis C drugs bring high cure rates in trial; 2012.
60. Poynard T, Bedossa P. Age and platelet count: a simple index for predicting the presence of histological lesions in patients with antibodies to hepatitis C virus. METAVIR and CLINIVIR Cooperative Study Groups. J Viral Hepat. 1997;4:199–208.
61. Selvin E, Parrinello CM, Sacks DB, et al. Trends in prevalence and control of diabetes in the United States, 1988–1994 and 1999–2010 trends in prevalence and control of diabetes in the United States. Ann Intern Med. 2014;160:517–25.
62. Guariguata L, Whiting DR, Hambleton I, et al. Global estimates of diabetes prevalence for 2013 and projections for 2035. Diabetes Res Clin Pract. 2014;103:137–49.
63. Howard AA, Arnsten JH, Gourevitch MN. Effect of alcohol consumption on diabetes mellitus: a systematic review. Ann Intern Med. 2004;140:211–9.
64. Ajani UA, Hennekens CH, Spelsberg A, et al. Alcohol consumption and risk of type 2 diabetes mellitus among US male physicians. Arch Intern Med. 2000;160:1025–30.
65. Koppes LLJ, Dekker JM, Hendriks HFJ, et al. Moderate alcohol consumption lowers the risk of type 2 diabetes: a meta-analysis of prospective observational studies. Diabetes Care. 2005;28:719–25.
66. Holmes MV, Dale CE, Zuccolo L, et al. Association between alcohol and cardiovascular disease: Mendelian randomisation analysis based on individual participant data. BMJ. 2014;349:g4164.
67. Knott CS, Coombs N, Stamatakis E, et al. All cause mortality and the case for age specific alcohol consumption guidelines: pooled analyses of up to 10 population based cohorts. BMJ. 2015;350:h384.
68. Engler PA, Ramsey SE, Stein MD. Brief alcohol intervention among diabetic patients: a pilot study; 2008.
69. Lee P, Greenfield JR, Campbell LV. Managing young people with Type 1 diabetes in a "rave" new world: metabolic complications of substance abuse in Type 1 diabetes. Diabet Med. 2009;26:328–33.
70. Lerman I. Adherence to treatment: the key for avoiding long-term complications of diabetes. Arch Med Res. 2005;36:300–6.
71. Shield KD, Parry C, Rehm J. Chronic diseases and conditions related to alcohol use. Alcohol Res Curr Rev. 2014;35:155–71.

72. Rosenblum A, Joseph H, Fong C, et al. Prevalence and characteristics of chronic pain among chemically dependent patients in methadone maintenance and residential treatment facilities. JAMA. 2003;289:2370–8.

73. Gourlay DL, Heit HA, Almahrezi A. Universal precautions in pain medicine: a rational approach to the treatment of chronic pain. Pain Med. 2005;6:107–12.

74. Savage SR, Kirsh KL, Passik SD. Challenges in using opioids to treat pain in persons with substance use disorders. Addict Sci Clin Pract. 2008;4:4–25.

75. Rupp T, Delaney KA. Inadequate analgesia in emergency medicine. Ann Emerg Med. 2004;43:494–503.

76. Manchikanti L, Manchukonda R, Pampati V, et al. Evaluation of abuse of prescription and illicit drugs in chronic pain patients receiving short-acting (hydrocodone) or long-acting (methadone) opioids. Pain Physician. 2005;8:257–61.

77. Broekmans S, Dobbels F, Milisen K, et al. Pharmacologic pain treatment in a multidisciplinary pain center: do patients adhere to the prescription of the physician? Clin J Pain. 2010;26:81–6.

78. Fishman SM, Wilsey B, Yang J, et al. Adherence monitoring and drug surveillance in chronic opioid therapy. J Pain Symptom Manage. 2000;20:293–307.

79. Lewis ET, Combs A, Trafton JA. Reasons for under-use of prescribed opioid medications by patients in pain. Pain Med. 2010;11:861–71.

80. Helmerhorst GTT, Vranceanu A-M, Vrahas M, et al. Risk factors for continued opioid use one to two months after surgery for musculoskeletal trauma. J Bone Joint Surg Am. 2014;96:495–9.

81. Bandura A. Social learning theory. Englewood Cliffs: Prentice Hall; 1977.

82. Hendershot CS, Witkiewitz K, George WH, et al. Relapse prevention for addictive behaviors. Subst Abuse Treat Prev Policy. 2011;6:17.

83. Miller WR, Rollnick S. Motivational interviewing: helping people change. New York: Guilford; 2012.

84. Dennis ML, Titus JC, White MK, et al. Global appraisal of individual needs: administration guide for the GAIN and related measures. Bloomington: Chestnut Health System; 2003.

85. McLellan AT, Kushner H, Metzger D, et al. The fifth edition of the addiction severity index. J Subst Abuse Treat. 1992;9:199–213.

86. Weiss RD, Griffin ML, Hufford C. Craving in hospitalized cocaine abusers as a predictor of outcome. Am J Drug Alcohol Abuse. 1995;21:289–301.

87. Kelly JF, Greene MC. Beyond motivation: initial validation of the commitment to sobriety scale. J Subst Abuse Treat. 2014;46:257–63.

88. Groshkova T, Best D, White W. The assessment of recovery capital: properties and psychometrics of a measure of addiction recovery strengths. Drug Alcohol Rev. 2013;32:187–94.

89. Spitzer RL, Kroenke K, Williams JBW, et al. A brief measure for assessing generalized anxiety disorder: the GAD-7. Arch Intern Med. 2006;166:1092–7.

90. Kroenke K, Spitzer RL, Williams JB. The PHQ-9: validity of a brief depression severity measure. J Gen Intern Med. 2001;16:606–13.

91. Magill M, Ray LA. Cognitive-behavioral treatment with adult alcohol and illicit drug users: a meta-analysis of randomized controlled trials. J Stud Alcohol Drugs. 2009;70:516–27.

92. Dutra L, Stathopoulou G, Basden SL, et al. A meta-analytic review of psychosocial interventions for substance use disorders. Am J Psychiatry. 2008;165:179–87.

93. Irvin JE, Bowers CA, Dunn ME, et al. Efficacy of relapse prevention: a meta-analytic review. J Consult Clin Psychol. 1999;67:563–70.

94. Curran PJ, Stice E, Chassin L. The relation between adolescent alcohol use and peer alcohol use: a longitudinal random coefficients model. J Consult Clin Psychol. 1997;65:130–40.

95. Li F, Jr MB, Hops H, et al. The longitudinal influence of peers on the development of alcohol use in late adolescence: a growth mixture analysis. J Behav Med. 2002;25:293–315.

96. Linehan M. Cognitive-behavioral treatment of borderline personality disorder. New York: Guilford; 1993.

97. Najavits LM. Seeking safety: a treatment manual for PTSD and substance abuse. 1st ed. New York: Guilford; 2001.
98. Marlatt GA. Buddhist philosophy and the treatment of addictive behavior. Cogn Behav Pract. 2002;9:44–50.
99. Clapp JD, Burke AC. Discriminant analysis of factors differentiating among substance abuse treatment units in their provision of HIV/AIDS harm reduction services. Soc Work Res. 1999;23:69–76.
100. MacMaster SA. Harm reduction: a new perspective on substance abuse services. Soc Work. 2004;49:356–63.
101. Hunt N, Ashton M, Lenton S, et al. A review of the evidence-base for harm reduction approaches to drug use. London: Forward Thinking on Drugs; 2003.
102. Spitzer RL, Kroenke K, Williams JB. Validation and utility of a self-report version of PRIME-MD: the PHQ primary care study. Primary Care Evaluation of Mental Disorders. Patient Health Questionnaire. JAMA. 1999;282:1737–44.
103. Larimer ME, Palmer RS, et al. Relapse prevention: an overview of Marlatt's cognitive-behavioral model. Alcohol Res Health. 1999;23:151–60.
104. Sampl, S., Kadden, R. (2001). Motivational Enhancement Therapy and Cognitive Behavioral Therapy for Adolescent Cannabis Users: 5 Sessions, Cannabis Youth Treatment Series, Volume 1. Rockville, MD: Center for Substance Abuse Treatment, Substance Abuse and Mental Health Services Administration. BKD384
105. Holmberg SD, Spradling PR, Moorman AC, Denniston MM. Hepatitis C in the United States. N Engl J Med. 2013;368(20):1859-1861. doi:10.1056/NEJMp1302973.
106. Yehia BR, Schranz AJ, Umscheid CA, et al. The Treatment Cascade for Chronic Hepatitis C Virus Infection in the United States: A Systematic Review and Meta-Analysis. PLoS ONE. 2014;9(7):e101554. doi:10.1371/journal.pone.0101554.

Part II
Chronic Conditions

Chapter 5
Cognitive Behavioral Therapy for Chronic Pain

Ana-Maria Vranceanu, Melissa Stone, Tim Wallace, and Ronald Kulich

Chronic pain, defined as persistent pain that lasts more than 3–6 months [1], has an estimated incidence of 100 million adults in the United States [2]. The total annual incremental cost of health care due to pain ranges from $560 billion to $635 billion (in 2010 dollars) in the United States, which combines the medical costs of pain care and the economic costs related to disability days and lost wages and productivity [2]. Among chronic pain conditions low back pain is the most common (27 %), followed by severe headache or migraine pain (15 %), neck pain (15 %), and facial ache or pain (4 %) [3].

5.1 Development and Evolution of the Cognitive Behavioral Model for Pain

The traditional model for the conceptualization of chronic pain was biomedical. Predicated on the mind–body dichotomy, the biomedical model enforced that pain had either a physical or psychological cause. The Gate Control Theory of Pain [4, 5] was pivotal in the transition from the biomedical ("find it and fix it") to the

A.-M. Vranceanu, Ph.D. (✉)
Behavioral Medicine Service, Department of Psychiatry, Institute of Brain Health,
Massachusetts General Hospital, Boston, MA 02174, USA
e-mail: avranceanu@mgh.harvard.edu

M. Stone • R. Kulich
Pain Medicine and Anesthesia, Harvard Medical School,
Massachusetts General Hospital, Boston, MA 02114, USA

T. Wallace
Behavioral Medicine Service, Department of Psychiatry, Massachusetts General Hospital,
Harvard Medical School, Boston, MA, USA

© Springer Science+Business Media New York 2017
A.-M. Vranceanu et al. (eds.), *The Massachusetts General Hospital Handbook of Behavioral Medicine*, Current Clinical Psychiatry,
DOI 10.1007/978-3-319-29294-6_5

biopsychosocial model of conceptualization and treatment of pain conditions. The Gate Control Theory of Pain emphasized that cognitive, emotional, and physiological/sensory factors are interrelated in the experience of pain and disability.

Fordyce later adapted and transferred the concepts of learning theory and operant conditioning principles to the conceptualization and treatment of pain [6]. He showed that similarly to other behaviors, pain behaviors could also be elicited and shaped by social and environmental contingencies. By shaping these behaviors, one can impact both pain and disability, in contrast with early operant programs, which viewed reports of pain as simply "pain behaviors," and specific function goals as the mainstay of treatment.

The development of the cognitive therapy for depression [7] further influenced the conceptualization of pain, leading first to a shift toward pain relief as a primary goal, while eventually to the blending of the cognitive and behavioral components [8, 9] into our current conceptualization of CBT for pain [10, 91]. McCracken [11] introduced third wave cognitive behavioral principles of acceptance and commitment into the conceptualization of pain, drawing attention to the importance of pain acceptance, and adjustment to current life situation. McCracken defines acceptance of chronic pain as "living with pain without reaction, disapproval, or attempts to reduce or avoid it" [12, p 198], thus enabling a shift in goal setting from pain control to increase function and quality of life.

5.2   Common Comorbid Psychological Factors

Chronic pain is a multidimensional construct. It is influenced by biological, psychological (cognitive, emotional, behavioral), and social factors, which are optimally managed when addressed concomitantly. Previous research has identified that depression [13–16], anxiety [17–20], ineffective coping including pain catastrophizing, pain anxiety, and fear avoidance [21–24], perceived stress [25–27], and health anxiety [20, 28, 29] are common in patients with pain, and also influence transition from acute to chronic pain [30–32].

Previously, well-compensated psychosocial factors may become problematic when one is confronted with pain and the stressors associated with pain [33]. For instance, a person who tends to worry may develop pain catastrophizing (a tendency to magnify the pain experience, to feel helpless when thinking about pain, and to ruminate on the pain experience). Someone who has a tendency to worry about his health may start viewing a benign pain condition as a sign of serious pathology and may have a difficult time internalizing reassurances that his condition is benign (heightened illness-concern, health anxiety, or hypochondriasis). A depressed patient may make internal ("It's my fault"), global ("Everything is going wrong"), and stable ("I will never get over this") attributions about the pain conditions. Pain may exacerbate a predisposition toward depression, may intensify an already existent depression, or may become a somatic focus for depressive symptoms [34]. A tendency toward negative thinking and appraisal of life situations may translate into a similar appraisal of the pain condition. All of this may convert into reports of increased pain and disability and may influence transition into chronic pain.

5.3   Efficacy of CBT for Chronic Pain

A large body of research including meta-analyses and reviews has evaluated the efficacy of CBT for chronic pain and related concomitant problems. This research has shown that CBT is generally superior to usual care or wait-list control in improving pain-related symptoms. Effect sizes are typically small to medium for improvements in pain intensity, pain catastrophizing, and mood (depression and anxiety), and small for pain-related disability and pain interference. Williams et al. [35] showed that CBT, compared with treatment-as-usual or wait-list control conditions, had significant but small effects on improving pain intensity and disability, and moderate effects on improving mood and pain catastrophizing immediately after treatment. By 6- to 12 months however, all treatment effects except for mood disappeared. When CBT is compared with active control conditions, it achieves similar effects, with no between-treatment statistical significant differences for pain intensity or mood outcomes. However, CBT is significantly better in improving disability and pain catastrophizing when compared to other active treatments at posttest. At 6- to 12-month follow-up, benefits maintain for disability only.

Although patients with chronic pain have a similar presentation regardless of where pain is located, research has also assessed efficacy of CBT for specific chronic pain conditions. For example, a meta-analysis of 22 randomized controlled trials (RCTs) of psychological treatments for chronic back pain indicated that psychological interventions, contrasted with various control conditions, had positive effects on pain, pain interference, health-related quality of life, and depression [36]. CBT was found to be superior to wait-list controls for improving only pain intensity post-treatment. More recently, a Cochrane review of behavioral treatments (including CBT) for chronic low back pain, which included 30 RCTs, concluded that behavioral treatments were more effective than usual care for pain post-treatment but not different in intermediate- to long-term effects on pain or functional status [37].

A review of behavioral treatments for headache [38] described CBT-based interventions (relaxation, biofeedback, and cognitive therapy) as reducing headache activity 30–60 % on average across studies. These effects surpassed those of various control conditions and were typically sustained over time, including years after treatment. Biofeedback interventions also are commonly used in treating chronic headaches, either as a stand-alone treatment or in conjunction with other CBT techniques [39]. Meta-analyses provide evidence of medium to large effects of biofeedback on improving migraine and tension-type headaches, including the frequency and duration of headaches, when compared with a variety of control (wait-list, placebo, pseudofeedback) conditions [40–42]. Biofeedback was comparable to relaxation training for migraine headaches [40] and superior for tension-type headaches [41, 42]. While behavioral interventions appear to have clear effect with persistent headache, studies demonstrate the greatest impact with recurrent migraine versus daily chronic tension-type headache. The salient behavioral treatment components remain unclear, while the cognitive interventions and lifestyle change have consistently demonstrated impact.

5.4 Cognitive Behavioral Therapy for Chronic Pain

CBT for pain management takes an active approach to tackling many challenges associated with the experience of chronic pain. CBT typically encourages patients to take control and reengage in activities with a focus on increasing functionality rather than decreasing pain intensity [9, 12].

Although CBT for pain is relatively short term in comparison to traditional psychotherapeutic techniques (5–20 sessions), duration depends on the complexity and severity of the presenting condition, length of time since onset (acute vs. chronic), and the patient's motivation level. Long-term therapy success is based on the continued utilization of skills after therapy ends, "booster" and relapse prevention sessions, and reinforcement of patient gains by the therapist and co-treating providers including primary care physicians.

CBT for chronic pain is complicated by multiple factors. First, in many situations, prior to referral for CBT patients have been managed with a narrow biomedical approach, with multiple medical procedures and medications. This approach often has iatrogenic effects and reinforces the search for a medical "cure," which may be detrimental for the majority of patients with chronic musculoskeletal pain [43]. Second, treatment non-engagement, missed sessions, and other adherence problems complicate care [44]. Third, patients may not be prepared to engage in an active treatment that requires participation and homework completion [45, 46]. Many patients do not adhere to pain management skills practice and homework [47]. As such, motivational interviewing (MI; [48]) may be applied to promote treatment engagement and adherence, wherein barriers to treatment are identified within the assessment process. Finally, medical subspecialists may unwittingly sabotage patient gains with additional unnecessary diagnostic studies, multiple referrals, and other strategies that deemphasize the importance of self-directed care and emphasize decrease in pain intensity. Especially, complex patients may require multiple ongoing sessions of treatment, especially where multiple providers are involved in care.

When return to work is a goal of CBT, time is of essence, with patients who have been out of work for less than 12 weeks having the highest chance to successfully return to work [49]. After 6 months of being out of work, the chance of returning to work drops to 40–55 % [49]. The CBT therapist has an important role in helping patients return to work through collaboration with the patient's medical team. Encouragement by the primary care doctor including a focus on active (e.g., exercise) rather than passive (e.g., massage) recommendations can enhance return to work rates and positive treatment outcomes [50, 51].

The success of CBT for pain is undoubtedly predicated upon a unified approach to treatment by all members of the treatment team. A recent survey of primary care

physicians has shown that patients with chronic pain are considered the most difficult to manage, with a patient doctor relationship described as "burdened" [52],
complicated by frustration and mutual lack of trust. Research has shown that primary care physicians often feel pressured to prescribe opioids, have a hard time
believing patient's pain, worry about secondary gain, and often find patients to be
"abusive" and "destructive" [53]. As the doctor–patient relationship is a predictive
factor of treatment success in chronic pain patients [53], it is particularly important
to work through these issues with both the patient and primary care physician, and
ensure mutual treatment goals and facilitate the success of the CBT treatment.

CBT for pain is not delivered uniformly. Rather, it is tailored to each patient
based on results of the initial assessment, patient presentation, and patient-specific
goals. A "tailored' CBT approach that employs a combination of motivational interviewing and patient-centered treatment modules is supported by research [54].

Below we present general CBT modules for pain management, and recommend
specific patient issues and/or comorbidities for which they can be used. Table 5.1
presents specific measures that may be employed in the assessment process, while
Table 5.2 presents the CBT modules and recommendations for specific patient
issues that they most often address. The number of sessions in each module varies.

Psychoeducation is a general and foundation module in which patient and provider first discuss the results of an initial biopsychosocial assessment, including any
self-report measures or rating scales. Typical measures (see Table 5.1) administered
include: measures of coping with pain, (e.g., The Pain Catastrophizing Scale [55],
The Pain Anxiety Sensitivity Scale [18], measures of pain interference and physical
functioning (e.g., PROMIS Pain Interference, Pain Interference Index [57], measures of pain intensity (Numerical Rating Scale, NRS), measures of pain behaviors
(e.g., The Pain Behavior Checklist, [64]), and measures of mood. Clinicians then
start building the therapeutic alliance, and discuss the general structure of treatment
and expectations, such as homework completion and practicing skills outside of
treatment sessions. During this module, the therapist and patient weigh the costs
and benefits of a CBT for pain intervention and decide together whether the intervention will be useful.

As part of this module patients also receive educational information on pain
including myths about pain [65] and an introduction to the conceptualization of pain
via the biopsychosocial model. One of the key components in pain management is
helping patients understand the concept of pain in the absence of or presence of
limited physical pathology. One simple strategy is comparing the changes that occur
in the body when a pain sensation occurs with the physiological changes that are
common in the fight or flight state. Just as the fight or flight can help signify danger,
the initial pain (or "pain alarm") also alerts the individual to potential danger. A
good example is removing ones hand from a hot stove to prevent damage from the
heat. The problem arises when pain sensations (e.g., "false alarms") that are not
dangerous such as those in chronic pain are interpreted as harmful and as a need for
protection. This is common as the brain is unable to differentiate between the pain
sensations that are dangerous or those that are not dangerous, which is one aspect
with which CBT can be helpful.

Table 5.1 Self-report assessments

Measure	Variable	Description
Pain Catastrophizing Scale [55]	Catastrophizing	13-item self-report scale measuring pain catastrophizing including metrics on Rumination, Magnification, and Helplessness
Pain Anxiety Sensitivity Scale—PASS [18, 56]	Pain-related anxiety	Four aspects of pain-related anxiety: cognitive anxiety, escape–avoidance behaviors, fear of pain, and physiological symptoms of anxiety
		Available in short (PASS-20) and long forms
PROMIS Pain Interference short-form [57]	Pain impact	Self-report questionnaire that measures the consequences of pain on the following aspects of one's life: social, cognitive, emotional, physical, and recreational
		Available in different forms in different lengths
Brief Pain Inventory [58]	Pain impact and pain intensity	Self-report questionnaire measures severity of pain, impact of pain on daily function, location of pain, pain medication, and the amount of pain relief in past 24 h
		Available in long and short form
Numerical Rating Scale [59]	Pain intensity	Self-report unidimensional pain scale that assesses pain on 0–10 scale
Patient Health Questionnaire (PHQ-9) [60]	Depression	Nine question self-report measures symptoms of depression
The Chronic Pain-Coping Inventory (CPCI) [61]	Coping	65-item measure of eight behavioral and cognitive coping strategies important for pain adaptation
World Health Organization Disability Assessment Schedule 2.0 (WHODAS 2.0) ([62]; WHODAS II 2001)	Disability/function	36-item self-report questionnaire that provides a global measure of disability and seven domain-specific scores
Roland Morris Disability Questionnaire (RMDQ or RMDI) [63]	Disability/function	Self-report 24-item questionnaire assessing physical disability due to pain

Table 5.2 CBT modules and recommendations for specific patient problems

Module	Strategies	Recommendations	Goals
Psychoeducation and goal setting	SMART goals	General module for all patients	Provide pain-specific educational information
			Provide educational information on CBT
			Delineate SMART goals
Acceptance versus control	Pros and cons	For patients unable to move away from an elusive goal of becoming pain free	Help patients understand the futility of searching for a cure for the pain
			Help patients move from pain control to increase functionality regardless of pain
Behavioral	Activity scheduling	For patients with depression	Help patients reengage in pleasant activities
	Quota-based activity pacing and aerobic exercise	For patients interested in increasing activity in spite of pain	Help patients increase activity regardless of pain status and break association between activity and pain
	Systematic desensitization	For patients with fear avoidance	Help patients gradually reengage in activities avoided due to fear of reinjury
Cognitive	Traditional cognitive restructuring	For patients with distorted negative pain. For patients with realistic negative thoughts that can't be problem solved	Help patients identify negative automatic thoughts, decide whether they are distorted or not, learn to choose between traditional cognitive restructuring and acceptance-based cognitive restructuring with or without problem solving
	Acceptance-based cognitive restructuring	For patients with realistic negative thoughts that can be problem solved	
	Problem solving		
Physiological	Breath awareness	For patients who are overly reactive to pain, or have comorbid anxiety and pain anxiety	Help patient elicit the relaxation response, decrease reactivity to pain, and improve the ability to "make the pain background"
	Guided imagery		
	Biofeedback		
	Progressive muscle relaxation		
	Mindfulness		
Pain and family dynamics	Partner education	For patient whose partners are solicitous or negative	Help decrease pain reinforcement
	Communication boundaries		Decrease amount of time spent talking about pain within the family to facilitate making the pain secondary within the relationship

Further, patient and therapist develop specific, measurable, attainable, realistic and time-specific (SMART; [66–69]) goals to be achieved during the course of therapy. Two to four SMART goals are typically set, and participants rate their current/ baseline status for each goal, and their expectations for goal attainment. Barriers to goal attainment are problem solved. Examples of such SMART goals include tapering ineffective medication on a specific schedule, increasing specific physical activities (e.g., walking to the grocery store three times per week), targeting a return to work date, and improving mood in certain settings. Close collaboration with co-treating physicians and other professionals involved in the patient's care remains critical to minimize mixed messages and sabotaging of treatment goals.

Next, the therapist typically draws the cognitive behavioral model and explains its components, completing a diagram with specific thoughts, behaviors, and feelings and sensations generated by the patient. A specific model for pain symptoms is next generated. This provides a general framework for treatment whereby patients not only see the interrelation among thoughts, behaviors, and feelings/sensations, but also learn about opportunities to improve quality of life by working at the level of each individual component. Different treatment modules (behavioral, cognitive, physiological) are explained using the CBT model. Based on the patient's symptom presentation, the therapist and patient together decide on main therapy modules to be used and the approximate number of sessions needed. The number and order of modules depends on patient's presentation and treatment goals.

Acceptance Versus Control Module. Acceptance refers to "a willingness to have pain without feeling the need to control or eliminate it," and is associated with "acknowledging that one has pain, giving up unproductive attempts to control pain, acting as if pain does not necessarily imply disability, and being able to commit one's efforts toward living a satisfying life, despite pain." [11, 70, 71]. This module is particularly beneficial for patients who are focused on finding a "cure" for their chronic pain (typically those with a long history of prior unsuccessful medical treatments), when such cure does not exist. The module includes several exercises aimed to raise awareness of failure from strategies aimed at pain reduction. One such as exercise is a pros and cons exercise in which patients recall what they have done so far to become pain free, whether those strategies have been successful, and whether they are living a life that is fulfilling. Next, patients are asked whether continuing on the same path would likely lead to different, positive results, and if not, they are asked to invest in a different approach that has worked well for other patients like themselves.

Behavioral Modules: Activity Scheduling, Quota-Based Activity, Exercise and Systematic Desensitization. Patients with chronic pain are typically avoidant of activities that are causing pain, likely due to incorrect beliefs about what they should be able or are currently able to do (e.g., a patient with chronic back pain who incorrectly believes that exercising will cause damage to his back). This often increases disability through physical changes including loss of muscle mass and flexibility, as well as psychological factors such as depression, as patients no longer participate in activities that they have previously enjoyed. Both depression and perception of symptoms are further exacerbated by avoidance.

Behavioral modules are aimed at increasing activity level, increasing conditioning and helping patients reengage in activities they previously enjoyed. A key component in ensuring the success of this module is communication with patient's medical team. Often patients get contradictory advice from health care professionals with regard to level of activity while in pain. When the medical team is aware of the goal of increasing activity despite pain, they can support the therapist and patient in their work toward this goal. Effective communication between providers can help provide a more comprehensive interdisciplinary treatment plan with greater consistency and follow through.

Activity scheduling and *activity pacing* are two behavioral pain management techniques that help patients return to activities that they previously enjoy and maximize their ability to participate in such activities.

Within an *activity scheduling module*, patients list activities that they previously enjoyed but have given up due to the chronic pain or depressed mood. Tools such as a "Positive Events Checklist" (e.g., [72, 73]) can be used to help the individuals identify pleasurable events and work to increase involvement in these activities. Often patients' misconceptions about the safety of such activities as well as guilt feeling about whether they deserve to enjoy themselves may interact with this module; patients should be informed that these issues will be addressed within the cognitive module.

Activity pacing involves patients learning to alternate activity with fixed periods of time for rest, rather than doing too much when they feel good and too little when they do not, i.e., pain contingent activity. Overall, they increase the amount of time they engage in activities despite the variability of their pain. *Quota-based activity pacing* involves teaching patients to engage in rested periods on a preset quota versus engaging in "rest" as a "pain behavior" contingent on exacerbation of pain. For patients with chronic pain, quota-based pacing exercises are also designed to help patients break the association between activity and pain, which has been established through classical conditioning by stopping all activities when in pain due to misconceptions about causing damage and making the problem worse. First, patients are asked to pick a meaningful activity, and assess the amount of time that they are able to engage in that activity without pain or with minimal pain. Using that baseline a quota-based pacing program is constructed in which activity blocks alternate with rest and patients are instructed to strictly adhere to this schedule. Over time, the blocks of activity are gradually increased while the fixed-schedule rest periods are decreased. Quota-based pacing typically involves patient self-monitoring and activity recording, generally monitoring of the activity versus the monitoring of pain. The daily logs are reviewed to identify trends, potential obstacles in pacing, and determine additional tools if needed (such as setting an alarm on the phone to signal a time for rest or activity). Quota-based pacing can also be used to help patients engage in *physical exercise*. Exercise is one of the most effective treatments for both mood and pain [74, 75] through the release of endorphins and increased muscle and tissue conditioning.

Systematic Desensitization is a behavioral strategy initially developed to treat anxiety disorders and phobias, and later adopted for the treatment of patients with chronic pain and fear avoidance issues (e.g., [76]). Systematic desensitization is particularly useful for patients with chronic pain who developed pain from an initial injury (e.g., work-related accident), and have difficulty re engaging in the activity that has caused the injury (e.g., working with a particular work tool) [77]. The fear avoidance is not only a large obstacle in the treatment of chronic pain, but is also predictive of poor physical and psychological treatment outcomes [78, 79]. The treatment consists of three main steps: establishing the fear hierarchy, learning the incompatible responses (relaxation techniques), and connecting the fearful experience to the incompatible response (exposure while in a state of relaxation). The patient and provider begin by collaboratively identifying the concerns and the specific goal of therapy, for example, returning to using a particular tool at work. Following, the patient and provider construct a fear hierarchy in session where each anxiety-provoking scenario is given a rating based on its perceived level of discomfort. The patient then learns relaxation techniques to utilize during the exposure work. Relaxation techniques may include progressive muscle relaxation, deep breathing, and visual imagery. Implementing systematic desensitization, the person is then gradually exposed to specific anxiety-producing stimuli by beginning with the less threatening exposures on the hierarchy and working toward the most anxiety-producing scenarios. Over several sessions (on average 6–10), the patient and therapist work up the hierarchy, experiencing feared stimuli while utilizing relaxation techniques. Most importantly, the experience of pain itself may be feared by the patient, and the exposure to exacerbations of pain utilizes the same desensitization principles. A key component is allowing sufficient time for the anxiety response to dissipate in each situation before moving ahead to the next scenario.

The approach may have minimal effect unless the "in vivo" practice is woven into the treatment plan from the onset, particularly when fears associated with return to work are present. Obtaining a targeted return-to-work document in collaboration with the attending physician is extremely important. This effort is often sabotaged by the patient's attorney, the employer, union contract rules, or even the patient himself. Even other coworkers can inhibit the best desensitization effort by ostracizing the patient who returns with a graded rather than full return to work plan. The process is complex, and the therapist's role has a risk of becoming marginalized as other factors appear. An open conversation about all these potential barriers and engaging in problem solving is particularly important when such issues are identified.

5.5   Cognitive Modules: Cognitive Restructuring and Problem Solving

Cognitive restructuring is a traditional CBT technique [7]. Within this module, patients become aware of their negative automatic thoughts, fit them into categories called cognitive distortions/errors, and restructure their automatic negative thoughts, replacing them with positive, realistic, adaptive thoughts. These negative related thoughts are triggered by pain or by outside events. The process of teaching cognitive restructuring occurs throughout several sessions. First, patients are asked to pay attention to their thoughts when in pain, or when experiencing negative emotions or physiological sensations and engaging in avoidant behaviors. Next, through the use of a thought record patients challenge specific negative thoughts and beliefs (about pain, disability, etc.). Through repetition, patients eventually learn to engage in cognitive restructuring immediately in situations that trigger negative thinking or interfere with activity scheduling or pacing. Pain coping measures such as Pain Catastrophizing Scale (PCS) can be very helpful in aiding patients in the process of identifying negative automatic pain thoughts. The therapist can work with the specific thoughts endorsed on the PCS, and teach cognitive restructuring and development of an adaptive response. The most common cognitive errors for patients with pain are pain catastrophizing (thinking of the worse when experiencing pain), black and white thinking (polarized thinking in which patients fail to see the gray), and control fallacies (feeling or thinking that one is more controlled by the outcomes of problems than one really is).

Acceptance-based cognitive restructuring occurs in situations where the negative thoughts generated by patients are actually rational/true (e.g., do not represent cognitive errors). In such situations, typical cognitive restructuring is unhelpful. Patients eventually understand that focusing on the negative thoughts can cause, exacerbate, and/or maintain negative mood states, inactivity, and, consequently, perceptions about pain. In many situations, patients are bewildered and shocked about the fact that chronic pain does not have a cure. Automatic ruminative thoughts such as "Why me?" or "I will have to have pain for the rest of my life" are common. In this module, patients are given time to grieve the loss/change, process feelings and thoughts about the pain, and work toward acceptance so that they can integrate this experience within their lives.

There are also situations in which the negative automatic thoughts are true but can be problem solved. Within the *problem-solving module* patients learn to intervene directly on the stressors, problem, behavior or rational negative thought. Often, when confronted with pain, patients experience greater difficulty solving problems than they did previously. In many situations, patients agonize over figuring out what is the best solution to a problem; other times, patients delay engaging in behaviors needed to manage their pain (i.e., procrastination) because thinking about a possible solution can cause anxiety and therefore make decision-making difficult. Hence, this intervention involves working with the patients through a process of relearning effective problem solving. Typical steps involve orienting the patient to the problem, generating alternative behavioral responses, reviewing decision-making practices, and determining how to implement the chosen solution(s) [80]. Turk [81] specified the following sequence to problem-solving for chronic pain [82]: (1) defining the source of distress or stress reaction as problems to be solved; (2) state the problem in changeable, behavioral terms; (3) generate a wide range of solutions; (4) imagine how others might react in the same situation; (5) evaluate pros and cons of each proposed solution and rank order the solutions; (6) try out the most feasible solutions; (7) expect failures, reward self for trying; (8) reconsider the original problem in light of attempted solution; and (9) recycle as needed. It is very important for the therapist to discuss with patients how the decisions they make are often personal, based on the information available at the time and in the specific context of their lives. This may relieve some of the pressure patients feel in picking the "best" solution. This module can be particularly useful for patients who have been out of work and are interested in returning to work but unsure how to find a job.

5.6   Physiological Module: Relaxation Training

Relaxation strategies are primarily focused on eliciting the relaxation response (RR; [83]), which has been found to counteract the negative effects of various stressors, including those associated with pain. The RR is a physiological state characterized by decreased arousal of the sympathetic nervous system and increased parasympathetic activity. The rationale for eliciting the RR among individuals with pain is that the changes associated with this response (e.g., decreases in oxygen consumption and carbon dioxide elimination and in heart rate, respiratory rate, and blood pressure [83] are considered to be the counterpart to the negative changes that occur during the stress response associated with the pain sensation. By eliciting the RR patients with pain can decrease reactivity to pain and quit the negative thinking that fuels pain intensity and disability. By consistent practice of the RR patients learn to "pain alarm," and "make the pain background" such that it no longer represents the center of their lives.

The RR occurs through a variety of strategies that have the common denominator of a sustained mental focus with an attitude of open receptive awareness. It is normally elicited in a two-step process—to help sustain focus one can (a) repeat a word, sound, prayer, or phrase and (b) disregard any unrelated thoughts that come to mind. To achieve the RR patients learn to pay gentle attention to their sensations, emotions, and pain activating thoughts, without getting fused with them or entertaining them. This is an exercise in paying attention and improving concentration and helps patients with pain cope with difficult emotions, physical sensations, and thoughts by giving them power to choose where to put their focus and how to react. The RR is particularly useful for patients with chronic pain who have pain anxiety or general anxiety, as well as those who have functional sleep disorders.

Breath Awareness/Diaphragmatic Breathing is a technique that teaches patients to become aware of how they breathe during times of stress or when in pain (e.g., shallow, irregularly, with incomplete exhalation) and learn to take deep, slow, and relaxing diaphragmatic breaths. One strategy to help patients learn diaphragmatic breathing is to encourage the patient to imagine that she has a balloon in her stomach, which inflates with every inhalation. Just as a balloon releases air, the patient is encouraged to allow her breath to simply release air with each exhalation. Diaphragmatic breathing elicits the RR, in part, through the mind–body connection. Just as the stress response signals the muscle fibers in the body to contract (shorten), diaphragmatic breathing stretches muscle fibers which then signals relaxation throughout the body and mind. Within this module, patients are encouraged to practice diaphragmatic breathing daily when calm; once they master this technique, they are encouraged to practice it also when they experience pain flare ups, and during activities that cause pain, anxiety, and stress.

Guided Imagery is an RR strategy where patients are led to imagine all of the details of a particular relaxing image, as vividly as possible. This can be a "joyful place" imagery, in which patients are guided to remember a special place from their past or present that is associated with peace, safety, and comfort. Patients are encouraged to visualize the details of that place, including imagining the joy they feel when in that place. Patients are encouraged to pay attention to how it feels to be safe, secure, and free of stress and worries, so that they have a memory of feeling peaceful and become able to return to this place in times of stress. This intervention can also be a specific pain-related guided imagery ([84]; UCLA free guided meditations at http://marc.ucla.edu/body.cfm?id=22).

Biofeedback is a form of eliciting the RR while getting immediate feedback on physiological signals (e.g., respiration rate, galvanic skin response, skin temperature), thus providing patients with clear evidence of the mind–body connection. Patients are taught to control various physiological signals that are thought to play a role in maintaining pain symptoms and disability. For example, patients with headaches may be taught to reduce the frequency of their attacks, particularly when it is comorbid with anxiety.

Progressive Muscle Relaxation (PMR) is an RR strategy in which patients are taught to systematically relax muscle groups throughout their bodies to reduce tension and anxiety. During the process, patients learn to alternate between tensing and relaxing various groups of muscles, which leads to overall reduction in tension throughout the body. PMR is helpful in teaching patients how to relax in situations that may cause stress or pain, and works well with patients who have difficulties with, or become hyperaroused during, diaphragmatic breathing.

Mindfulness, defined as "paying attention in a particular way: on purpose, in the present moment, and nonjudgmentally" [84] allows patients to observe their sensations, thoughts, and feelings as they occur without responding or reacting. The two main components of mindfulness are an active awareness and a nonjudgmental stance. Throughout this module, chronic pain patients learn to pay attention to the pain with curiosity and without judgment, and to let go of expectations and pain relief-related goals. By bringing awareness to the pain, patients often learn that pain is not constant, as typically thought of, but has valleys and sometimes completely subsides, which often relieves frustration. Through practicing mindfulness patients learn to make the pain background, so that it is no longer on the front of their minds, constantly impacting their mood, thoughts, and behaviors. In the treatment of chronic pain, mindfulness training is frequently incorporated into cognitive behavioral therapy as a skill that facilitates awareness [85–87], in conjunction with the acceptance module.

5.7 Relationships and Pain

Chronic pain can significantly impact relationships. In turn, pain and disability can also be influenced by relationships. Significant others and family members can play a critical role in a patient's journey with pain. Two types of partners can be particularly detrimental to a patient's treatment, the overly solicitous partner and the neglectful partner. The overly solicitous partner tends to take on a caretaker role that facilitates the maintenance of the patient role and the identity of a "disabled" person, contradicting the treatment goals of improving functioning and activity. Just as harmful is the neglectful partner who is unsupportive and discouraging. Effective assessment and treatment must include the partner in the treatment plan to ensure proper encouragement and support of treatment goals throughout therapy [88, 89]. Typically, partners learn about the negative role of solicitous and negative behaviors and are taught how to engage in neutral non-reinforcing behaviors that are consistent with the goal of improving patient's function. Patient and partner are also taught to pick a specific time weekly when they discuss patient's pain and refrain from making the pain the main focus of the relationship.

5.8 Case Example

5.8.1 Background

Andrea is a woman in her mid-50s who was referred for a behavioral medicine intervention by her orthopedic surgeon. Andrea had experienced several episodes of back pain over the past 20 years, following a period of intense training for a marathon in her early 30s. All her prior episodes improved, and she was treated successfully with physical therapy and nerve blocks at that time. In all instances, testing revealed no pathology. The pain was considered to have a myofascial component and also referred to as "idiopathic" (vague, diffuse, with little or no objective abnormality). The most recent episode was the most severe and disabling, and she failed to get relief with biomedical treatments. Further, although passive physical therapy was recommended, Andrea reported difficulties adhering to treatment due to intense pain.

Upon the first meeting, a detailed psychosocial assessment was conducted. Andrea rated her pain at rest, on a scale of 1–10, as a "3" on a good day and "7" on a bad day. With activity, she rated her pain as a "10." She described her pain as "unbearable" and reported frustration with the fact that she was not given a "proper diagnosis." The pain was localized to her low back region. She noted that although she was relieved that her medical tests showed that there was no serious pathology, she was also frustrated and felt that her pain was being considered "in my head" by her physician. Further, she was concerned that treatments that had worked in the past no longer helped her. She was convinced that there was something seriously wrong with her back that had been missed, as her pain was more intense than during previous episodes. She noted that pain interfered with activities of daily living, and that her husband was currently doing all the household chores. She noted that she was no longer able to run, which had been her main source of stress relief all her life. She also revealed recent high stress at work, in the context of multiple lay-offs and stressed coworkers. When asked how she coped with the pain, Andrea noted that she received some relief from ibuprofen 1800 mg daily, but that it upset her stomach and she was concerned about its long-term effects. She noted that her mood was down, and she felt worried about her future. She was unable to sleep as the moment she laid down she felt overwhelmed by negative thoughts, worries, and anxiety. Andrea had mild pressured speech and was in obvious distress. Although she was alert, oriented, and well-groomed, she appeared disheveled, wearing oversized, baggy clothes, which the therapist discovered later was due to her depressed mood.

5.8.2 Case Conceptualization

Andrea was faced with another back pain episode at a time when things were going fairly well within her primary relationship. However, Andrea found her job stressful, was worried she would be laid off, and had trouble negotiating a stressful work environment. She worried that her back pain interfered with her ability to fulfill her duties both at work and at home. She felt that she was no longer able to engage in physical exercise, which had been her primary coping mechanism in the past. Because all her previous back pain episodes were treated biomedically, she felt that she needed more medical tests in order to discover why her current back pain episode was more severe than in the past. She was concerned that her pain was a sign of something pathologically wrong that, if not found, would get worse with the passage of time.

Andrea had great social support from family and friends. A careful analysis of relationship issues revealed that her husband, albeit well intentioned, was reinforcing her pain and avoidance by taking over her household responsibilities. In describing her feelings of being useless, dependent, and scared, she stated, "I can't do anything." She was also worried about the fact that her husband might get tired of doing so much and might leave her. Andrea experienced intense fear of worsening her pain and spent a lot of time monitoring her symptoms and paying attention to her back. Instead of running, she spent time at home watching TV and ruminating on her pain condition. Her mood was depressed and anxious. She was not suicidal, and showed no risk to herself or others. Fortunately, she was not self-medicating with alcohol or other substances. Andrea's symptoms fit well within a cognitive behavioral case conceptualization. She endorsed negative thoughts about pain, such as, "My pain will never get better"; "My pain is awful and overwhelming"; and "There must be something seriously wrong with my back"—and she avoided activities that might cause pain, including physical therapy exercises and running. This, in turn, negatively influenced her pain sensation and mood.

5.8.3 Treatment

After the assessment session, which consisted of interview with the patient and spouse, self-report measures, a review of medical records, and discussion with her treating physician, Andrea underwent ten treatment sessions utilizing a cognitive behavioral approach. The first two sessions of the treatment was *psychoeducational* and was focused on normalizing the low back pain condition and Andrea's diagnosis. Content of the session focused on educational information about the mind–body relationship as it relates to pain and how stress, depression, and anxiety symptoms are common correlates of pain. Andrea learned that depression and anxiety symptoms (e.g., low energy, difficulties concentrating, decreased motivation, psychomotor retardation, decreased appetite, fatigue, fears, increased heartbeat, shortness of breath, avoidance) are correlates of pain that occur in most people, in different degrees. This session was also focused on helping Andrea understand how the CBT intervention could help her, and on increasing her confidence in treatment. In the first session, she also learned the results of the assessment. Specifically, Andrea learned that her scores on two coping measures, Pain Catastrophizing [55] and Pain Anxiety Sensitivity [18], were high. This meant that compared to most people, Andrea attributed negative and "catastrophic" consequences to the experience of pain, and had more anxiety about her pain.

This session also focused on discussing the rationale for psychosocial treatment in the context of an episode of idiopathic pain, and how addressing the psychosocial factors related to pain might benefit her pain condition and related concomitants of the pain, i.e., depression, anxiety, disability, and fear avoidance. A motivational interview exercise was conducted to help Andrea move away from wanting a medical diagnoses and a cure to acceptance and management of symptoms. A pros and cons exercise was conducted for working on her pain within the behavioral medicine intervention framework versus continuing a purely biomedical treatment. Finally, SMART treatment goals were established.

During the following three sessions, Andrea learned about the CBT model and the connection between thoughts, feelings, and behaviors. This was done using specific examples pertaining to Andrea's responses to pain. During these three *cognitively* focused sessions, Andrea learned how her negative pain-related thoughts, low mood, and avoidance behaviors were interrelated, and that these placed her at risk for more disability over time. Andrea also learned to identify her negative pain thoughts, fit them into cognitive errors, and cognitively reframe her pain-related negative thoughts. For example, when she noted thoughts like, "pain is awful and overwhelming," she learned to replace that thought with a more adaptive one: "I can do many things in spite of pain." This helped Andrea change the manner in which she construed herself. Instead of thinking of herself as "a victim of her pain," Andrea began to experience herself as someone who was learning and employing strategies to cope with her pain. When she noted thinking that, "I feel pain, therefore there must be something seriously wrong," she learned to tell herself that "my doctor thoroughly checked me out, I have had pain before and eventually it went away; there is no evidence that there is something seriously wrong with my back." This showed a high level of understanding that one can have pain without a physiological cause, as it is the case in most chronic back pain conditions. Andrea also learned to reframe negative thoughts associated with her job and the possibility of losing it.

The next session was focused on relaxation training. Andrea learned about the relaxation response, and how pain initiates and maintains a stress response. She learned to engage in diaphragmatic breathing during her physical therapy exercises, and the fact that she was in a relaxed state allowed her to progress with her exercises. She also learned to engage in relaxation strategies during times of stress at work.

Next, Andrea underwent two *behavioral sessions* focused on pacing and activity scheduling. Within the pacing module, Andrea learned to reengage in activities that she previously enjoyed but was now avoiding, including running. Through her quota-based exercise, she slowly increased the amount of time she was able to run with specific benchmarks, so that eventually she managed to return to 45 min sessions several times a week. Activity scheduling was done in conjunction with quota-based exercise to help Andrea return to activities she previously enjoyed, such as meeting friends, going to see movies, as well as engaging in household activities that she had previously avoided. Eventually, as part of her specific treatment plan timeline she and her husband returned to equally sharing household chores.

The last two sessions were focused on reinforcing progress and relapse prevention. A focus of these sessions was developing an acceptance that pain may return, particularly in times of stress, but that Andrea now has the tools to adaptively cope.

5.8.4   Treatment Outcome

At the time of termination, Andrea's self-reported pain intensity at rest and with repetitive activity had decreased, as had her disability. With support from her clinician, attending physician and husband, she continued to work throughout the treatment process, a good prognostic indicator. Her mood and her scores on the pain scales had decreased as well. At the end of treatment, Andrea was still bothered by intermittent pain, but the pain no longer consumed her. She accepted that her pain was "real," but would not be responsive to multiple medical treatments. She was no longer avoidant of activities that she enjoyed. She had returned to doing her share of household chores, was exercising and was slowly building up to her past level of physical activity. Andrea had not sought medical treatment since the end of therapy several months ago, while she was encouraged to have regular visits with her primary care physician to offer her assurance about her gains, a plan of care engineered along with her treating behavioral therapist.

Conclusion: Changes in behavior, cognitions, and lifestyle can improve quality of life and reduce symptom burden in patients with chronic pain. Clinical practice and research have shown that CBT interventions can help patients with chronic pain feel better physically and emotionally, improve their health status, increase their activity, and improve their ability to live with chronic illness. Outcomes for the treating clinicians can be greatly enhanced by active collaboration with other treating providers, family members, and others who have a stake in the patient's success. Improvements in chronic pain outcomes are predicated on developing strategies to identify patients at risk for chronicity and providing interventions early on in the acute phase. There is evidence that short-term CBT is more efficacious than usual care in reducing pain and disability and improving coping and mood in patients with acute orthopedic trauma [24, 30, 33].

References

1. International Association for the Study of Pain. Classification of chronic pain. Seattle: IASP Press; 1994.
2. Institute of Medicine (US). Relieving pain in America: a blueprint for transforming prevention, care, education and research. Washington, DC: National Academies Press (US); 2011.
3. National Centers for Health Statistics. Chartbook on Trends in the Health of Americans. Special feature: pain. 2006. http://www.cdc.gov/nchs/data/hus/hus06.pdf.
4. Melzack R, Casey KL. Sensory, motivational, and central control determinants of pain. In: Kenshalo DR, editor. The skin senses. Springfield: Thomas; 1968. p. 423–39.
5. Melzack R, Wall PD. Gate control theory of pain. In: Soulairoc A, Cahn J, Charpentier J, editors. Pain. New York: Academic; 1968. p. 11–31.
6. Fordyce WE. Behavioral methods for chronic pain and illness. St. Louis: The CV Mosby Company; 1976.
7. Beck AT, Rush AJ, Shaw BF, Emery G. Cognitive behavioral therapy for depression. New York: Guilford; 1979.
8. Turner JA, Romano JM. Cognitive-behavioral therapy for chronic pain. In: Loesser JD, editor. Bonica's management of pain. Philadelphia: Lippincott Williams & Wilkins; 2001. p. 1751–8.
9. Turk DC, Meichenbaum DH, Genest M. Pain and behavioral medicine: theory, research, and clinical guide. New York: Guilford; 1983.
10. Turk DC, Kerns RD. Conceptual issues in the assessment of clinical pain. Int J Psychiatry Med. 1983;13:15–26.
11. McCracken LM. Learning to live with the pain: acceptance of pain predicts adjustments in persons with chronic pain. Pain. 1998;74:21–7.
12. McCracken LM, Eccleston C. Coping or acceptance: what to do about chronic pain? Pain. 2003;105:197–204.
13. Crombez G, Eccleston C, van Hamme G, Vlieger P. Attempting to solve the problem of pain: a questionnaire study in acute and chronic pain. Pain. 2008;137:556–63.
14. Ericsson M, Poston II WS, Linder J, Taylor JE, Haddock CK, Foreyt JP. Depression predicts disability in long-term chronic pain patients. Disabil Rehabil. 2002;24:334–40.
15. Keogh E, McCracken LM, Eccleston C. Gender moderates the association between depression and disability in chronic pain. Eur J Pain. 2006;10:413–22.
16. Asmundson GJ, Norton PJ, Vlaeyen JWS. Fear-avoidance models of chronic pain: an overview. In: Asmundson GJ, Vlaeyen JW, Crombez G, editors. Understanding and treating fear of pain. Oxford: Oxford University Press; 2004. p. 1–36.
17. Dersh J, Polatin PB, Gatchel RJ. Chronic pain and psychopathology: reading findings and theoretical considerations. Psychosom Med. 2002;64:773–86.
18. McCracken LM, Zayfert C, Gross RT. The pain anxiety symptoms scale: development and validation of a scale to measure fear of pain. Pain. 1992;50:67–73.
19. Vlaeyen JW, Linton SJ. Fear-avoidance and its consequences in chronic musculoskeletal pain: a state of the art. Pain. 2000;85:317–32.
20. Vranceanu AM, Safren SA, Cowan J, Ring DC. Health concerns and somatic symptoms explain perceived disability and idiopathic hand and arm pain in an orthopedics surgical practice: a path-analysis model. Psychosomatics. 2010;51:330–7.
21. De Das S, Vranceanu AM, Ring D. Contribution of kinesophobia and catastrophic thinking to upper-extremity-specific disability. J Bone Joint Surg Am. 2013;95:76–81.
22. Fordyce WE, Shelton JL, Dundore DE. The modification of avoidance learning pain behaviors. J Behav Med. 1982;5:405–14.
23. Phillips HC. Avoidance behavior and its role in sustaining chronic pain. Behav Res Ther. 1987;25:273–9.
24. Vranceanu AM, Barsky A, Ring D. Psychosocial aspects of disabling musculoskeletal pain. J Bone Joint Surg Am. 2009;91:2014–8.

25. Keefe FJ, Rumble ME, Scipio CD, Giordano LA, Perri LM. Psychological aspects of persistent pain: current state of the science. J Pain. 2004;5:195–211.
26. Turner JA, Holtzman S, Mancl L. Mediators, moderators, and predictors of therapeutic change in cognitive-behavioral therapy for chronic pain. Pain. 2007;127:276–86.
27. Varni JW, Rapoff MA, Waldron SA, Gragg RA, Bernstein BH, Lindsley CB. Effects of perceived stress on pediatric chronic pain. J Behav Med. 1996;19:515–28.
28. Barsky AJ, Orav J, Bates DW. Somatization increases medical utilization and costs independent of psychiatric and medical comorbidity. Arch Gen Psychiatry. 2005;62:903–10.
29. Nicholas MK, Linton SJ, Watson PJ, Main CJ. Early identification and management of psychological risk factors ("yellow flags") in patients with low back pain: a reappraisal. Phys Ther. 2011;91(5):737–53.
30. Vranceanu AM, Bachoura A, Weening A, Vrahas M, Smith RM, Ring D. Psychological factors predict disability and pain intensity after skeletal trauma. J Bone Joint Surg Am. 2014;96(3):e20.
31. Fransen M, Woodward M, Norton R, Coggan C, Dawe M, Sheridan N. Risk factors associated with the transition from acute to chronic occupational back pain. Spine. 2002;27:92–8.
32. Casey CY, Greenberg MA, Nicassio PM, Harpin RE, Hubbard D. Transition from acute to chronic pain and disability: a model including cognitive, affective, and trauma factors. Pain. 2008;134:69–79.
33. Vranceanu AM, Hageman M, Strooker J, ter Meulen D, Vrahas M, Ring D. A preliminary RCT of a mind body intervention addressing mood and coping strategies in patients with acute orthopedic trauma. Injury. 2015;46(4):552–7.
34. Sullivan MJ, Adams H, Tripp D, Stanish WD. Stage of chronicity and treatment response in patients with musculoskeletal injuries and concurrent symptoms of depression. Pain. 2008;135:151–9.
35. Williams ACC, Eccleston C, Morley S. Psychological therapies for the management of chronic pain (excluding headache) in adults. Cochrane Database Syst Rev. 2012;11:CD007407.
36. Hoffman BM, Papas RK, Chatkoff DK, Kerns RD. Meta-analysis of psychological interventions for chronic low back pain. Health Psychol. 2007;26:1–9.
37. Henschke N, Ostelo RW, van Tulder MW, Vlaeyen JWS, Morley S, Assendelft WJJ, Main CJ. Behavioural treatment for chronic low-back pain. Cochrane Database Syst Rev. 2010;(7):CD002014.
38. Andrasik F. What does the evidence show? Efficacy of behavioural treatments for recurrent headaches in adults. Neurol Sci. 2007;28:70–7.
39. Turk DC, Swanson KS, Tunks ER. Psychological approaches in the treatment of chronic pain patients—when pills, scalpels, and needles are not enough. Can J Psychiatry. 2008;53:213–23.
40. Nestoriuc Y, Martin A. Efficacy of biofeedback for migraine: a meta-analysis. Pain. 2007;128:111–27.
41. Nestoriuc Y, Martin A, Rief W, Andrasik F. Biofeedback treatment for headache disorders: a comprehensive efficacy review. Appl Psychophysiol Biofeedback. 2008;33:125–40.
42. Nestoriuc Y, Rief W, Martin A. Meta-analysis of biofeedback for tension-type headache: efficacy, specificity, and treatment moderators. J Consult Clin Psychol. 2008;76:379–96.
43. Sharp TJ. Chronic pain: a reformulation of the cognitive-behavioural model. Behav Res Ther. 2001;39:787–800.
44. Turk DC, Rudy TE. Neglected topics in the treatment of chronic pain patients—relapse, noncompliance, and adherence enhancement. Pain. 1991;44:5–28.
45. Jensen MP, Nielson WR, Turner JA, Romano JM, Hill ML. Changes in readiness to self-manage pain are associated with improvement in multidisciplinary pain treatment and pain coping. Pain. 2004;111:84–95.
46. Kerns RD, Habib S. A critical review of the pain readiness to change model. J Pain. 2004;5:357–67.
47. Jensen M. Enhancing motivation to change in pain treatment. In: Turk D, Gatchel R, editors. Psychological treatment for pain: a practitioner's handbook. 2nd ed. New York: Guilford; 2002. p. 71–93.

48. Miller WR, Rollnick S. Motivational interviewing: preparing people for change. New York: Guilford; 2002.
49. Linton SJ. The manager's role in employees' successful return to work following back injury. Work Stress. 1991;5:3.
50. Dasinger L, Krause N, Thompson P, Brand R, Rudolph L. Doctor proactive communication, return to work recommendations, and duration of disability after a workers' compensation low back injury. J Occup Environ Med. 2001;43:515–25.
51. Kosny A, MacEachen E, Ferrier S, Chambers L. The role of health care providers in long term and complicated workers' compensation claims. J Occup Rehabil. 2011;21:582–90.
52. Bieber C, Muller KG, Blumenstiel K, Schneider A, Richter A, Wilke S, et al. Long-term effects of a shared decision-making intervention on physician-patient interaction and outcome in fibromyalgia: a qualitative and quantitative 1 year follow-up of a randomized controlled trial. Patient Educ Couns. 2006;63:357–66.
53. Matthias MS, Bair MJ. The patient-provider relationship in chronic pain management: where do we go from here? Pain Med. 2010;11:1747–9.
54. Kerns RD, Burns JW, Shulman M, Jensen MP, Nielson WR, et al. Can we improve cognitive-behavioral therapy for chronic back pain treatment engagement and adherence? A controlled trial of tailored versus standard therapy. Health Psychol. 2014;33:938–47.
55. Sullivan MJL, Bishop SR, Pivik J. The pain catastrophizing scale: development and validation. Psychol Assess. 1995;7:524.
56. McCracken LM, Dhingra L. A short version of the Pain Anxiety Symptoms Scale (PASS-20): preliminary development and validity. Pain Res Manag. 2002;7:45–50.
57. Amtmann D, Cook KF, Jensen MP, Chen WH, Choi S, Revicki D, et al. Development of a PROMIS item bank to measure pain interference. Pain. 2010;150:173–82.
58. Cleeland CS, Ryan KM. Pain assessment: global use of the brief pain inventory. Ann Acad Med. 1994;23:129–38.
59. McCaffery M. Pain: clinical manual for nursing practice. 2nd ed. St. Louis: Mosby; 1989.
60. Kroenke K, Spitzer RL, Williams JBW. The Phq-9. J Gen Intern Med. 2001;16:606–13.
61. Jensen MP, Turner JA, Romano JM, Strom SE. The chronic pain coping inventory: development and preliminary validation. Pain. 1995;60:203–16.
62. Garin O, Ayuso-Mateos JL, Almansa J, Nieto M, Chatterji S, Vilagut G, et al. Validation of the "World Health Organization Disability Assessment Schedule, WHODAS-2" in patients with chronic diseases. Health Qual Life Outcomes. 2010;8:51.
63. Roland M, Morris R. A study of the natural history of back pain: part I: development of a reliable and sensitive measure of disability low-back pain. Spine. 1983;8:141–4.
64. Kerns RD, Haythornthwaite J, Rosenberg R, Soutwick S, Giller EL, Jacob MC. The pain behavior check list (PBCL): factor structure and psychometric properties. J Behav Med. 1991;14:155–67.
65. Turk DC, Winter F. The pain survival guide: how to reclaim your life. Washington, DC: American Psychological Association; 2006.
66. Khan F, Pallant JF, Turner-Stokes L. Use of goal attainment scaling in inpatient rehabilitation for persons with multiple sclerosis. Arch Phys Med Rehabil. 2008;89:652–9.
67. Locke EA, Latham GP. Building a practically useful theory of goal setting and task motivation. A 35 year-old odyssey. Am Psychol. 2002;57:705–17.
68. Siegert RJ, McPherson KM, Taylor WJ. Toward a cognitive-affective model of goal-setting in rehabilitation: is self-regulation theory a key step? Disabil Rehabil. 2004;26:1175–83.
69. Turner-Stokes L. Goal attainment scaling (GAS) in rehabilitation: a practical guide. Clin Rehabil. 2009;23:362–70.
70. McCracken LM, Spertus IL, Janeck AS, Sinclair D, Wetzel FT. Behavioral dimensions of adjustment in persons with chronic pain: pain-related anxiety and acceptance. Pain. 1999;80:283–9.

71. McCracken LM, Vowles KE. Acceptance of chronic pain. Curr Pain Headache Rep. 2006;10:90–4.

72. Linehan M. Cognitive-behavioral treatment of borderline personality disorder. New York: Guilford; 1993.

73. Safren SA, Gonzalez JS, Soroudi N. Coping with chronic illness: a cognitive-behavioral approach for adherence and depression. New York: Oxford University Press; 2008.

74. Nichols DS, Glenn TM. Effects of aerobic exercise on pain perceptions, affect, and level of disability in individuals with fibromyalgia. Phys Ther. 1994;74:327–32.

75. Wigers SHR, Stiles TC, Vogel PA. Effects of aerobic exercise versus stress management treatment in fibromyalgia. Scand J Rheumatol. 1996;25:77–86.

76. Vlaeyen JW, de Jong J, Geilen M, Heuts P, Van Breukelen G. The treatment of fear of movement/(re) injury in chronic low back pain: further evidence on the effectiveness of exposure in vivo. Clin J Pain. 2002;18:251–61.

77. Woods MP, Asmundson GJG. Evaluation the efficacy of graded in vivo exposure for the treatment of fear in patients with chronic back pain: a randomized controlled clinical trial. Pain. 2008;136:271–80.

78. Asmundson GJ, Norton PJ, Norton GR. Beyond pain: the role of fear and avoidance in chronicity. Clin Psychol Rev. 1999;19:97–119.

79. Waddell G, Newton M, Henderson I, Somerville D, Main CJ. A Fear-Avoidance Beliefs Questionnaire (FABQ) and the role of fear avoidance beliefs in chronic low back pain and disability. Pain. 1993;52:157–68.

80. Nezu AM, Nezu CM, D'Zurilla TJ. Problem-solving therapy: a treatment manual. New York: Springer; 2013.

81. Turk DC, Meichenbaum D. A cognitive-behavioral approach to pain management. In: Textbook of pain. 3rd ed. 1999. p. 1337–48.

82. D'Zurilla TJ, Nezu AM, Maydeu-Oliveras A. Social problem solving: theory and assessment. In: Chang EC, D'Zurilla TJ, Sanna LJ, editors. Social problem solving: theory, research and training. Washington, DC: American Psychological Association; 2004.

83. Benson H, Klipper MZ. The relaxation response. London: Collins; 1976.

84. Kabat-Zinn J. Wherever you go, there you are: mindfulness meditation in everyday life. New York: Hyperion; 1994.

85. Chiesa A, Serretti A. A systematic review of neurobiological and clinical features of mindfulness meditations. Psychol Med. 2010;40:1239–52.

86. Chiesa A, Serretti A. Mindfulness-based interventions for chronic pain: a systematic review of the evidence. J Altern Complement Med. 2011;17:83–93.

87. McCracken LM, Vowles KE. Acceptance and commitment therapy and mindfulness for chronic pain: model, process, and progress. Am Psychol. 2014;69:178–87.

88. Delvey J, Hopkins L. Pain patients and their partners; the role of collusion in chronic pain. J Marital Fam Ther. 1982;8:135–42.

89. Kerns RD, Turk DC. Depression and chronic pain: the mediating role of the spouse. J Marriage Fam. 1984;46:845–52.

90. Kerns and Habit was meant to be: Kerns RD, Habib S. A critical review of the pain readiness to change model. J Pain. 2004; 5: 357–367.

91. Turk DC, Meichenbaum D. A cognitive –behavioral approach to pain management. Textbook of pain 3. 1999; 1337–1348.

92. Casey CY, Greenberg MA, Nicassio PM, Harpin RE, Hubbard D. Transition from acute to chronic pain and disability: A model including cognitive, affective, and trauma factors. Pain. 2008; 134: 69–79.

93. McCracken LM, Dhingra L. A short version of the Pain Anxiety Symptoms Scale (PASS-20): Preliminary development and validity. Pain Res manag; 2002

Resources

Turk DC, Winter F. The pain survival guide: how to reclaim your life. Washington, DC: American Psychological Association; 2006.

http://www.health-psych.org/

http://www.sbm.org/

http://www.psychosomatic.org/home/index.cfm

American Pain Society (APS). http://www.americanpainsociety.org/

International Association for the Study of Pain (IASP). http://www.iasp-pain.org/

UCLA Free Guided Meditation. http://marc.ucla.edu/body.cfm?id=22

Insight LA Free Mindfulness Meditation. www.insightla.org

Chapter 6
Cognitive Behavioral Therapy for Adherence and Depression in Diabetes

Jeffrey S. Gonzalez, Naomi S. Kane, and Trina E. Chang

Approximately 14.3 % of the nationally representative population of noninstitutionalized adults was estimated to have diabetes in 2012, and slightly over one-third were unaware of their diagnosis. Strikingly, an additional 38 % were estimated to have significantly elevated blood sugars (glucose), or prediabetes, placing them at risk for the development of type 2 diabetes. Prevalence has been steadily increasing over the last 20–30 years in the overall population and across ethnic groups, education levels, and levels of income [1]. Type 2 diabetes accounts for 90–95 % of total cases of diabetes and involves a combination of decreased response to insulin, or insulin resistance, and relative insulin deficiency. It is usually diagnosed in adulthood and is associated with obesity, which contributes to insulin resistance and poor glucose control. Thus, weight loss, involving changes in diet and physical activity, is important to managing blood glucose levels and slowing disease progression [2, 3]. Type 1 diabetes is characterized by an absolute insulin deficiency, prompted by an autoimmune response that destroys the insulin-manufacturing beta cells in the pancreas. Thus, it requires the regular administration of exogenous insulin, through multiple daily injections or an electronic insulin pump. Between 5 and 10 % of those diagnosed with diabetes have type 1 [4], which is usually diagnosed in childhood or young adulthood.

J.S. Gonzalez, Ph.D. (✉)
Ferkauf Graduate School of Psychology, Yeshiva University, Bronx, NY 10461, USA

Diabetes Research Center, Albert Einstein College of Medicine, Yeshiva University, Bronx, NY 10461, USA
e-mail: jeffrey.gonzalez@einstein.yu.edu

N.S. Kane, M.A.
Ferkauf Graduate School of Psychology, Yeshiva University, Bronx, NY 10461, USA

T.E. Chang, M.D., M.P.H.
Depression Clinical and Research Program, Department of Psychiatry, Massachusetts General Hospital, 1 Bowdoin Square, 6th floor, Boston, MA 02114, USA
e-mail: techang@partners.org

© Springer Science+Business Media New York 2017
A.-M. Vranceanu et al. (eds.), *The Massachusetts General Hospital Handbook of Behavioral Medicine*, Current Clinical Psychiatry,
DOI 10.1007/978-3-319-29294-6_6

In both type 1 and type 2 diabetes, the goal of treatment is to achieve tight control of glucose levels and associated cardiovascular risk factors—blood pressure and cholesterol—to prevent or delay the development of diabetes complications, such as cardiovascular disease, nephropathy, neuropathy, and retinopathy. Landmark trials established clinically significant reduction in risk for diabetes complications among patients with type 1 and type 2 diabetes who were intensively treated to keep glucose levels close to the normal range [5, 6]. Results have had a dramatic impact on the management of diabetes in clinical practice from the mid-1990s to the present.

Current standards of care from the American Diabetes Association (ADA) recommend lowering HbA1c, a form of hemoglobin measured in blood to quantify average plasma glucose concentrations over approximately 3 months, to 7.0 % or less for most adults. More stringent goals (e.g., $\leq 6.5 \%$) may be appropriate for some adults if they can be achieved without significant adverse effects of treatment. Less stringent goals (e.g., $\leq 8.0 \%$) may also be appropriate for older adults, who may be frail or have limited life expectancy, as well as those with advanced complications or comorbid conditions. Less stringent targets are also appropriate for adolescents [7]. The flexibility in these targets and the importance of tailoring to the individual reflect the trade-off between treatment-associated reductions in hyperglycemia and increased risk of hypoglycemia, or low blood sugars, which when severe can cause accidents, coma, and death. ADA recommendations also include targets for control of blood pressure and cholesterol, which are considered at least as important as those for glycemic control given the increased risk for cardiovascular disease in diabetes [7].

A complex set of behaviors is required to meet blood glucose goals. These behaviors include medication taking, self-monitoring of blood glucose via finger-stick and analysis with a glucose meter, changes in nutrition and exercise, regular inspection of feet for early signs of ulceration, and regular preventive appointments with healthcare providers. Suboptimal self-management is associated with higher blood glucose levels [8, 9] and increased risk for diabetes complications, hospitalization, and mortality [10]. Difficulties with self-management are common, with diabetes having one of the lowest rates of treatment adherence among various chronic illnesses [11]. This finding likely reflects the difficulty of diabetes lifestyle changes related to diet and physical activity [12]. Self-management is burdensome to many patients; basic self-care is estimated to require approximately 2 h of work per day [13]. Roughly half of adults with diabetes in the USA meet recommendations for A1c, blood pressure or cholesterol, with less than 20 % meeting criteria for all three biomarkers [14]. The demands of treatment provide a context for understanding diabetes-associated stressors, including regimen-related stress.

6.1 Psychological and Psychiatric Issues in Diabetes

Studies consistently demonstrate elevations in the prevalence of several psychiatric disorders, as well as subclinical diabetes-related emotional distress, among individuals diagnosed with diabetes. Diabetes-related distress, or emotional distress that is specifically related to the burdens of living with this chronic, difficult-to-manage, and life-threatening health condition, appears to be common and closely related to difficulties with self-management and suboptimal glycemic control.

Depression. Meta-analyses suggest that the risk for depression is 1.6–2.0 times higher in those with diabetes compared to those who do not have diabetes [15, 16]. However, few studies have used structured clinical interviews to diagnose depressive disorders. The vast majority of studies in this literature rely on screening cutoffs on self-report questionnaires to identify cases of depression. This is a significant limitation of the literature, as a review reported that over 50 % of diabetes patients with positive screens on these instruments will be false-positives [17]. One study using a widely used self-report questionnaire (Center for Epidemiological Studies Depression Scale (CESD)) to screen for depression in adults with type 2 diabetes showed that approximately 70 % of those who screened positive (CESD ≥ 16) did not meet diagnostic criteria for MDD or dysthymia based on a semi-structured interview [18]. Thus, although it is clear that adults with diabetes have significantly increased risk for experiencing clinical depression compared to those without diabetes, prevalence estimates will vary considerably depending on method of assessment. That said, elevations in depressive symptoms may be important even when diagnostic criteria are not met, given the relationships between symptoms of depression that would not meet criteria for a diagnosis and poor diabetes self-management and control [19] (see also: Diabetes-related Distress, below).

Anxiety. Although fewer studies are available, evidence suggests that prevalence of anxiety disorders is also increased among adults with diabetes. A national survey showed the age-adjusted prevalence of lifetime diagnosis of an anxiety disorder was 19.5 % in adults with self-reported, previously diagnosed diabetes and 10.9 % in those without diabetes [20]. Fisher et al. found 85 % higher rates of panic disorder and 123 % higher rates of GAD relative to national estimates, using structured clinical interviews in a sample of adults with type 2 diabetes [21]. International data based on structured clinical interviews suggest that the prevalence of GAD (odds ratio [OR] 1.6), panic disorder (OR 1.5), social phobia (OR 1.3), and PTSD (OR 1.3) is significantly increased among adults diagnosed with diabetes [22].

Eating Disorders. Disordered eating appears to be more prevalent among adolescent females with type 1 diabetes than those without diabetes although few studies are available. A systematic review of studies of females with diabetes compared to nondiabetic controls found that the prevalence of anorexia nervosa was not significantly increased but that bulimia nervosa was significantly more common among those with diabetes (1.73 %) than among controls (0.06 %) [23]. Among people with type 2 diabetes, estimates of the prevalence of binge eating disorder (BED) vary considerably, ranging from 1.4 to 25.6% [24–30]. One study of 3000 primary care patients showed that individuals with diabetes were 2.4 times more likely to have BED than those without diabetes [31]. Due to the small sample sizes of most studies and the variability of methods used to assess binge eating, questions remain about the heterogeneity and generalizability of these estimates. Subclinical presentations, including some disordered eating behaviors or attitudes, are more commoh and may also complicate diabetes management, given the importance of diet in achieving and maintaining glycemic control.

Serious Mental Illness. Bipolar disorder and schizophrenia are each associated with increased risk for development of type 2 diabetes, most likely through exposure to specific psychotropic medications and shared environmental and behavioral risk factors. Estimates from a range of national and international epidemiological studies have shown the prevalence of diabetes in patients with schizophrenia to be 1.5–2.5 times greater than that found in the general population, with the difference particularly striking among younger patients [32, 33]. A study of more than 4000 Veterans Health Administratiori patients with bipolar disorder found the prevalence of diabetes to be over 17% [34].

Diabetes-Related Distress. While the data are clear in showing consistent links between diabetes and psychopathology, especially depressive and anxiety disorders, evidence also emphasizes the importance of non-psychopathological levels of emotional distress stemming from the burdens of living with diabetes and managing its treatment. Measures developed to assess diabetes-related distress have established its independence distress have established its independence from depressive symptoms in predicting diabetes treatment outcomes (e.g., [35]). Data from a multinational study of almost 9000 adults with type 1 or type 2 diabetes showed that across 17 countries, 44.6% expressed significant diabetes-related distress (28% in the USA), as compared with 13.8% of participants who screened positive for depression (19% in the USA) [12].

Data suggest that depressive symptoms and diabetes distress, and not MDD per se, may be particularly enduring. In an 18-month longitudinal study with three assessment points of 508 adults with type 2 diabetes, approximately 11% met criteria for MDD at baseline and 19.8% during at least one visit during the study. Of those who had MDD at one assessment, or wave, 28% continued to meet criteria for MDD at the next; 14% of those with MDD at two waves also met criteria at a third [21]. Elevations in depressive symptoms were more common and much more persistent: 76% of those with elevated depressive symptoms at one wave reported elevations at another, and 77% of these also scored similarly at a third wave. Of those with high diabetes distress at one wave, 50% had high diabetes distress at the second, and 86% of these patients had high diabetes distress at the third wave [21]. Longitudinal data from the Montreal Evaluation of Diabetes Treatment Study of 1691 adults with type 2 diabetes demonstrate a reciprocal relationship between increases in diabetes distress and depressive symptoms over time, suggesting bidirectional [36].

6.2   Treatment of Psychopathology in Diabetes

Too few rigorous treatment studies are available for anxiety, eating disorders or severe mental illness to offer specific recommendations for applications in patients with diabetes. In clinical practice, clinicians should consider the context of diabetes and its management when evaluating and treating psychological conditions in individuals with diabetes. For example, patients with diabetes may experience significant anxiety related to insulin injections [37] or may keep blood glucose levels high due to excessive fear and avoidance of hypoglycemia [38]. Treatment approaches to psychopathology in diabetes should be sensitive to the burdens of illness and treatment and to the chronically stressful nature of diabetes self-management. A more detailed review of the wider treatment literature is available elsewhere [39, 40]. Here, we focus on the treatment of depression and emotional distress in diabetes, two of the most common psychological issues in patients with diabetes. Clinicians should also be aware that individuals who do not meet the diagnostic threshold for major depressive disorder but do experience symptoms of significant emotional distress are also at risk for poorer self-care, glucose control, and health outcomes [18, 41, 42]; thus, subclinical symptoms may warrant treatment.

6.3   Mechanisms Linking Emotional Distress and Depression to Health in Diabetes

Depression and emotional distress may affect diabetes health outcomes through behavioral (treatment nonadherence and self-management) [41] and/or biological pathways (hormonal abnormalities, increased immuno-inflammatory activation, dysregulation of the HPA axis) [43–45]. Previous studies have examined the psychological factors influencing self-management and health outcomes. Patients' beliefs about illness and the utility of treatment show a relationship to health behavior [46]. For instance, a consistent link has been found between greater treatment adherence and both greater belief in one's personal need for treatment and fewer concerns about negative side effects [47]. More symptoms and disease-related burden, perception of less ability to influence or control diabetes, greater diabetes-related consequences, and diabetes-specific emotional distress have each been associated with worse glycemic control [48]. Additionally, significant psychosocial stressors may be more common in individuals with diabetes, including sedentary lifestyle, unemployment, lower socioeconomic status, disparities in access to and quality of healthcare, and experiences of chronic stress [49]. Given the close association between emotional distress, treatment characteristics and diabetes outcomes, the directionality of these relationships is unclear, and more evidence is needed to inform causal models.

6.4   Treatments for Depression in Diabetes

Selective serotonin reuptake inhibitors (SSRIs) are among the safest and most efficacious pharmacological treatment options for patients with diabetes and depression [50, 51] because along with their antidepressant properties, some of them may reduce blood glucose and result in weight loss [52]. For example, fluoxetine may reduce weight and improve glycemic control [53]. Bupropion, a norepinephrine/dopamine reuptake inhibitor, is as effective as SSRIs for depression [54] and also may reduce weight and blood glucose [55]. However, other pharmacological treatments may be contraindicated in individuals with diabetes. Monoamine oxidase inhibitors (MAOIs) can cause weight gain while tricyclic antidepressants (TCAs) can cause hyperglycemia [56]. Furthermore, atypical antipsychotics approved by the FDA for treatment of unipolar depression [57] can result in weight gain [58] and decrease glycemic control in patients with diabetes; they likely also cause glycemic abnormalities among those at risk for diabetes [59].

Various psychological interventions to address clinical and subclinical depression have been investigated in adults with type 2 diabetes [60]. Cognitive Behavioral Therapy (CBT) and related approaches have received the most attention in this research [60]. Most of these treatments have been effective in improving depression and mood-related outcomes, but they often are less successful in affecting diabetes self-management and glycemic control [60]. The treatment of depression and emotional distress in diabetes may be necessary but not sufficient to improve self-management and health outcomes. Thus, integrating cognitive and behavioral strategies to directly target diabetes self-management into therapy approaches may be necessary for behavioral medicine approaches to have maximal impact. In a review of 72 studies examining self-management training, positive results were shown for blood glucose self-monitoring, dietary habits, and glycemic control for short-term (<6 month) interventions [61]. Thus, there is an evidence base on which the psychologist or other behavioral medicine service provider can draw when developing comprehensive approaches to depression and diabetes.

As problem-solving skills are an integral component of diabetes self-management, problem-solving therapy may be a promising intervention approach in the context of diabetes self-management, particularly for distress related to the burden of the treatment regimen [62]. Problem-solving skill building is a core component of diabetes self-management education and overlaps considerably with problem-solving treatment (PST), an evidence-based therapy for preventing and treating depression in a variety of populations [63]. The patient generates strategies to resolve problems, chooses and implements a strategy and examines the effectiveness of this strategy [64]. PST is adaptable and has been used by variety of clinicians (e.g., nurses, diabetes educators, bachelor-level health workers, mental health professionals) through multiple modes of delivery (computer administration, phone, primary care, group support group, peer leaders). For now, the evidence on problem-solving training for improving diabetes outcomes is intriguing but still mixed and subject to methodological issues [65]. In a systematic review of 24 studies that used problem solving for children, adolescent and adult patients with diabetes, only 38 % of studies showed a meaningful improvement in glycemic control; however, studies did tend to have positive effects on a number of psychosocial outcomes [65].

Cognitive Behavioral Therapy for Adherence and Depression (CBT-AD) is an evidence-based, integrative approach to treating depression and improving disease self-management and treatment adherence in the context of chronic illness [66]. CBT-AD has received empirical support in improving depression, diabetes self-management and glycemic control among clinically depressed adults with type 2 diabetes [67] and has also been piloted in individual [68] and group formats with adults with type 1 diabetes [69]. CBT-AD was originally developed for patients with HIV to address both symptoms of depression and treatment adherence and has been demonstrated to have similarly consistent effects on depression severity, treatment adherence, and indicators of disease control in depressed adults treated for HIV/AIDS [70–75].

6.5 Description of CBT-AD for Diabetes

CBT-AD treatment is grounded in the idea that there are cognitive and behavioral connections between depression and problems in the management of diabetes; interventions that improve patients' ability to successfully manage diabetes will result in an improved sense of self-efficacy that will in turn benefit depression. Conversely, cognitive and behavioral changes associated with depression treatment can improve the patient's approach to diabetes self-management and provide tools for coping with challenges. These linkages are made explicitly as part of orientation to treatment. CBT strategies are directly applied to problems with depression and to problems with self-management. CBT-AD consists of six modules (see Table 6.1). The sequence of modules and the number of sessions spent on each module are flexible for tailoring to patient problems though the treatment is intended to be approximately 10–12 sessions in total. Below we provide brief descriptions of each module; the treatment is elaborated in greater detail in the published therapist guide and client workbook [66, 76].

6.6 Psychoeducation and Motivational Interviewing for Behavior Change

In the first module, the therapist and patient review the cognitive behavioral model of depression in the context of diabetes. Together, they apply the model to the patient's unique presentation of symptoms. The aim is to orient the patient to CBT and to promote the patient's understanding of this approach to treat depression and improve diabetes self-management. The therapist and patient discuss the cycle of

Table 6.1 CBT modules and recommendations for specific patient problems

MODULE	Strategies	Recommendations	Goals
Psychoeducation and motivation interviewing for behavior change	Introduce the cognitive behavioral model of depression in context of diabetes	For the patient with depression	Help patients to understand reasons for participating in treatment
	Pros and cons of change	For the patient who has difficulty motivating themselves to change	Discuss potential difficulties with treatment, address ambivalence
			Generate patient's personal reasons for change
Life-steps	AIM framework	General module for all patients	Provide information about importance of medication adherence
	Articulate goals		Reduce burden of self-management, discuss potential barriers, and make a plan
	Identify potential barriers		Spark patient's interest about effects of behavior change
	Make a plan and back-up plan		
Activity scheduling	Behavioral activation	For the patient who experiences a lack of pleasurable activities	Help patient to evaluate role of behavioral avoidance with attention to role of diabetes self-management
		For the patient who uses diabetes as avoidance	Help patient generate list of pleasurable activities
			Help patient to reinforce skills through activity, mood, and blood glucose records
Adaptive thinking	Cognitive restructuring	For the patient who struggles with diabetes distress	Help patient endorse more balanced thinking related to self-blame, labeling, and black and white thinking
		For the patient with realistic negative thoughts that can't be problem solved	Implement use of thought record to identify negative automatic thoughts
Problem solving	Articulate problem	For the patient who has trouble managing the day-to-day tasks of self-care	Help patient to identify and elaborate on problems related to self-management
	Set a goal		Help patient to implement and assess strategies
	Brainstorm solutions		Rehearse skills learned in this session in future sessions
	Weigh pros and cons		
	Rate solutions		
	Develop a plan		
	Review and evaluate		
Relaxation training	Diaphragmatic breathing	For the patient interested in helping to manage physical symptoms, ease pain or help with sleep	Assist patient in learning relaxation techniques
	Slowed breathing		Help patient to manage physical symptoms (i.e., ease distress associated with medical procedures)
	Progressive muscle relaxation		Rehearse relaxation skills in future sessions

depression, in which thoughts, behaviors, emotions, and physiological symptoms interact to worsen mood, functioning, and self-care, thereby influencing quality of life and physical health.

The therapist uses elements of a motivational interviewing (MI) intervention focused on making changes for depression and diabetes self-care. MI, developed by Miller and Rollnick [77], has been used as a stand-alone treatment approach in diabetes [78]. In CBT-AD, the therapist uses MI to strengthen the patient's own internal motivation to change and to practice the skills learned in future modules. Pros and cons of change are examined, and the therapist assists the patient in articulating personal reasons and goals for change.

6.7 Life-Steps

The second module, Life-Steps, consists of a single session designed to address medication adherence. As a stand-alone intervention, Life-Steps has received support in improving medication adherence in HIV [79] and has been adapted for use in diabetes. Life-Steps identifies 11 informational, problem-solving, and cognitive behavioral steps, using the AIM framework to teach patients to Articulate goals, Identify potential barriers, and Make a plan and a back-up plan at each stage.

The first step is to provide education about the critical role of medication adherence in diabetes. Patients then articulate one to four goals for adherence, several potential barriers, and a plan and backup plan for increasing adherence. The therapist emphasizes that large problems can be broken down into a series of smaller tasks.

In subsequent steps, the therapist introduces problem-solving and rehearsal techniques to address such issues as getting to medical appointments, communicating with healthcare providers, coping with side effects of medications, storing medications, implementing cues for taking medications, managing slips in adherence and preventing relapse. The AIM method helps the patient and therapist begin to explore depression and distress-related factors affecting diabetes self-care. Self-monitoring and interpretation of feedback from blood glucose are reviewed in an attempt to increase the patient's curiosity about the potential effects of behavioral change and to provide a means for observing short-term effects of his or her efforts at behavior change. Rather than identifying good vs. bad behaviors or good vs. bad glucose values, the therapist models curiosity about the factors that may influence fluctuations in glucose values in a way that will parallel the examination of fluctuations in mood, medication adherence, and self-care behaviors. Maladaptive cognitive distortions (e.g., labeling, black and white thinking) are also identified as common barriers to success. The therapist reinforces these steps by reviewing the plans using guided imagery and role-plays, creating a follow-up plan and checking in with the patient at the next session to obtain feedback and further refine the plan.

6.8   Activity Scheduling

Behavioral activation is key in addressing the lack of pleasurable activities and events experienced by individuals with depression. The therapist should evaluate the presence of any health impairments or diabetes-related complications (e.g., retinopathy, neuropathy) that might require attention in adapting activation plans. Evaluation of the role that diabetes may play in behavioral avoidance is also necessary. For example, patients may avoid going out to eat at restaurants or attending family get-togethers because they feel they cannot eat healthfully in these situations. Finally, the therapist should also take opportunities to integrate diabetes self-management in delivering the rationale for this skill and in developing and evaluating activity schedules. For example, there is an important parallel between the rationales for self-monitoring of blood glucose and mood. A similar mindset is useful for each: Evaluate the feedback with curiosity and a desire to be informed, rather than with self-criticism and labeling. Identifying environmental and behavioral factors that are associated with fluctuations in feedback informs the development of effective activation plans. Activities that provide opportunities for positive mood states and also lower blood glucose (e.g., exercise, walking, hiking) deserve prioritization. This module is usually introduced in one session, with subsequent sessions reinforcing skills through review of activity, mood and blood glucose records.

In the first session, the patient lists activities that he or she used to enjoy but has stopped doing since becoming depressed. The therapist encourages the patient to identify what was pleasurable about these activities, whether it is possible to reincorporate these activities back into his or her life, and how he or she could resume the activities. Using a list of pleasurable events [80], the therapist and patient highlight potentially enjoyable activities. Patients are asked to participate in two enjoyable activities over the next week and to monitor the influence of behavior on mood.

6.9   Adaptive Thinking

The adaptive thinking module is designed to last approximately five sessions and is typically introduced after activity scheduling. An understanding of the often stressful context of diabetes—the demands of self-management, changes in functioning associated with complications, the threat of hypoglycemia and fear of death—is important for tailoring this module. These individuals often have negative beliefs about themselves related to common cognitive distortions, such as labeling, self-blame, black and white thinking, and "should statements." They may also have unrealistic expectations for the changes required for successful self-management. Alternatively, some patients are fatalistic about their ability to influence the course of their diabetes and may express hopelessness, sometimes masked by denial and avoidance. Evaluating the evidence for these thoughts and their effects on mood and diabetes self-management is an important part of the integrative approach to depression and diabetes-related distress.

After introducing a list of cognitive distortions and providing examples for each, the patient is asked to generate examples from his/her own life. Thought records are used to track stressful situations and build skills in identifying automatic thoughts and challenging distortions. The therapist encourages the patient to think about "*what was going through your mind?*" during periods of low mood. Such negative beliefs frequently lead to maladaptive coping such as avoidance, feelings of helplessness and hopelessness, and poor adherence to self-care activities. Throughout the next few sessions, the patient learns to recognize that a negative mood can be a "red flag" or cue for an unbalanced or distorted thought. Restructuring an automatic thought involves changing thinking patterns and beliefs, using evidence-based strategies for cognitive therapy for depression [81, 82].

6.10 Problem Solving

Diabetes requires the patient to take an active role in managing the day-to-day tasks of self-care, which can conflict with other goals and compete for attention and motivational resources. Problem solving involves a series of steps to effectively address problems related to depression and diabetes self-management [83].

Similar to PST in Primary Care, the CBT-AD problem-solving module reviews the following steps: (1) articulate a clear description of a problem on which to work, (2) set a clear and achievable goal, (3) brainstorm as many solutions as possible (i.e., don't rule anything out), (4) consider the advantages and disadvantages of each solution, including the option of making no change, (5) rate the solutions and chose the best option in terms of time, effort, money, and effects on other people, (6) develop an action plan in which the patient describes step-by-step *what* he/she will do and *when* he/she will do it, and (7) review and evaluate progress throughout the remaining sessions. Problem solving is flexible and should be used for a variety of diabetes self-management challenges.

6.11 Relaxation Training

Relaxation training and breathing retraining are widely used in behavioral medicine interventions to teach patients to relax during times of stress, ease muscle tension and manage physical symptoms such as headache, pain, and nausea [84–86]. The module has been adapted for diabetes to help manage physical symptoms (e.g., pain, side-effects of medication) and to help with disturbed sleep. This module is usually completed in one session but rehearsed in other sessions, as appropriate.

Patients learn to distinguish between chest breathing and diaphragmatic breathing. Similarly, the therapist also provides training and opportunities for modeling and practice with progressive muscle relaxation [87, 88]. As part of the session's homework, participants are to practice daily and record their level of tension before and after each exercise for review in the next session.

6.12   Assessment and Monitoring

6.12.1   Psychological Symptoms

Careful assessment of the psychological symptoms and the behavioral and cognitive mechanisms that maintain them is a foundation of CBT-AD (see Table 6.2). It is crucial to be attuned to how diabetes-related distress may influence depressive symptoms (and vice versa) in order to conceptualize the patient's clinical presentation and treatment plan [89, 90]. Comprehensive and consistent assessment of depression severity, medication adherence, and blood glucose values is an integral part of CBT-AD.

   Depression: A structured clinical interview is recommended for diagnosing depression or identifying subthreshold symptoms in diabetes. Clinician-rated scales such as the 10-item Montgomery-Åsberg Depression Rating Scale (MADRS) may serve as supplemental tools for systematic symptom measurement throughout treatment, though they do not replace a diagnostic interview.

   Diabetes-Related Distress. There are a number of measures that are commonly used to assess diabetes-related distress and the perception of problem severity, such as the patient-rated Diabetes Distress Scale (DDS) [35]. Participants rate their experienced distress across four domains: the emotional burden of diabetes, physician-related distress, regimen-related distress, and interpersonal distress [35, 91, 92].

6.12.2   Diabetes Treatment Adherence and Self-Management

Behaviors: One scale that can be used to measure diabetes self-management behaviors in the past 1–2 months is the 15-item Self-Care Inventory-Revised (SCI-R) (e.g., "check blood glucose with monitor" and "exercise") [93, 94] with higher scores indicating better self-care. The measure has been validated in samples of patients with type 1 and type 2 diabetes [93, 94]; however, not all items are relevant to patients with type 2 diabetes [95].

   Medication Adherence: In the efficacy trial for CBT-AD in diabetes, medication adherence was assessed using electronic pill caps. If electronic monitors are not available, clinicians should use validated self-reports, with the understanding that these reports may inflate true adherence and are subject to reporting biases [96, 97]. Additionally, clinicians may review blood glucose records from meter downloads or diaries; other technologies may also be incorporated (continuous blood glucose monitoring, apps that link changes in blood glucose to behavior) [98].

   Biological Markers. Finally, we recommend that clinicians be aware of their patient's glycemic control when beginning treatment. HbA1c (glycosylated hemoglobin) is a blood test that measures blood glucose control over approximately 2–3 months. Evidence suggests a link between glycemic control and developing future complications [14].

Table 6.2 Assessment measures

Measure	Variable	Description
Montgomery-Åsberg Depression Rating Scale MADRS [107]	Depression severity	10-item clinician-rated depression severity structured clinical interview: apparent sadness, reported sadness, inner tension, reduced sleep, reduced appetite, concentration difficulties, lassitude, inability to feel, pessimistic thoughts, suicidal thoughts
Diabetes Distress Scale—DSS [35]	Diabetes-related distress	Self-report questionnaire that measures four aspects of diabetes-related distress: emotional burden, physician-related distress, regiment-related distress and interpersonal distress
		Also available as a brief screening instrument [21, 91]
Self-care inventory-revised [93]	Diabetes self-care behaviors	15-item self-report questionnaire that measures behaviors specific to diabetes self-management including checking blood glucose levels with monitor, eating correct food portions, exercise, going to clinic for medical appointments
Medication Adherence Questionnaires [99]	Medication adherence	Self-report questionnaire measures that assess diabetes medication/insulin adherence within the last 30 days (including days missed at least one dose, how good of a job taking medicines the way supposed to, how often taken medication the way supposed to)
Biological markers	HbA1c (glycosylated hemoglobin)	A blood test that measures average blood glucose over the last 2–3 months, which has been linked to the risk of developing future complications

6.13   Case Illustration

Robert was a married, college-educated and self-employed, non-Hispanic White male in his early 40s with a baseline HbA1c of 12 % and a BMI of 41.9. Diagnostic interview indicated that he met criteria for major depressive disorder—current, recurrent, and dysthymia (Clinical Global Impression of 5; markedly ill) with an MADRS of 27 (moderate depression). He also met diagnostic criteria for panic disorder with agoraphobia and obsessive-compulsive disorder (obsessions only). Robert reported taking three oral medications for diabetes and no psychiatric medications. Baseline medication adherence data from electronic monitoring caps (MEMS) indicated that he took approximately 57 % of his prescribed doses for one of his oral diabetes medications, and adherence to nurse-recommended frequency of self-monitoring of blood glucose was 0 %, based on downloaded data from his glucometer. Robert was diagnosed with diabetes 2 years before study enrollment.

Conceptualization. Robert reported a number of maladaptive cognitions about diabetes including self-blame about his inability to have enough "willpower" to control his dietary choices or to be consistent with glucose monitoring and medications. Robert viewed attempts at better self-care as unlikely to be enough to make an appreciable change in diabetes outcome (e.g., all-or-nothing thinking). He was also quite resistant to beginning insulin therapy, despite considerable efforts from his providers to convince him that insulin therapy would be necessary to achieve a lower HbA1c. He reported that he did not have confidence in his ability to manage insulin self-administration, feared becoming hypoglycemic and had concerns that the injections would be painful and leave marks on his skin. Frustration with frequently high blood sugar readings had led to an avoidance of blood glucose self-monitoring. These patterns of avoidance were supported by beliefs that there was nothing he could do to make a difference anyway. Intermediate beliefs and automatic thoughts related to viewing himself as fundamentally incompetent and believing that anything less than perfect was inadequate were paralleled by similar distortions relating to Robert's relationship with his wife, which had deteriorated over the last years. He reported significant distress and rumination about dissatisfaction with their sexual and emotional relationship. Finally, stressors related to his business were also prominent in Robert's depression. A similar pattern of all-or-nothing thinking about his performance led to self-criticism, negative affect, and behavioral avoidance. While the use of avoidance led to short term but significant reductions in anxiety and distress, the longer term effects included worsening of depression and diabetes control.

Treatment. CBT-AD sessions began with a review of monitoring data on blood glucose values, depression symptom severity scores and medication adherence. Robert's depression severity was quite marked when he began treatment. He had been mostly disengaged from diabetes self-management, although he was trying to avoid sweets based on his understanding that sugary foods were the most important dietary factor to consider in the management of blood glucose. He was also doing other things that he thought were healthy for diabetes management but that in fact were significant contributors to weight gain and high blood sugars. For example, he reported drinking one gallon of whole milk each day as he thought that milk was natural and low in sugar, as compared to the sodas he drank prior to his diagnosis.

Reviewing the importance of diabetes self-management and the goals of treatment in the Life-Steps was an important part of enhancing motivation for change. The therapist also began to identify barriers to self-management from the perspective of the CBT model. Fear of complications was a major part of Robert's diabetes-related distress. However, he acknowledged that he viewed self-management as a burden that demanded more discipline than he had. The behavioral consequences of these thoughts and beliefs (e.g., avoiding self-care, forgetting to take medications) were identified as important targets of CBT-AD. Black and white thinking was challenged in this first session through an interactive discussion about the implications of results from Diabetes Control and Complications Trial and the UK Prospective Diabetes Study about the benefits of a 1-point reduction in HbA1c in reduced risk of developing complications [5, 100]. Rather than talking about good or bad glycemic control, the therapist and Robert agreed to think about a continuum of change. Psychoeducation also emphasized the message that factors outside of one's control influence glycemic control—even patients who are effective in self-management often have to change medications as diabetes progresses. Beliefs about insulin as representing failure were questioned in light of this new information.

Organizing Robert's symptoms of depression into a graphical representation of the relationships among cognitive, emotional, and behavioral aspects was important in orienting Robert to CBT-AD as a structured, skill-based approach to depression and diabetes self-management. Relating symptoms to the context of diabetes self-management supported a rationale for targeting depression and diabetes self-management in each session. Beliefs about insulin therapy and the burdens of diabetes self-management identified in Life-Steps were also incorporated into this model, which was described as representing a vicious cycle of negative thinking, distress, and avoidance that required making active efforts to change. Modules of CBT-AD that target each aspect of this cycle were briefly reviewed. Through an examination of the pros and cons of change, Robert noted that though there would be short-term negative consequences to engaging in the treatment in terms of time, work, and exposure to uncomfortable emotions and thoughts, these cons were offset by major positive consequences for his long-term health and quality of life. Robert was particularly motivated to avoid or at least delay the development of diabetes complications that would limit his functioning, such as blindness and kidney failure. Robert was interested in learning more about insulin therapy and how it had changed since he observed a grandparent self-inject when he was a child.

Based on this conceptualization, treatment was focused primarily on cognitive restructuring and on behavior change that would decrease the use of avoidance and secondarily on providing corrective feedback for distorted cognitions related to depression and diabetes self-management. Problem-solving skills were applied to improve the likelihood that Robert would choose approach-oriented coping responses when facing stressful circumstances related to his diabetes or other life stressors. Examination of feedback—about mood and glucose values—in the context of environmental situations and health behaviors was used test beliefs in each session. Problem-solving steps were applied directly to situations in which feedback indicated that goals were not being reached or when the feedback was confusing. Examples of feedback included data from blood glucose meter downloads, a calendar of missed doses of medication identified by electronic monitoring, and daily mood ratings. The rationale for relaxation training was similarly based on the observation that Robert's tension ratings decreased from pre- to post-practice.

Over time, Robert became interested in the interpretation of this feedback and became more consistent in recording his mood and activities and testing his blood sugars. As patterns emerged, he became motivated to better understand the factors contributing to his blood glucose. Behavioral experiments were applied as a tool for cognitive restructuring. For example, the belief that "nothing I do will make a difference" could be tested by committing to several days of more intensive physical activity and then comparing blood glucose and mood values to days when he was less physically active. Making a plan to talk with his wife about how to improve the quality of their time together could test the same belief. Cognitive restructuring and problem-solving steps were applied for various life stressors, with decreasing direction from the therapist over time, as Robert became more proficient in applying skills.

In consultation with a dietitian from our multidisciplinary team, Robert tested the effect of replacing his whole milk, first with low-fat milk, then skim and finally a non-sweetened beverage or water. Similarly, Robert tested the effect of his favorite restaurant meal and was surprised to learn that his blood glucose was over 450 mg/dL 2 h later. Still, Robert observed that his overall pattern was one of consistently high blood glucose values, even when fasting. Although he was motivated by the feedback associated with these dietary and physical activity changes, he also began to accept that insulin might be required to reduce his blood sugars further. He spoke with his provider and began taking insulin about one-third of the way through the program. After he began insulin, with the attitude that this too was an experiment and not necessarily a commitment, he began to notice dramatic improvements in his blood glucose with no significant hypoglycemia and with only minimal discomfort.

Outcomes. Robert improved on all measures of adherence and depression between baseline and post-treatment assessment and agreed to begin insulin therapy, which he had refused in the past. His acceptance of insulin therapy was directly related to cognitive restructuring to challenge maladaptive beliefs about the risks of and the meaning associated with taking insulin (e.g., "If I have to take insulin, that means I failed at managing my diabetes on my own"). He experienced a striking decrease in HbA1c, most likely due to beginning and remaining adherent to insulin therapy. His depression improvements were similarly clinically significant. Self-reported frequency of diabetes self-management behaviors showed improvement in all components of self-care. Glucose self-monitoring was consistent with recommendations at post-treatment and medication adherence had improved, although he continued to miss doses occasionally (see Table 6.3).

Summary. Although this patient achieved improvements that were more dramatic than the average participant in the CBT-AD trial, the domains in which significant improvements were achieved—depression severity, medication adherence, glucose self-monitoring and HbA1c—were each significantly affected by CBT-AD in the efficacy trial [67]. Still, therapists should not expect such large reductions in HbA1c to result from modest health behavior changes. Rather than focus on the application of core skills of CBT, this case was meant to emphasize the importance of systematic collection and interpretation of feedback for behavior change and cognitive restructuring applied to diabetes-related and non-diabetes-related stressors. A further unique element is the equal weight given to diabetes management and the management of depression as targets of the intervention.

Finally, it is important to note that effects of CBT-AD were achieved with a multidisciplinary team of nurse educators, dietitians, and psychotherapists working collaboratively. The expertise of the therapist in understanding the pathophysiology of diabetes and the goals of its treatment and self-management is a final important consideration when adapting CBT-AD for application in real-world clinical settings, where such a multidisciplinary approach may be challenging to implement.

6.14   Future Directions

Cognitive-behavioral approaches for patients with subclinical distress and diabetes continue to be piloted and adapted in other formats. For instance, DIAMOS, a cognitive-behavioral approach was delivered in a group format for patients with subclinical depression; this intervention showed promising results in reducing diabetes-related distress and the likelihood of developing future depression [101]. Furthermore, we have modified CBT-AD as a telephonic intervention for patients with poorly controlled diabetes through collaboration with the New York City Department of Health (ClinicalTrials.gov identifier: NCT02137720).

At the same time, work is continuing on the development of other psychological interventions that might hold promise for improving psychological well-being and diabetes outcomes. For example, the REDEEM trial found reductions in diabetes-related distress and improvements in self-management behaviors with three computer-assisted interventions (self-management, self-management with problem solving, and supportive intervention) [62]. In the DYNAMIC trial, which used nurse care managers trained in motivational interviewing to work with high-risk patients with type 2 diabetes, intervention patients experienced greater improvements in depressive symptoms [102, 103]. Other researchers have proposed studying a combination of problem-solving treatment and motivational interviewing [104], positive psychology [105], and family or community interventions [106]. The next generation of psychological intervention studies in diabetes will need to attend to issues of sustainability and reach in order to have the widest impact on the growing number of patients who could benefit from intervention.

Table 6.3   Robert's results

		Pre	Post
Diabetes measures	HbA1c	12.0	7.7
	MEMS (%)	57	71
	Glucose monitoring	0	100
Depression	MADRS	27	5
	CGI	5	2
	BDI	22	6
Diabetes self-care activities	General diet	0	6.5
	Specific diet	2.3	6
	Exercise	0	7
	BG testing	0	7
	Foot care	2.8	5.6
	Activities	4	5

Note: MEMS and Glucose Monitoring figures refer to % of prescribed medication taken and glucose tests completed over the past week. All data in this table represent the mean number of days per week that the patient was adherent to each type of diabetes self-care activity based on a standardized questionnaire

References

1. Menke A, Casagrande S, Geiss L, Cowie CC. Prevalence of and trends in diabetes among adults in the United States, 1988–2012. JAMA. 2015;314:1021–9. doi:10.1001/jama.2015.10029.
2. Glasgow RE, Boles SM, McKay HG, et al. The D-Net diabetes self-management program: long-term implementation, outcomes, and generalization results. Prev Med. 2003;36:410–9. doi:10.1016/S0091-7435(02)00056-7.
3. Newman S, Steed L, Mulligan K. Self-management interventions for chronic illness. Lancet. 2004;364:1523–37.
4. U.S. Centers for Disease Control and Prevention. National diabetes fact sheet: national estimates and general information on diabetes and prediabetes in the United States, 2011. US Dep Heal Hum Serv Centers Dis Control Prev. 2011;3:1–12.
5. Diabetes Control and Complications Trial Research Group. Effect of intensive diabetes management on macrovascular events and risk factors in the diabetes control and complications trial. Am J Cardiol. 1995;75:894–903. doi:10.1016/S0002-9149(99)80683-3.
6. Stratton IM, Adler AI, Neil HAW, et al. Association of glycaemia with macrovascular and microvascular complications of type 2 diabetes (UKPDS 35): prospective observational study. Br Med J. 2000;321:405–12.
7. American Diabetes Association. Standards of medical care in diabetes-2015. Diabetes Care. 2015;38:S1–94.
8. Feldman BS, Cohen-Stavi CJ, Leibowitz M, et al. Defining the role of medication adherence in poor glycemic control among a general adult population with diabetes. PLoS One. 2014;9:e108145.
9. Hood KK, Peterson CM, Rohan JM, Drotar D. Association between adherence and glycemic control in pediatric type 1 diabetes: a meta-analysis. Pediatrics. 2009;124:e1171–9. doi:10.1542/peds.2009-0207.
10. Ho PM, Rumsfeld JS, Masoudi FA, et al. Effect of medication nonadherence on hospitalization and mortality among patients with diabetes mellitus. Arch Intern Med. 2006;166:1836–41. doi:10.1001/archinte.166.17.1836.
11. DiMatteo MR. Variations in patients' adherence to medical recommendations: a quantitative review of 50 Years of research. Med Care. 2004;42:200–9. doi:10.1097/01.mlr.0000114908.90348.f9.
12. Nicolucci A, Kovacs Burns K, Holt RIG, et al. Diabetes attitudes, wishes and needs second study (DAWN2TM): cross-national benchmarking of diabetes-related psychosocial outcomes for people with diabetes. Diabet Med. 2013;30:767–77. doi:10.1111/dme.12245.
13. Russell LB, Dong-Churl S, Safford MA. Time requirements for diabetes self-management: too much for many? J Fam Pract. 2005;54:52–6.
14. Casagrande SS, Fradkin JE, Saydah SH, et al. The prevalence of meeting A1C, blood pressure, and LDL goals among people with diabetes, 1988–2010. Diabetes Care. 2013;36:2271–9. doi:10.2337/dc12-2258.
15. Anderson RJ, Freedland KE, Clouse RE, Lustman PJ. The prevalence of comorbid depression in adults with diabetes. Diabetes Care. 2001;24:1069–78. doi:10.2337/diacare.24.6.1069.
16. Ali S, Stone MA, Peters JL, et al. The prevalence of co-morbid depression in adults with type 2 diabetes: a systematic review and meta-analysis. Diabet Med. 2006;23:1165–73. doi:10.1111/j.1464-5491.2006.01943.x.
17. Roy T, Lloyd CE, Pouwer F, et al. Screening tools used for measuring depression among people with Type 1 and Type 2 diabetes: a systematic review. Diabet Med. 2012;29:164–75. doi:10.1111/j.1464-5491.2011.03401.x.
18. Fisher L, Skaff MM, Mullan JT, et al. Clinical depression versus distress among patients with type 2 diabetes. Diabetes Care. 2007;30:542–8. doi:10.2337/dc06-1614.

19. Gonzalez JS, Safren SA, Cagliero E, et al. Depression, self-care, and medication adherence in type 2 diabetes: relationships across the full range of symptom severity. Diabetes Care. 2007;30:2222–7. doi:10.2337/dc07-0158.
20. Li C, Barker L, Ford ES, et al. Diabetes and anxiety in US adults: findings from the 2006 behavioral risk factor surveillance system. Diabet Med. 2008;25:878–81. doi:10.1111/j.1464-5491.2008.02477.x.
21. Fisher L, Skaff MM, Mullan JT, et al. A longitudinal study of affective and anxiety disorders, depressive affect and diabetes distress in adults with type 2 diabetes. Diabet Med. 2008;25:1096–101. doi:10.1111/j.1464-5491.2008.02533.x.
22. Lin EHB, Von Korff M, Alonso J, et al. Mental disorders among persons with diabetes— results from the World Mental Health Surveys. J Psychosom Res. 2008;65:571–80. doi:10.1016/j.jpsychores.2008.06.007.
23. Jones JM, Lawson ML, Daneman D, et al. Eating disorders in adolescent females with and without type 1 diabetes: cross sectional study. BMJ. 2000;320:1563–6. doi:10.1136/bmj.320.7249.1563.
24. Papelbaum M, Appolinário J, Moreira R, et al. Prevalence of eating disorders and psychiatric comorbidity in a clinical sample of type 2 diabetes mellitus patients. Rev Bras Psiquiatr. 2005;27:135–8.
25. Hudson J, Hiripi E, Pope HJ, Kessler R. The prevalence and correlates of eating disorders in the National Comorbidity Survey Replication. Biol Psychiatry. 2007;61:348–58. doi:10.1016/j.biopsych.2006.03.040.
26. Herpertz S, Albus C, Wagener R, et al. Comorbidity of diabetes and eating disorders: does diabetes control reflect disturbed eating behavior? Diabetes Care. 1998;21:1110–6. doi:10.2337/diacare.21.7.1110.
27. Crow S, Kendall D, Praus B, Thuras P. Binge eating and other psychopathology in patients with type II diabetes mellitus. Int J Eat Disord. 2001;30:222–6.
28. Mannucci E, Tesi F, Ricca V, et al. Eating behavior in obese patients with and without type 2 diabetes mellitus. Int J Obes Relat Metab Disord. 2002;26:848–53. doi:10.1038/sj.ijo.0801976.
29. Carroll P, Tiggemann M, Wade T. The role of body dissatisfaction and bingeing in the self-esteem of women with type II diabetes. J Behav Med. 1999;22:59–74. doi:10.1023/A:1018799618864.
30. Allison K, Crow S, Reeves R, et al. Binge eating disorder and night eating syndrome in adults with type 2 diabetes. Obesity (Silver Spring). 2007;15:1287–93.
31. Goodwin RD, Hoven CW, Spitzer RL. Diabetes and eating disorders in primary care. Int J Eat Disord. 2003;33:85–91.
32. Rouillon F, Sorbara F. Schizophrenia and diabetes: epidemiological data. Eur Psychiatry. 2005;20 Suppl 4:S345–8. doi:10.1016/S0924-9338(05)80189-0.
33. Schoepf D, Potluri R, Uppal H, et al. Type-2 diabetes mellitus in schizophrenia: Increased prevalence and major risk factor of excess mortality in a naturalistic 7-year follow-up. Eur Psychiatry. 2012;27:33–42. doi:10.1016/j.eurpsy.2011.02.009.
34. Kilbourne AM, Cornelius JR, Han X, et al. Burden of general medical conditions among individuals with bipolar disorder. Bipolar Disord. 2004;6:368–73. doi:10.1111/j.1399-5618.2004.00138.x.
35. Polonsky WH, Fisher L, Earles J, et al. Assessing psychosocial distress in diabetes: development of the diabetes distress scale. Diabetes Care. 2005;28:626–31.
36. Deschês SS, Burns RJ, Schmitz N. Associations between diabetes, major depressive disorder and generalized anxiety disorder comorbidity, and disability: findings from the 2012 Canadian Community Health Survey-Mental Health (CCHS-MH). J Psychosom Res. 2015;78:137–42.
37. Mollema ED, Snoek FJ, Heine RJ, Van Der Ploeg HM. Phobia of self-injecting and self-testing in insulin-treated diabetes patients: opportunities for screening. Diabet Med. 2001;18:671–4. doi:10.1046/j.1464-5491.2001.00547.x.

38. Weinger K, Lee J. Psychosocial and psychiatric challenges of diabetes mellitus. Nurs Clin North Am. 2006;41:667–80. doi:10.1016/j.cnur.2006.07.002.
39. Gonzalez JS, Esbitt SA, Schneider HE, et al. Psychological issues in adults with type 2 diabetes. Psychological co-morbidities of physical illness. New York: Springer; 2011. p. 73–121.
40. Gonzalez JS, Hood KK, Esbitt SA, et al. Psychiatric and psychosocial issues among individuals living with diabetes. Diabetes in America. 2nd ed. NIDDK; in press.
41. Gonzalez JS, Peyrot M, McCarl LA, et al. Depression and diabetes treatment nonadherence: a meta-analysis. Diabetes Care. 2008;31:2398–403. doi:10.2337/dc08-1341.
42. Aikens JE. Prospective associations between emotional distress and poor outcomes in type 2 diabetes. Diabetes Care. 2012;35:2472–8. doi:10.2337/dc12-0181.
43. Tsigos C, Chrousos GP. Hypothalamic-pituitary-adrenal axis, neuroendocrine factors and stress. J Psychosom Res. 2002;53(4):865–71.
44. Zanoveli JM, de Morais H, de Silva Dias IC, et al. Depression associated with diabetes: from pathophysiology to treatment. Curr Diabetes Rev. 2015;11:1–11.
45. Stetler C, Miller GE. Depression and hypothalamic-pituitary-adrenal activation: a quantitative summary of four decades of research. Psychosom Med. 2011;73:114–26.
46. Leventhal H, Leventhal EA, Contrada RJ. Self-regulation, health, and behavior: a perceptual-cognitive approach. Psychol Health. 1998;13:717–33. doi:10.1080/08870449808407425.
47. Horne R, Chapman SCE, Parham R, et al. Understanding patients' adherence-related beliefs about medicines prescribed for long-term conditions: a meta-analytic review of the Necessity-Concerns Framework. PLoS One. 2013;8(12):e80633. doi:10.1371/journal.pone.0080633.
48. Mc Sharry J, Moss-Morris R, Kendrick T. Illness perceptions and glycaemic control in diabetes: a systematic review with meta-analysis. Diabet Med. 2011;28:1300–10. doi:10.1111/j.1464-5491.2011.03298.x.
49. Brown AF, Ettner SL, Piette J, et al. Socioeconomic position and health among persons with diabetes mellitus: a conceptual framework and review of the literature. Epidemiol Rev. 2004;26:63–77. doi:10.1093/epirev/mxh002.
50. Sclar DA, Robison LM, Skaer TL, Galin RS. Trends in the prescribing of antidepressant pharmacotherapy: office-based visits, 1990–1995. Clin Ther. 1998;20:871–84. doi:10.1016/S0149-2918(98)80148-3.
51. MacGillivray S, Arroll B, Hatcher S, et al. Efficacy and tolerability of selective serotonin reuptake inhibitors compared with tricyclic antidepressants in depression treated in primary care: systematic review and meta-analysis. BMJ. 2003;326:1014. doi:10.1136/bmj.326.7397.1014.
52. Goodnick PJ, Henry JH, Buki VM. Treatment of depression in patients with diabetes mellitus. J Clin Psychiatry. 1995;56:128–36.
53. Ye Z, Chen L, Yang Z, et al. Metabolic effects of fluoxetine in adults with type 2 diabetes mellitus: a meta-analysis of randomized placebo-controlled trials. PLoS One. 2011;6(7):e21551. doi:10.1371/journal.pone.0021551.
54. Thase ME, Haight BR, Richard N, et al. Remission rates following antidepressant therapy with bupropion or selective serotonin reuptake inhibitors: a meta-analysis of original data from 7 randomized controlled trials. J Clin Psychiatry. 2005;66:974–81.
55. Lustman PJ, Williams MM, Sayuk GS, Nix BD, Clouse RE. Factors influencing glycemic control in type 2 diabetes during acute-and maintenance-phase treatment of major depressive disorder with bupropion. Diabetes Care. 2007;30(3):459–66.
56. Goodnick P. Use of antidepressants in treatment of comorbid diabetes mellitus and depression as well as in diabetic neuropathy. Ann Clin Psychiatry. 2001;13:31–4.
57. Philip NS, Carpenter LL, Tyrka AR, Price LH. Augmentation of antidepressants with atypical antipsychotics: a review of the current literature. J Psychiatr Pract. 2008;14:34–44. doi:10.1097/01.pra.0000308493.93003.92.
58. Lett TAP, Wallace TJM, Chowdhury NI, et al. Pharmacogenetics of antipsychotic-induced weight gain: review and clinical implications. Mol Psychiatry. 2012;17:242–66. doi:10.1038/mp.2011.109.
59. Haddad PM, Sharma SG. Adverse effects of atypical antipsychotics: differential risk and clinical implications. CNS Drugs. 2007;21:911–36. doi: 21114 [pii].

60. Markowitz SM, Gonzalez JS, Wilkinson JL, Safren SA. A review of treating depression in diabetes: emerging findings. Psychosomatics. 2011;52:1–18. doi:10.1016/j.psym.2010.11.007.
61. Norris SL, Engelgau MM, Narayan KM. Effectiveness of self-management training in type 2 diabetes: a systematic review of randomized controlled trials. Diabetes Care. 2001;24:561–87. doi:10.2337/diacare.24.3.561.
62. Fisher L, Hessler D, Glasgow RE, et al. REDEEM: a pragmatic trial to reduce diabetes distress. Diabetes Care. 2013;36:2551–8. doi:10.2337/dc12-2493.
63. Bell AC, D'Zurilla TJ. Problem-solving therapy for depression: a meta-analysis. Clin Psychol Rev. 2009;29:348–53. doi:10.1016/j.cpr.2009.02.003.
64. Hill-Briggs F, Gemmell L. Problem solving in diabetes self-management and control: a systematic review of the literature. Diabetes Educ. 2007;33:1032–50. doi:10.1177/0145721707308412; discussion 1051–2.
65. Fitzpatrick SL, Schumann KP, Hill-Briggs F. Problem solving interventions for diabetes self-management and control: a systematic review of the literature. Diabetes Res Clin Pract. 2013;100:145–61. doi:10.1016/j.diabres.2012.12.016.
66. Safren SA, Gonzalez JS, Soroudi N. Coping with chronic illness, therapist guide. New York: Oxford University Press; 2007.
67. Safren SA, Gonzalez JS, Wexler DJ, et al. A randomized controlled trial of cognitive behavioral therapy for adherence and depression (CBT-AD) in patients with uncontrolled type 2 diabetes. Diabetes Care. 2014;37:625–33. doi:10.2337/dc13-0816.
68. Markowitz SM, Carper MM, Gonzalez JS, Delahanty LM, Safren SA. Cognitive-behavioral therapy for the treatment of depression and adherence in patients with type 1 diabetes: pilot data and feasibility. Prim Care Companion CNS Disord. 2012;14(2).
69. Esbitt SA, Batchelder AW, Tanenbaum ML, et al. "Knowing That You're Not the Only One": perspectives on group-based cognitive-behavioral therapy for adherence and depression (CBT-AD) in adults with type 1 diabetes. Cogn Behav Pract. 2014;22(3):393–406. doi:10.1016/j.cbpra.2014.02.006.
70. Soroudi N, Perez GK, Gonzalez JS, et al. CBT for Medication Adherence and Depression (CBT-AD) in HIV-infected patients receiving methadone maintenance therapy. Cogn Behav Pract. 2008;15:93–106. doi:10.1016/j.cbpra.2006.11.004.
71. Safren SA, O'Cleirigh C, Tan JY, et al. A randomized controlled trial of cognitive behavioral therapy for adherence and depression (CBT-AD) in HIV-infected individuals. Health Psychol. 2009;28:1–10. doi:10.1037/a0012715.
72. Gonzalez JS, McCarl LA, Wexler DJ, et al. Cognitive–behavioral therapy for adherence and depression (CBT-AD) in type 2 diabetes. J Cogn Psychother. 2010;24:329–43. doi:10.1891/0889-8391.24.4.329.
73. Safren SA, O'Cleirigh CM, Bullis JR, et al. Cognitive behavioral therapy for adherence and depression (CBT-AD) in HIV-infected injection drug users: a randomized controlled trial. J Consult Clin Psychol. 2012;80:404–15. doi:10.1037/a0028208.
74. Simoni JM, Wiebe JS, Sauceda JA, et al. A preliminary RCT of CBT-AD for adherence and depression among HIV-positive latinos on the U.S.-Mexico border: the Nuevo Dia study. AIDS Behav. 2013;17:2816–29. doi:10.1007/s10461-013-0538-5.
75. Berg C, Raminani S, Greer J, et al. Participants' perspectives on cognitive-behavioral therapy for adherence and depression in HIV. Psychother Res. 2008;18:271–80. doi:10.1080/10503300701561537.
76. Safren SA, Gonzalez JS, Soroudi N. Coping with chronic illness, workbook. New York: Oxford University Press; 2007.
77. Miller W, Rollnick S. Motivational interviewing, helping people change. 3rd ed. New York: Guilford; 2013.
78. Harvey JN. Psychosocial interventions for the diabetic patient. Diabetes Metab Syndr Obes. 2015;8:29–43.
79. Safren SA, Otto MW, Worth JL, et al. Two strategies to increase adherence to HIV antiretroviral medication: life-steps and medication monitoring. Behav Res Ther. 2001;39:1151–62. doi:10.1016/S0005-7967(00)00091-7.

80. Linehan M. Skills training manual for treating borderline personality disorder. New York: Guilford; 1993.
81. Beck AT. Cognitive therapy of depression. New York: Guilford; 1979.
82. Beck JS. Cognitive behavior therapy: basics and beyond. 2nd ed. New York: Guilford; 2011.
83. D'Zurilla TJ. Problem-solving therapy: a positive approach to clinical intervention. 3rd ed. New York: Springer; 2007.
84. Cotanch P. Relaxation training for control of nausea and vomiting in patients receiving chemotherapy. Cancer Nurs. 1983;6:277–83.
85. Turner J, Chapman C. Psychological intervention for chronic pain: a critical review-relaxation and biofeedback. Pain. 1982;12:1–221.
86. Smith W. Biofeedback and relaxation training: the effect on headache and associated symptoms. Headache. 1987;27:511–4.
87. Ost L. Applied Relaxation: manual for a behavioral coping technique. Department of Psychology, Stockholm University.
88. Otto M, Jones J, Craske M, Barlow D. Stopping anxiety medication: panic control therapy for benzodiazepine discontinuation (therapist guide). San Antonio: Psychological Corporation; 1996.
89. Tanenbaum ML, Ritholz MD, Binko DH, et al. Probing for depression and finding diabetes: a mixed-methods analysis of depression interviews with adults treated for type 2 diabetes. J Affect Disord. 2013;150:533–9. doi:10.1016/j.jad.2013.01.029.
90. Tanenbaum ML, Gonzalez JS. The influence of diabetes on a clinician-rated assessment of depression in adults with type 1 diabetes. Diabetes Educ. 2012;38:695–704. doi:10.1177/0145721712452795.
91. Fisher L, Glasgow RE, Mullan JT, et al. Development of a brief diabetes distress screening instrument. Ann Fam Med. 2008;6:246–52. doi:10.1370/afm.842.
92. Fisher L, Hessler D, Polonsky WH, Mullan J. When is diabetes distress meaningful? Establishing cut points for the diabetes distress scale. Diabetes Care. 2012;35:259–64.
93. Weinger K, Butler HA, Welch GW, La Greca AM. Measuring diabetes self-care: a psychometric analysis of the Self-Care Inventory-Revised with adults. Diabetes Care. 2005;28:1346–52.
94. La Greca A. Manual for the self care inventory. Miami: University of Miami; 2004.
95. Khagram L, Martin CR, Davies MJ, Speight J. Psychometric validation of the Self-Care Inventory-Revised (SCI-R) in UK adults with type 2 diabetes using data from the AT. LANTUS follow-on study. Health Qual Life Outcomes. 2013;11:24. doi:10.1186/1477-7525-11-24.
96. Gonzalez JS, Schneider HE. Methodological issues in the assessment of diabetes treatment adherence. Curr Diab Rep. 2011;11(6):472–9.
97. Gonzalez JS, Schneider HE, Wexler DJ, et al. Validity of medication adherence self-reports in adults with type 2 diabetes. Diabetes Care. 2013;36:831–7. doi:10.2337/dc12-0410.
98. Chomutare T, Fernandez-Luque L, Arsand E, Hartvigsen G. Features of mobile diabetes applications: review of the literature and analysis of current applications compared against evidence-based guidelines. J Med Internet Res. 2011;13(3):e65. doi:10.2196/jmir.1874.
99. Wilson IB, Fowler Jr FJ, Cosenza CA, Michaud J, Bentkover J, Rana A, Kogelman L, Rogers WH. Cognitive and field testing of a new set of medication adherence self-report items for HIV care. AIDS Behav. 2014;18(12):2349–58.
100. United Kingdom Prospective Diabetes Study (UKPDS) Group. United Kingdom Prospective Diabetes Study (UKPDS). 13: Relative efficacy of randomly allocated diet, sulphonylurea, insulin, or metformin in patients with newly diagnosed non-insulin dependent diabetes followed for three years. BMJ. 1995;310:83–8. doi:10.1136/bmj.310.6972.83.
101. Hermanns N, Schmitt A, Gahr A, et al. The effect of a diabetes-specific cognitive behavioral treatment program (DIAMOS) for patients with diabetes and subclinical depression: results of a randomized controlled trial. Diabetes Care. 2015;38(4):551–60. doi:10.2337/dc14-1416.
102. Chen S, Creedy D, Lin H, Wollin J. Effects of motivational interviewing intervention on self-management, psychological and glycemic outcomes in type 2 diabetes: a randomized controlled trial. Int J Nurs Stud. 2012;49:637–44.

103. Gabbay RRA, Añel-Tiangco R, Dellasega C, et al. Diabetes nurse case management and motivational interviewing for change (DYNAMIC) results of a 2-year randomized control pragmatic trial. J Diabetes. 2013;5:349–57.
104. Welschen L, van Oppen P, Dekker J, et al. Effects of a cognitive behavioural treatment in patients with type 2 diabetes when added to managed care; a randomised controlled trial. BMC Public Health. 2007;7:74.
105. Huffman JC, DuBois CM, Millstein RA, et al. Positive psychological interventions for patients with type 2 diabetes: rationale, theoretical model, and intervention development. J Diabetes Res. 2015;2015:428349. doi:10.1155/2015/428349.
106. Fisher L, Gonzalez JS, Polonsky WH. The confusing tale of depression and distress in patients with diabetes: a call for greater clarity and precision. Diabet Med. 2014;31:764–72. doi:10.1111/dme.12428.
107. Montgomery SA, Asberg MA. A new depression scale designed to be sensitive to change. The British journal of psychiatry. 1979 Apr 1;134(4):382–9.

Additional Resources

Safren S, Gonzalez J, Soroudi N. Coping with chronic illness: a cognitive-behavioral approach for adherence and depression therapist guide. New York: Oxford University Press; 2008.
Safren S, Gonzalez J, Soroudi N. Coping with chronic illness: a cognitive-behavioral approach for adherence and depression client workbook. New York: Oxford University Press; 2007.
Lloyd CE, Pouwer F, Hermanns N, editors. Screening for depression and other psychological problems in diabetes: a practical guide. New York: Springer; 2012.
Katon W, Maj M, Sartorius N, editors. Depression and diabetes, vol. 16. New York: Wiley; 2011.
Polonsky W. Diabetes burnout: what to do when you can't take it anymore. Alexandria: American Diabetes Association; 1999.
Rubin R. Psyching out diabetes: a positive approach to your negative emotions. Los Angeles: Lowell House; 1993.
Young-Hymam D, Peyrot M. Psychosocial care for people with diabetes. Washington, DC: American Diabetes Association; 2012.
American Diabetes Association. American Diabetes Association complete guide to diabetes. New York: McGraw-Hill/Contemporary; 2011.
American Diabetes Association (ADA). http://www.diabetes.org/
National Diabetes Education Program's (NDEP). http://ndep.nih.gov/
Behavioral Diabetes Institute. http://www.behavioraldiabetesinstitute.org/
Promoting Medication Adherence in Diabetes (NDEP Web Resource): https://www.niddk.nih.gov/health-information/health-communication-programs/ndep/health-care-professionals/medication-adherence/Pages/default.aspx

Chapter 7
Gastrointestinal Disorders

Jonathan A. Lerner and Julianne G. Wilner

7.1 Introduction

Gastrointestinal (GI) disorders constitute an interfering and costly portion of the behavioral medicine disorders, affecting 60–70 million US citizens annually. Spending on GI diseases in the United States has been estimated at $142 billion per year in direct and indirect costs [1]. From 2009 to 2010, the number of medical visits to physician offices, hospital outpatient, and emergency departments with the primary diagnosis of diseases of the digestive system was estimated to be 51.0 million [2]. The consequential morbidity of GI disorders is substantial; in 2009, 10 % of US deaths were attributable to an underlying GI cause [1]. A particular concern within the treatment of GI disorders is the negative effect that psychopathology has for quality of life, treatment interference and adherence [3] (Table 7.1).

There are a number of distinct gastrointestinal disorders frequently seen in GI clinics, primary care, and outpatient behavioral medicine settings. These GI disorders are classified as structural and functional. Structural disorders, such as Crohn's disease and ulcerative colitis (UC), also known as inflammatory bowel disorders (IBD), involve an abnormal response by the body's immune system, in which food, bacteria, and other materials are mistaken for foreign or invading substances [42]. The resulting immune response causes chronic inflammation and ulcerations of the lining of the intestine. Functional GI disorders are not typically

J.A. Lerner, Ph.D. (✉) • J.G. Wilner, M.A.
Behavioral Medicine Service, Department of Psychiatry, Massachusetts General Hospital,
Harvard Medical School, Boston, MA, USA
e-mail: jalerner@mgh.harvard.edu; jgwilner@mgh.harvard.edu

© Springer Science+Business Media New York 2017
A.-M. Vranceanu et al. (eds.), *The Massachusetts General Hospital
Handbook of Behavioral Medicine*, Current Clinical Psychiatry,
DOI 10.1007/978-3-319-29294-6_7

Table 7.1 Cognitive Behavioral Therapeutic Skills, Techniques, and Goals

CBT skill	Techniques	Goals
Psychoeducation	Three component model	Increase awareness of interplay among thoughts, behavior, and physical symptoms
	Treatment rationale	Enhance motivation, build rapport, and foster therapeutic alliance
	Goal setting	Clearly define realistic expectations for therapy
Cognitive	Cognitive restructuring	Identify and challenge maladaptive thought patterns and beliefs
	Hypothesis testing	Break down overwhelming tasks into more manageable pieces to decrease avoidance and increase mastery and self-efficacy
	Problem solving	
Behavioral	Behavioral exposure	Provide opportunity to refute erroneous beliefs and develop evidence for use in cognitive restructuring
	Behavioral experiments	Increase engagement in pleasurable activities to enhance quality of life and provide opportunities for naturalistic reinforcement
	Behavioral activation	
Mind-body	Diaphragmatic breathing	Decrease physiological reactivity to stress
	Progressive muscle relaxation	Enhance ability to tolerate negative affect and physical discomfort
	Mindfulness	Increase ability to be present in the moment without judgment
	Meditation	
Lifestyle	Adherence	Decrease behaviors with potential to exacerbate disease symptoms
	Diet	Enhance overall physical health and well-being, with associated psychological benefits
	Exercise	
	Sleep hygiene	

detected by normal diagnostic tests (e.g., endoscopy, X-ray), have a variable and unpredictable course of symptoms, and are often influenced by multiple factors. Examples of functional GI disorders include, but are not limited to, gastroparesis, gastroesophageal reflux disease (GERD), cyclical vomiting syndrome (CVS), and irritable bowel syndrome (IBS). GI disorders are heterogeneous, each with their own unique challenges, including symptom presentation, psychological comorbidity, and psychotherapeutic treatment interventions. This chapter aims to highlight these disease-specific challenges and provide a psychosocial context for the treatment of GI disorders in clinical practice.

7.2 Structural Disorders

7.2.1 Crohn's Disease

Crohn's disease (CD) is commonly characterized by chronic gastrointestinal inflammation in the small bowel and GI tract. As with other GI disorders, there is evidence suggesting comorbidity of psychopathology and CD [4]. For example, a study by Cámara et al. [5] found the association between perceived stress and exacerbation of CD to be fully attributable to anxiety and depression. Specifically, for every one standard deviation of perceived stress, the odds of exacerbation of CD symptoms increased by 1.85 times (95% confidence interval 1.43–2.40, $P < 0.001$). Another study of young patients with CD ($n = 2144$) compared with healthy controls ($n = 10,720$) found that after adjusting for patient characteristics, individuals with CD had significantly greater risks of developing persistent anxiety and depressive disorders (HR [95% CI] = 4.35 [2.22–8.50] and 2.75 [1.73–4.38], respectively; [6]). Additionally, a prospective study by Persoons et al. [7] found major depressive disorder predictive of a lower remission rate in CD patients (OR = 0.166, 95% CI = 0.049–0.567, $P = 0.004$), and at 9 month follow-up (HR = 2.271, 95% CI: 1.36–3.79, $P = 0.002$).

CBT interventions specific to CD and psychopathology are quite limited, and most focus on a more general IBD diagnosis. While these studies may not differentiate in treatment outcome for CD in comparison to other IBD disorders, many do identify patients with CD in their methods, thereby providing some evidence that those with CD may benefit from reductions in anxious and depressive symptoms through CBT interventions.

7.2.2 Ulcerative Colitis

In Ulcerative Colitis (UC), inflammation is limited to only the innermost lining of the intestinal tract, between the large intestine and rectum. Studies have demonstrated that UC and psychiatric disorders co-occur at high rates [8]. For instance, Porcelli et al. [9] found that patients with active UC reported statistically significantly higher scores for psychological distress, somatization, obsessive-compulsive, depression, phobic anxiety, and psychotocisim than patients with non-active UC. A more recent study showed that in a sample with mild to moderately severe UC, greater disease activity was associated with greater depressive symptoms [10]. Another study of patients with UC revealed moderate to strong associations between psychological distress (depression and health anxiety) and disease activity, with support for a psychobiological interaction of the perinuclear antineutrophil cytoplasmic antibody (pANCA), an indicator of UC disease status [11].

Psychosocial interventions have been developed to aid in relief of psychological distress in patients with UC. For example, a study examined a group-based patient education program for high-anxiety patients with CD or UC and found that while the eight-session intervention was helpful in relaying information about disease-related topics, there were no significant improvements in anxiety or UC symptoms [12]. Cognitive-behavioral interventions may be more effective in reducing these symptoms. For instance, a prospective study by Mussell et al. [13] found that after 12 weekly group sessions of CBT for patients with UC or CD, disease-related worries and concerns significantly decreased in those with UC [13]; however, future studies should look at such interventions through randomized, controlled methodologies.

Psychosocial interventions have been developed to aid in relief of psychological distress in patients with UC. For example, a study examined a group-based patient education program for high-anxiety patients with CD or UC and found that while the eight-session intervention was helpful in relaying information about disease-related topics, there were no significant improvements in anxiety or UC symptoms [12]. Cognitive-behavioral interventions may be more effective in reducing these symptoms. For instance, a prospective study by Mussell et al. [13] found that after 12 weekly group sessions of CBT for patients with UC or CD, disease-related worries and concerns significantly decreased in those with UC [13]; however, future studies should look at such interventions through randomized, controlled methodologies.

7.3   Functional Disorders

7.3.1   Gastroparesis

Gastroparesis is characterized by delayed gastric emptying that occurs in the absence of any sort of obstruction or blockage [14]. Individuals with gastroparesis feel full after eating very little (called early satiety), and may also experience nausea, vomiting, abdominal pain, and bloating [14]. This condition can be present for a number of different reasons, and when the etiology is unknown, the diagnosis of idiopathic gastroparesis is made. While idiopathic gastroparesis is the most common form, some of the causes of non-idiopathic gastroparesis include diabetes and complications from abdominal surgery. In both cases, damage to the nerve that controls stomach contractions, the vagus nerve, seems to be the mechanism of action. Unfortunately, as with many GI disorders, there is no cure for gastroparesis, and treatment focuses primarily on management of symptoms and avoidance of some of the more serious potential consequences of the disorder (e.g., malnutrition, dehydration, and formation of hard masses of undigested food called bezoars). Treatment of gastroparesis typically includes dietary changes, such as eating smaller but more frequent meals, chewing food more thoroughly, and avoiding certain types of food, such as raw fruits and vegetables [14].

Pharmacologic treatments for gastroparesis usually aim to either increase gastric motility or control nausea and vomiting [15]. Finally, there is some early evidence that acupuncture may help reduce symptoms of gastroparesis [16]. While psychological factors are not thought to cause or maintain gastroparesis, they can play a significant role in managing the disease, adhering to treatment, and influencing the subjective experience of pain. Studies have found anxiety or depression to be associated with more severe gastroparesis symptoms [17, 18]. One study found that elevated levels of anxiety, depression, and neuroticism were each independently associated with nearly double the prevalence of GI symptoms in diabetic patients, even when controlling for age, gender, duration and type of diabetes, and glycemic control [19].

There is some evidence suggesting psychosocial treatments for gastroparesis may be helpful in relieving symptoms, particularly in instilling hope and self-care, as well as assisting patients focus on aspects of their life they can control [20, 21]. Clinical psychologists can be an important part of the patient's care by emphasizing psychobiological/psychosocial education, and facilitating social support with family and friends [21, 22].

7.3.2 Gastroesophageal Reflux Disease

Gastroesophageal reflux disease (GERD) involves the backflow of gastric contents into the esophagus, which leads to irritation of the esophageal lining. This irritation can range from mild to severe, with the latter causing structural tissue damage. The underlying cause of GERD is relaxation of the lower esophageal sphincter (LES), which typically keeps the stomach contents from travelling back up the esophagus. Individuals suffering with GERD often report that symptoms worsen during periods of increased stress and anxiety. Studies have shown that stress does not lead to increased acid production, but does increase the sensitivity of the esophagus [23, 24]. Treatment for GERD can involve medications (both over-the-counter and prescription) that target acid production; dietary modification to eliminate foods that lead to LES relaxation or increased acid production; and in some cases, surgery. Evidence from psychosocial interventions suggests relaxation training may be helpful in conjunction with traditional therapies (i.e., antireflux therapy) for those whose GERD symptoms are exacerbated under stress [25]. Moreover, for those who have undergone surgical treatment for stress-related GERD symptoms, psychological interventions may augment the surgical outcome [26].

7.3.3 Cyclical Vomiting Syndrome

Cyclical Vomiting Syndrome (CVS) is characterized by episodic vomiting and associated intense nausea interspersed amongst nausea-free intervals [27]. Due to the unique symptomatology of CVS, the disease has significant morbidity risks, with up to 50 % of patients requiring multi-week hospitalizations and intravenous hydration during each episode [27]. Therefore, it is a highly interfering disease with a heavy economic burden, especially in terms of work loss. Multiple studies have demonstrated that individuals with CVS are at an increased risk for psychiatric disorders, particularly anxiety in children [28, 29], and that the anxiety may be a predisposing factor to CVS episodes. For instance, in a study of 85 children and adolescents with CVS, 47% met criteria for an anxiety disorder and 14% met for an affective disorder, much higher than rates in the general population [30]. Panic attacks are also particularly common in CVS patients, as demonstrated through a study by Fleisher et al. [31]. Researchers found 68% of adults in the study had four or more panic symptoms during the prodromal and emetic phases of their episodes [31].

There is some preliminary evidence of effective cognitive behavioral treatments for CVS. For example, a recent case presentation examined CBT and heart rate variability (HRV) biofeedback training for a 13-year-old boy with CVS [32]. Triggers for vomiting episodes for the patient centered on anticipatory anxiety related to school, family, and health concerns. Treatment was focused on this anxiety and autonomic dysregulation, and outcome was indicative of more effective management of psychological stressors, self-efficacy, and control in regard to vomiting cycles [32]. Although further research with controlled, randomized interventions is necessary to evaluate the effectiveness of CBT for CVS, studies such as the case presentation provide initial evidence for the feasibility and acceptability of CBT for CVS.

7.3.4   Irritable Bowel Syndrome

Irritable Bowel Syndrome (IBS), characterized by chronic cramping, abdominal pain, bloating, gas, diarrhea, and constipation, is associated with co-occurring psychopathology such as anxiety and depression. For example, research has shown that anxiety and depression are more common in patients with IBS, and that anxious and depressive symptoms are elevated during active periods of disease [33]. One study found a significantly higher lifetime prevalence of major depression for the IBS cases compared to cases in the community (27% vs. 12%). These findings were similar for 12-month prevalence rates (9.1% for IBS vs. 5.5% for community), with a trend toward significance (odds ratio [OR] 1.53, 95% confidence interval [CI] 0.96–2.45). Lifetime prevalence of panic disorder for those with IBS was also demonstrated (8.0% vs. 4.7%, OR 1.59, 95% CI 0.96–2.63; [34]). Another study examined two nationally representative Canadian health surveys [35] and found 12-month depression rates to be 14 and 16% amongst participants reporting IBS symptoms for each survey, nearly triple the rate of depression in Canada. Moreover, it has been demonstrated that the course of IBS is worse in depressed patients, and there is evidence to suggest that the psychopathology may actually mediate poorer health outcomes in IBS patients [33].

Evidence-based, cognitive-behavioral interventions have been shown to improve anxiety, depression, and GI-related symptoms in IBS patients. An open trial and consequential randomized controlled trial (RCT) demonstrated cognitive behavior therapy (CBT) to be effective in treating adolescents with IBS and depression [36–38]. For those adolescents with comorbid anxiety, there was a significant reduction in anxiety as well. While the open trial did not find any change in IBS symptom severity posttreatment, the RCT demonstrated a decrease in the number of individuals with moderate to severe disease posttreatment (29 % pre- vs. 15 % posttreatment). Although the findings were not statistically significant, treatment gains were maintained at 12-month follow-up [37]. Another randomized controlled trial with adults with IBS found clinically significant reductions in anxiety and depression from a CBT program emphasizing relaxation training, distraction, and cognitive restructuring, and treatment gains were maintained through 12-month follow-up [39]. Overall, there is limited but promising evidence suggesting that CBT interventions are accepted and effective in depressed or anxious patients with IBS.

Gastrointestinal disorders are a heterogeneous group of illnesses with varied etiologies, symptoms, and impacts. Accordingly, there is no single psychotherapeutic protocol that can be applied across disorders. Nevertheless, as described above, the research shows that psychosocial interventions based on cognitive behavioral principles can help individuals cope more effectively with symptoms, improve quality of life, and interrupt the feedback loop that often exists between symptoms of anxiety and depression and exacerbation of GI symptoms.

7.3.5   Approach

While there is a wide variety of disorders and symptoms within the GI disorders, a behavioral medicine approach has some commonalities across patients. Psychological treatment of GI disorders begins with a careful assessment, including both the details of the medical condition and functional impairments, limitations, and restrictions, but also psychiatric symptoms or diagnoses, such as anxiety or depression. Each patient will have specific ways in which their GI symptoms are impacting their level of functioning and level of distress, and specific emotional and behavioral responses to their symptoms. It is important to get a clear picture so as to be able to target problem areas most effectively, especially if the allotted time frame is short. When working in a GI clinic or other primary medical setting, with patients who have GI disorders but not co-occurring Axis I disorders, the length of treatment may be quite short, such as 4–6 sessions. For patients with more significant co-occurring psychiatric symptoms, length of treatment will be longer, averaging 12–20 sessions. If the patient has a full diagnosis of an Axis I disorder, such as MDE or GAD, he or she may need to be referred for further outpatient treatment or a medication evaluation.

When possible, a multidisciplinary approach to the treatment of the individual with chronic GI difficulties is ideal. In addition to a health psychologist, a typical multidisciplinary team might include primary care physicians, gastroenterologists, nurse practitioners, registered dieticians, and physical therapists.

After the initial evaluation, the next step is psychoeducation and introducing the 3-component CBT model of how thoughts, feelings, and behaviors interact. Informing this initial discussion is the fact that GI problems are, unlike some other medical issues, at least somewhat familiar to most people. Also the relationship between mood and GI symptoms is something that most of us have experienced. When children are nervous or anxious, they talk about being sick to their stomach. When we think about going onstage to speak or perform in front of a group, we experience "butterflies in the stomach," and sometimes when we hear very bad news we have the sensation of our stomach dropping or a "pit in the stomach." This conversation can pave the way to a more formal introduction of the CBT model, which illustrates the interconnectedness of thoughts, feelings, and behaviors and is a core concept for psychological treatment of GI disorders.

One concern often expressed by GI patients who have been referred for CBT by their PCP or gastroenterologist is that the referring physician does not take the patients symptoms seriously, or "think it's all in their head." This concern can be readily addressed as part of providing psychoeducation and a treatment rationale during the first session. When presenting the model, the therapist explains to the patient that physical and psychological factors interact to exacerbate the disease process, and by targeting the factors under their control, they may experience less distress and better coping with their disease.

Given the chronic and relapsing nature of some GI disorders, it can be difficult to adjust after initial diagnosis. It is not surprising that individuals often present with symptoms of depression, if not a full episode of major depression. This is especially true when the disorder has led to significant restrictions in normal activities, functional impairment, physical pain, new dietary habits, etc. In these cases, targeting depressive symptoms directly with CBT strategies can be helpful, as can helping patients work towards acceptance of these changes. When discussing acceptance, it is important to clarify that acceptance is not the same as giving up. Instead, acceptance means acknowledging the fact that their situation has changed and then working to adapt to these changes and develop new habits and attitudes that allow the patient to continue to move forward with life.

7.3.6 Goals

While this general approach tends to apply to many patients with GI disorders, their specific goals for therapy may be quite varied and individualized. There are a number of specific goals that may apply to behavioral medicine work in GI disorders, and any patient may have one or more of these goals. In the initial assessment, it is important to inquire specifically about the patient's own goals, and work with what the patient presents, so the treatment is most focused and helpful. Some common goals include, but are not limited to, the following:

- Fewer GI episodes or flares
- Increasing awareness of the interrelationship between GI symptoms and anxiety/ stress
- Identifying behavioral and environmental triggers for GI episodes

- Decreasing avoidance of normal/usual activities (e.g., with limited bathroom access)
- Decreasing mobility restrictions (actual vs. feared needs)
- Improving social interactions
- Obtaining appropriate support and accommodations
- Decreasing embarrassment (invisible disability)
- Decreasing anxiety about long-term consequences of disorder
- Acceptance of chronicity, importance of management
- Improved adherence (diet, medication, etc.)
- Improved assertiveness skills (limits on energy)

7.3.7 Skills for Cognitive Behavioral Therapy for GI Disorders

There are a number of different cognitive behavioral skills that can be useful for individuals diagnosed with GI disorders. Specific skills detailed below include cognitive restructuring, structured problem solving, adherence interventions, relaxation and mindfulness, and pain management. Depending on GI symptom presentation and an individual's subjective experience, some skills may be more relevant than others, and the order in which the clinician introduces each skill will also vary.

7.3.8 Cognitive Restructuring

Cognitive restructuring focuses on identifying negative, and often unrealistic, automatic thoughts (ATs) that can lead to increased anxiety or depression, and then critically evaluating the ATs and developing a more balanced and realistic alternative thought or rational response (RR). In many of the GI disorders patients have ATs about the meaning of the disorder, the impact it will have on their life, and the impact treatment may have. Given the varied nature of ATs, the first step in cognitive restructuring is identifying the specific ATs the patient is having, and teaching the patient how to recognize and identify them as well. Socratic questioning and a downward arrow approach can be helpful in accomplishing this, as is assigning between-session monitoring and recording of automatic thoughts and the situations in which they occur. After learning to readily identify ATs, the focus shifts to identifying cognitive errors and disputing the AT that the patient has identified. Finally, it is important to look for evidence that both supports and refutes the thought, after which one can then develop a rational response.

For example, a common area of concern for many GI patients is eating in social situations, such as business lunches, parties, or dinners. Patients are worried that friends and coworkers may notice that their eating habits have changed, and question or judge them. These fears can lead to either increased anxiety, avoidance of these situations, or both. Cognitive restructuring, as described above, can help a patient identify the cognitive errors (e.g., mind reading, magnification) and allow the patient to put these concerns in perspective. Additionally, patients can be encouraged to gather evidence and test the hypothesis that others are scrutinizing their eating behavior; often patients will find that people are not, but if they are, the patient can typically cope effectively by providing simple answers to any questions or comments that may arise.

7.3.9 Structured Problem Solving

There are a number of areas in which structured problem solving (SPS) can be helpful to patients with GI disorders, such as accommodating to new, often more complex, dietary regimens; making travel arrangements for business or pleasure; and/or requesting and implementing accommodations at work. SPS entails several steps, the first of which is defining the problem area clearly and specifically. Once the problem has been defined, the next step is to list all of the possible solutions to the problem without regard for practicality or effectiveness, after which the pros and cons of each solution are enumerated with the end result being a rank ordered list of solutions from best to worst. The final step in SPS is to break the best solution down into discrete, manageable tasks that the patient can incorporate into his or her day.

For example, as noted above, many individuals with GI disorders have concerns around continence. Depending on the type of GI disorder, severity can range from mild, occasional diarrhea, gas and cramping to episodes of intense urgency and lack of control of bowel function. As a result, individuals with GI disorders may fear or avoid situations where bathroom access is unknown or limited. In conducting problem solving, this avoidance will be evaluated as a possible solution and compared to other possible solutions.

In discussing avoidance in this context, it will often become apparent that avoidance may help to decrease anxiety in the short term, but precludes testing the hypothesis or gathering evidence to support or counter the patient's prediction, as well as reinforcing both anxiety and avoidance in the long term. There is also the objective cost of missed opportunities, experiences, and activities. As other potential solutions are evaluated, their relative costs and benefits may be preferable. For example, having backup clothing at hand and noting the locations of public restrooms on arrival may be preferable to completely avoiding an entire event or experience. In addition to helping GI patients more accurately assess their options, another benefit of problem solving is that it often leads to exposure to the feared situation, which in turn provides patients with opportunities to use their other CBT tools.

7.3.10   Adherence Interventions

GI disorders, depending on the type, are more or less influenced by day-to-day behavior and by medications. For disorders like CVS, there is not yet a medication or dietary regimen that can manage symptoms, so the typical approach is to decrease the likelihood of an occurrence in the first place by managing stress, identifying and modifying or avoiding environmental triggers, and engaging in good self-care and healthy behaviors in general. Management of other disorders, such as Crohn's disease, may rely heavily on regular and consistent use of medications that affect the underlying biological processes of the disorder. For many GI disorders, diet is an important aspect of disease management, and specific diets exist for specific disorders (e.g., gluten-free for Celiac disease; Fermentable, Oligo-, Di-, Monosaccharides And Polyols (FODMAP) for IBS, gastroparesis, and other functional GI disorders). While the modality, costs, and benefits of treatment differ across GI disorders and individuals, adherence is important to maximize treatment effectiveness.

Medication adherence is relevant to almost all chronic medical conditions, and GI disorders are no exception. Two common barriers to medication adherence include difficulties with ingestion or administration, and negative side effects. Biologic medications for IBD such as Humira and Remicade are administered either subcutaneously or intravenously, which for some can be a minor barrier to adherence due to discomfort, while for others (e.g., individuals with injection phobia) it can halt treatment completely. Breathing and relaxation techniques can help to manage some of the pain and anxiety associated with injections, and for those with a clinical phobia, there are well-documented, empirically validated cognitive behavioral treatments to address the problem [40].

Oral steroids are another commonly used treatment for GI disorders, but many patients experience affective dysregulation including irritability, anxiety, and depression when taking these medications. Basic education about the effect of steroids on mood can be helpful for many patients, as can mindfulness training to help individuals increase affective awareness, and cognitive restructuring to identify automatic thoughts and distortions.

As briefly mentioned above, diet is another area which individuals can find especially difficult to manage and adhere to. Even with the support of a nutritionist, many patients can still feel overwhelmed by the prospect of changing their diet, and factors such as cost, preparation time, convenience, enjoyment, and social isolation can all contribute to the problem of adherence to a dietary regimen.

Food serves as a primary reinforcer from the time we are born and is tightly woven into the fabric of day-to-day life, as well as being associated with celebrations, socialization, and emotional support and comfort. For this reason, dietary adherence can be especially difficult for many individuals. Oftentimes, the best place to start is to identify triggers for eating, including specific situations, occasions, types of food, and strong emotions. Enhancing awareness of when dietary challenges are most likely to occur allows the patient to develop a plan for dealing with these situations (e.g., bringing one's own food, eating a small meal prior to arrival, using alternative coping strategies such as relaxation and meditation). Structured problem solving around shopping, meal preparation, and food access can also facilitate adherence to a particular dietary regimen. For example, patients can create and use a grocery list; prepare several servings of a particular meal at once to decrease preparation time during the week; and build time into their schedule to allow for eating.

7.3.11 Relaxation and Mindfulness

Relaxation and mindfulness techniques fall under the general heading of mind-body interventions, and can be an important focus of treatment because they address thoughts, behavior, and physical sensations in an integrative way. There are a number of methods for enhancing relaxation, including progressive muscle relaxation and diaphragmatic breathing. Mindfulness, while it can lead to relaxation, is a broader construct, and can be defined as, "the awareness that emerges through paying attention on purpose, in the present moment, and nonjudgmentally to the unfolding of experience moment by moment" [41, p 145]. Specifically, these techniques can decrease the subjective experience of pain, decrease reactivity to symptoms, provide a respite from ruminative worry, and ameliorate some of the physical symptoms of anxiety. Since many patients report a worsening of GI symptoms with increased anxiety, these techniques can potentially interrupt the negative feedback loop between anxiety symptoms and GI symptoms.

7.3.12 Pain Management

While the subjective experience of pain is unique to the individual, almost all of the GI disorders are associated with at least some pain and discomfort. Not surprisingly, abdominal pain is often the focus of attention, but pain or discomfort can be experienced anywhere along the digestive tract, including, for example, esophageal pain, pain associated with bowel movements, and the experience of nausea. Other causes of pain can include constipation, pancreatitis, irritation due to diarrhea, postprandial pain (sometimes in response to specific types of food), and pain and cramping associated with gas. Sometimes GI pain worsens with movement. It is important for patients to be in regular contact with their gastroenterologist since pain can sometimes be a sign of serious problems that require immediate attention (e.g., development of fistulae). In addition to variations in location, the quality of the pain among GI disorders varies, and may be acute and episodic or chronic and sustained.

In working with pain and GI disorders, typical strategies include relaxation and breathing, meditation and mindfulness, distraction, and biofeedback. In addition, behavioral medicine can help patients with pain management by helping them to adhere to optimal practices advised by physicians or other members of the health-care team. For example, the patient's nutritionist may recommend avoiding certain foods that are fibrous and more difficult to digest, or foods that tend to produce gas and bloating. Patients with GERD may be advised to elevate the head of their bed so as to sleep at an angle and decrease reflux. Patients may need to eat multiple small meals across the day as opposed to three larger meals. When there are practical or emotional barriers to following these practices, a psychologist can help with a combination of motivational interviewing, problem solving, cognitive restructuring, and psychoeducation.

7.3.13 Case Illustration

Ruth was a 42-year-old married white female on temporary medical leave as a result of ulcerative colitis. Ruth worked as an accountant at a medium-size firm, and was very high achieving and goal oriented with strong perfectionistic tendencies. The patient had multiple surgeries related to her UC, which is what necessitated her taking a leave of absence from work. Ruth was referred for CBT within the GI clinic by her gastroenterologist for "stress and anxiety," and completed an initial evaluation with the results being diagnoses of panic disorder and generalized anxiety disorder. Based on her report, both of these diagnoses predated her UC diagnosis, although after her diagnosis, issues around UC became the primary trigger for her anxiety symptoms. She was naïve to psychotherapy, and was somewhat anxious about the prospect of meeting with a psychologist.

7.3.14 Session 1

The first session focused on establishing rapport, collaboratively setting treatment goals, providing a brief explanation of CBT in general, and then introducing the 3-component cognitive behavioral model of anxiety. The therapist presented the model using a Socratic style, and drew from the patient's own day-to-day experiences to illustrate the components of the model. When working with a patient who has a chronic GI disorder, it is important to integrate the signs and symptoms of the disorder into the 3-component model. In Ruth's case, the therapist pointed out that some of her UC symptoms were similar to some of the GI symptoms that arise as a normal part of the anxiety response. The therapist then went on to explain how this can create a negative feedback loop in which the anxiety response exacerbates the GI symptom, which in turn increases anxiety. The patient found this explanation fit with her own experience, and was able to provide several of her own examples. The therapist also explained that because of the treatment setting (GI specialty clinic), therapy would be a short-term, skills-based approach of four to six sessions that would be spaced out over a number of weeks. For homework, the therapist asked the patient to monitor her thoughts, behavior, and physical symptoms prior to the next session, and to bring her monitoring forms in with her to her next appointment.

7.3.15   Session 2

Session 2 focused primarily on introducing the concept of cognitive restructuring, specifically, identifying automatic thoughts and cognitive distortions. After defining automatic thoughts, the therapist used some of the thoughts from Ruth's completed monitoring homework as examples. Two of the thoughts the patient had recorded were, "I will never be able to go back to work again, and my friends and coworkers will be disappointed in me and think of me as a failure," and, "I will never be healthy again, and my partner will leave me because I am sick and cannot pull my own weight." The therapist then explained cognitive distortions and went through the list of distortions with the patient, having her indicate whether a distortion fit with either of the thoughts she had recorded.

The therapist also allotted enough time to introduce diaphragmatic breathing and relaxation and conduct a brief, 5-min guided relaxation. This was important, because Ruth was having difficulty managing her ruminative worry, especially at night, which was negatively affecting her sleep. As is the case with most patients, it was helpful to provide Ruth with some basic behavioral stress management skills early on to use while learning techniques such as cognitive restructuring. Ruth was assigned as homework to complete the *automatic thought* and *cognitive distortion* columns of the monitoring form, and to practice diaphragmatic breathing and relaxation for 5 min, one to two times per day.

7.3.16   Session 3

During session 3 the homework from the previous meeting was reviewed and the patient reported that she had not had a chance to practice relaxation. The therapist responded nonjudgmentally, and asked the patient what she thought had gotten in the way of her practicing. The patient reported that she had been too busy, and it had slipped her mind. The therapist and patient looked at her schedule together and identified blocks of time that would work well for practicing relaxation. The therapist then asked the patient to physically add relaxation practice to her daily schedule and set a reminder for it on her phone. ·

The patient and therapist then moved on to reviewing the automatic thoughts the patient had recorded. One prominent thought was "My friends think that I am lazy because I am taking a leave of absence from work." The patient and therapist then continued to complete the remaining columns of the thought monitoring record together, identifying cognitive errors, generating evidence for and against the automatic thought, and using Socratic questioning to challenge the automatic thought. During this process the patient identified that the thought she had recorded was an example of *mind reading* and *jumping to conclusions*, and was unable to generate any evidence to support the AT that her friends thought she was lazy. In fact, when prompted, the patient was able to recall information *inconsistent* with her AT, including the fact that her friends had specifically told her how impressed they were with her ability to simultaneously manage her health, taking graduate classes, and organizing her parents' 50th anniversary party. After reviewing the evidence for and against the AT, the patient asked herself if she would label a good friend in the same situation as "lazy," and concluded that she would not. More importantly, the patient reported that she was more open to the notion that perhaps her friends did not, in fact, perceive her as lazy.

The therapist asked the patient to continue practicing breathing and relaxation. Additionally, the patient was asked to continue monitoring and recording automatic thoughts, and to complete the entire cognitive restructuring form for each thought identified.

7.3.17   Session 4

Session 4 began with a review of the patient's relaxation practice and cognitive restructuring homework. The patient reported practicing relaxation at least once most days, and indicated that adding this to her schedule and setting phone reminders had been very helpful. Overall, the patient reported a decrease in anxiety and tension associated with relaxation and diaphragmatic breathing; however, she also noted that the diaphragmatic breathing was physically uncomfortable when she was experiencing gas and bloating. The therapist explained to the patient that this was sometimes a problem for individuals with abdominal pain, and that guided relaxation could still be accomplished without the benefit of diaphragmatic breathing during those times when the diaphragmatic breathing was uncomfortable.

The review of the Ruth's cognitive monitoring forms showed that she had been able to recognize, identify, and challenge several automatic thoughts and cognitive distortions related to her beliefs about being lazy and being judged by others. Moreover, the patient reported being better able to "let the thoughts go," and ruminate less after restructuring. However, she had also had an experience that was more overwhelming and resistant to cognitive restructuring. Specifically, the patient was running late for class due to heavy traffic, and after arriving on campus was only able to find parking in an overflow lot that was a 10–15 min walk from her class. Ruth started to feel abdominal discomfort and cramping, and worried that she would not be able to sit through class without having to run to the bathroom and would feel "completely humiliated." Ultimately, the patient decided to get back into her car and return home, missing class altogether.

The therapist had the patient start a new cognitive restructuring form, and walked her though the process, step by step. The automatic thought the patient arrived at was, "I will have to drop out of school completely because of my UC, and I will be a failure." After considering the evidence for this belief and thinking through the realistic worst-case scenario, the patient was able to generate several alternative, more adaptive thoughts. In addition, the patient was able to use problem solving to identify steps she could take to address some of the practical aspects of the situation, including leaving earlier for class, and contacting the administration at her college to see about getting a handicap placard.

For homework Ruth was to continue to use relaxation strategies, cognitive restructuring, and reach out to the school administration to find out about reasonable accommodations.

7.3.18   Session 5

The first thing the therapist did was to review the homework from the previous session with the patient. Ruth reported that she had been using breathing and relaxation several times per day with good benefit. The patient also reported that, although she experienced significant anticipatory anxiety prior to her next class, she was able to make the drive and use the cognitive restructuring and breathing skills to manage her anxiety and get to class without incident. In addition, she was able to obtain a parking accommodation to park closer to campus. Ruth noted that over the next few weeks there was a significant decrease in anticipatory anxiety prior to class, and that she was also able to apply some of the cognitive restructuring techniques to her perfectionistic concerns around timeliness.

Given that sessions had been at approximately alternate week intervals, it had been 11 weeks since the start of therapy, and the patient had made good progress in achieving the goals agreed on at the initial session. The remainder of the session was devoted to a review of the patient's progress to date, with a focus on the specific strategies used. In reviewing each strategy, the therapist made sure to discuss potential challenges the patient might face, and how to cope with and respond to challenges that arise. The therapist and patient agreed to have an additional follow-up session in 1 month.

7.3.19   Session 6

As in prior sessions, the therapist began by reviewing the period since the last meeting. Ruth reported that she had maintained the gains she had made and continued to regularly use the strategies she had learned during the active phase of treatment. The therapist was supportive and reinforced the patient's use of strategies, and also asked if there had been any challenges or difficulties. The patient acknowledged that she had experienced pain and discomfort related to her UC, and that she continued to have automatic thoughts similar to the ones she had identified previously, however, she also reported that she was better able to manage both her physical symptoms and anxiety, and that the frequency and intensity of negative automatic thoughts had decreased. The therapist encouraged Ruth to be thoughtful about anticipating stressful situations and triggers, so that she could apply her new skills to prevent small lapses from becoming relapses. Overall, Ruth reported that she was coping much better with her UC, and that her quality of life had improved in consequence.

7.4   Conclusion

Cognitive behavioral therapy can be an important adjunct to standard medical treatment for gastrointestinal disorders. CBT can help individuals with GI disorders cope with the emotional impact of chronic illness, as well as facilitate behavioral changes that can decrease functional impairment, improve quality of life, and increase treatment adherence. Moreover, since the experience of anxiety can include GI symptoms, using CBT to manage anxiety may decrease symptom burden overall.

References

1. Everhart JE, Ruhl CE. Burden of digestive diseases in the United States part I: overall and upper gastrointestinal diseases. Gastroenterology. 2009;136(2):376–86. http://doi.org/10.1053/j.gastro.2008.12.015.
2. Center for Disease Control and Prevention. FastStats: digestive diseases. 2010. http://www.cdc.gov/nchs/fastats/digestive-diseases.htm.
3. López San Román A, Bermejo F, Carrera E, Pérez-Abad M, Boixeda D. Adhesión al tratamiento en la enfermedad inflamatoria intestinal. Rev Esp Enferm Dig. 2005;97(4):249–57.
4. Mardini HE, Kip KE, Wilson JW. Crohn's disease: a two-year prospective study of the association between psychological distress and disease activity. Dig Dis Sci. 2004;49(3):492–7. http://doi.org/10.1023/B:DDAS.0000020509.23162.cc.
5. Cámara RJA, Schoepfer AM, Pittet V, Begré S, von Känel R, The Swiss Inflammatory Bowel Disease Cohort Study (SIBDCS) Group. Mood and nonmood components of perceived stress and exacerbation of Crohn's disease. Inflamm Bowel Dis. 2011;17(11):2358–65. http://doi.org/10.1002/ibd.21623.
6. Loftus EV, Guérin A, Yu AP, Wu EQ, Yang M, Chao J, Mulani PM. Increased risks of developing anxiety and depression in young patients with Crohn's disease. Am J Gastroenterol. 2011;106(9):1670–7. http://doi.org/10.1038/ajg.2011.142.
7. Persoons P, Vermeire S, Demyttenaere K, Fischler B, Vandenberghe J, Van Oudenhove L, Pierik M, Hlavaty T, Van Assche G, Norman M, Rutgeerts P. The impact of major depressive disorder on the short- and long-term outcome of Crohn's disease treatment with infliximab. AlimPharmacolTherap.2005;22(2):101–10.http://doi.org/10.1111/j.1365-2036.2005.02535.x.
8. Schwarz SP, Blanchard EB, Berreman CF, Scharff L, Taylor AE, Greene BR, Suls JM, Malamood HS. Psychological aspects of irritable bowel syndrome: comparisons with inflammatory bowel disease and nonpatient controls. Behav Res Ther. 1993;31(3):297–304.
9. Porcelli P, Zaka S, Centonze S, Sisto G. Psychological distress and levels of disease activity in inflammatory bowel disease. Ital J Gastroenterol. 1994;26(3):111–5.
10. Maunder RG, Lancee WJ, Hunter JJ, Greenberg GR, Steinhart AH. Attachment insecurity moderates the relationship between disease activity and depressive symptoms in ulcerative colitis. Inflamm Bowel Dis. 2005;11(10):919–26. http://doi.org/10.1097/01.mib.0000179468.78876.2d.
11. Maunder RG, Greenberg GR, Hunter JJ, Lancee WJ, Steinhart AH, Silverberg MS. Psychobiological subtypes of ulcerative colitis: pANCA status moderates the relationship between disease activity and psychological distress. Am J Gastroenterol. 2006;101(11):2546–51. http://doi.org/10.1111/j.1572-0241.2006.00798.x.
12. Larsson K, Sundberg Hjelm M, Karlbom U, Nordin K, Anderberg UM, Lööf L. A group-based patient education programme for high-anxiety patients with Crohn disease or ulcerative colitis. Scand J Gastroenterol. 2003;38(7):763–9. http://doi.org/10.1080/00365520310003309.
13. Mussell M, Böcker U, Nagel N, Olbrich R, Singer MV. Reducing psychological distress in patients with inflammatory bowel disease by cognitive-behavioural treatment: exploratory study of effectiveness. Scand J Gastroenterol. 2003;38(7):755–62. http://doi.org/10.1080/00365520310003110.

14. Ali T, Hasan M, Hamadani M, Harly RF. Gastroparesis. South Med J. 2007;100(3):281–6. doi:10.1097/SMJ.0b013e31802f3795.
15. Camilleri M, Parkman HP, Shafi MA, Abell TL, Gerson L. Clinical guideline: management of gastroparesis. Am J Gastroenterol. 2013;108(1):18–37. http://doi.org/10.1038/ajg.2012.373.
16. Kim KH, Lee MS, Choi T-Y, Kim T-H, Ernst E. Acupuncture for symptomatic gastroparesis. Cochrane Database Syst Rev. 2012. http://onlinelibrary.wiley.com/doi/10.1002/14651858. CD009676/abstract.
17. Hasler WL, Parkman HP, Wilson LA, Pasricha PJ, Koch KL, Abell TL, Snape WJ, Farrugia G, Lee L, Tonascia J, Unalp-Arida A, Hamilton F. Psychological dysfunction is associated with symptom severity but not disease etiology or degree of gastric retention in patients with gastroparesis. Am J Gastroenterol. 2010;105(11):2357–67. http://doi.org/10.1038/ajg.2010.253.
18. Maleki D, Locke III G, Camilleri M, et al. GAstrointestinal tract symptoms among persons with diabetes mellitus in the community. Arch Intern Med. 2000;160(18):2808–16. http://doi.org/10.1001/archinte.160.18.2808.
19. Talley SJ, Bytzer P, Hammer J, Young L, Jones M, Horowitz M. Psychological distress is linked to gastrointestinal symptoms in diabetes mellitus. Am J Gastroenterol. 2001;96(4):1033–8. http://doi.org/10.1111/j.1572-0241.2001.03605.x.
20. Abell TL, Bernstein VK, Cutts T, Farrugia G, Forster J, Hasler WL, Mccallum RW, Oldn KW, Parkman HP, Parrish CR, Pasricha PJ, Prather CM, Soffer EE, Twillman R, Vinik AI. Treatment of gastroparesis: a multidisciplinary clinical review. Neurogastroenterol Motil. 2006;18:263–83. doi:10.1111/j.1365-2982.2006.00760.x.
21. Drossman DA, Talley NJ, Leserman J, Olden KW, Barriero MA. Sexual and physical abuse in gastrointestinal illness. Review and recommendations. Ann Intern Med. 1995;123:782–94.
22. Wagner EH, Glasgow RE, Davis C, Bonomi AE, Provost L, McCulloch D, Carver P, Sixta C. Quality improvement in chronic illness care: a collaborative approach. Jt Comm J Qual Improv. 2001;27:63–80.
23. Fass R, Naliboff BD, Fass SS, Peleg N, Wendel C, Malagon IB, Mayer EA. The effect of auditory stress on perception of intraesophageal acid in patients with gastroesophageal reflux disease. Gastroenterology. 2008;134(3):696–705. http://doi.org/10.1053/j.gastro.2007.12.010.
24. Yoshida N. Inflammation and oxidative stress in gastroesophageal reflux disease. J Clin Biochem Nutr. 2007;40(1):13–23. http://doi.org/10.3164/jcbn.40.13.
25. McDonald-Halie J, Bradley LA, Bailey MA, Schan CA, Richter JE. Relaxation training reduces symptom reports and acid exposure in patients with gastroesophageal reflux disease. Gastroenterology. 1994;107(1):61–9.
26. Kamolz T, Granderath FA, Bammer T, Pasiut M, Pointner R. Psychological intervention influences the outcome of laparoscopic antireflux surgery in patients with stress-related symptoms of gastroesophageal reflux disease. Scand J Gastroenterol. 2001;36(8):800–5. doi:10.1080/00365520117106.
27. Talley N, Napthali K. Cyclical vomiting syndrome. In: Lacy B, Crowell M, DiBaise J, editors. Functional and motility disorders of the gastrointestinal tract. New York: Springer; 2015. p. 101–10.
28. Magagna J. Psychophysiologic treatment of cyclic vomiting. J Pediatr Gastroenterol Nutr. 1995;21 Suppl 1:S31–6.
29. Reinhart JB, Evans SL, McFadden DL. Cyclic vomit in children: seen through the psychiatrist's eye. Pediatrics. 1977;59(3):371–7.
30. Tarbell S, Li BU. Psychiatric symptoms in children and adolescents with cyclic vomiting syndrome and their parents. Headache. 2008;48(2):259–66. http://doi.org/10.1111/j.1526-4610.2007.00997.x.
31. Fleisher DR, Gornowicz B, Adams K, Burch R, Feldman EJ. Cyclic vomiting syndrome in 41 adults: the illness, the patients, and problems of management. BMC Med. 2005;3(1):20. http://doi.org/10.1186/1741-7015-3-20.
32. Slutsker B, Konichezky A, Gothelf D. Breaking the cycle: cognitive behavioral therapy and biofeedback training in a case of cyclic vomiting syndrome. Psychol Health Med. 2010;15(6):625–31. http://doi.org/10.1080/13548506.2010.498893.
33. Graff LA, Walker JR, Bernstein CN. Depression and anxiety in inflammatory bowel disease: a review of comorbidity and management. Inflamm Bowel Dis. 2009;15(7):1105–18. http://doi.org/10.1002/ibd.20873.

34. Walker JR, Ediger JP, Graff LA, Greenfeld JM, Clara I, Lix L, Rawsthorne P, Miller N, Rogala L, McPhail CM, Bernstein CN. The Manitoba IBD cohort study: a population-based study of the prevalence of lifetime and 12-month anxiety and mood disorders. Am J Gastroenterol. 2008;103(8):1989–97. http://doi.org/10.1111/j.1572-0241.2008.01980.x.
35. Fuller-Thomson E, Sulman J. Depression and inflammatory bowel disease: findings from two nationally representative Canadian surveys. Inflamm Bowel Dis. 2006;12(8):697–707. http://doi.org/10.1097/00054725-200608000-00005.
36. Szigethy E, Carpenter J, Baum E, Kenney E, Baptista-Neto L, Beardslee WR, Demaso DR. Case study: longitudinal treatment of adolescents with depression and inflammatory bowel disease. J Am Acad Child Adolesc Psychiatry. 2006;45(4):396–400. http://doi.org/10.1097/01.chi.0000198591.45949.a4.
37. Szigethy E, Kenney E, Carpenter J, Hardy DM, Fairclough D, Bousvaros A, Keljo D, Weisz J, Beardslee WR, Noll R, DeMaso DR. Cognitive-behavioral therapy for adolescents with inflammatory bowel disease and subsyndromal depression. J Am Acad Child Adolesc Psychiatry. 2007;46(10):1290–98. http://doi.org/10.1097/chi.0b013e3180f6341f.
38. Szigethy E, Whitton SW, Levy-Warren A, DeMaso DR, Weisz J, Beardslee WR. Cognitive-behavioral therapy for depression in adolescents with inflammatory bowel disease: a pilot study. J Am Acad Child Adolesc Psychiatry. 2004;43(12):1469–77. http://doi.org/10.1097/01.chi.0000142284.10574.1f.
39. Díaz Sibaja MA, Comeche Moreno MI, Mas Hesse B. Tratamiento cognitivo-conductual protocolizado en grupo de las enfermedades inflamatorias intestinales. Revista Española de Enfermedades Digestivas 2007;99(10). http://doi.org/10.4321/S1130-01082007001000006.
40. Ost LG, Sterner U. Applied tension. A specific behavioral method for treatment of blood phobia. Behav Res Ther. 1987;25(1):25–9.
41. Kabat-Zinn J. Mindfulness-based interventions in context: past, present, and future. Clin Psychol Sci Pract. 2003;10(2):144–56. doi:10.1093/clipsy/bpg016.
42. Lee SJ, Maizels RM. Inflammatory Bowel Disease. Evolution, Medicine, and Public Health. 2014;2014(1):95. doi:10.1093/emph/eou017.

Resources (Websites, Books, etc.)

International Foundation for Functional Gastrointestinal Disorders (IFFGD). A nonprofit organization whose mission is to inform, assist, and support people affected by gastrointestinal disorders of function and motility, like gastroparesis. www.aboutGastroparesis.org

Digestive Health Alliance (DHA). The grassroots arm of IFFGD where individuals can interact and take action to improve treatments and help find cures for functional GI and motility disorders, like gastroparesis, through coordinated fundraising, advocacy, and awareness efforts. www.dha.org

Crystal Zaborowski Saltrelli CHC. Living (well!) with gastroparesis—answers, advice, tips and recipes for a healthier, happier life. This book is a comprehensive and easy to follow guide to navigating life after a gastroparesis diagnosis. Amazon.com

Gastroparesis Patient Association for Cures and Treatments (G-PACT). A nonprofit organization dedicated to increasing awareness of gastroparesis and chronic intestinal pseudo-obstruction. www.g-pact.org

The Oley Foundation. A nonprofit organization whose mission is to enrich the lives of patients dependent on home intravenous (parenteral) and tube feeding (enteral) through education, outreach, and networking. www.oley.org

The National Institutes of Health (NIH), Gastroparesis Clinical Research Consortium (GpCRC). A network of medical centers, sponsored by the National Institute of Diabetes and Digestive and Kidney Diseases (NIDDK), established to improve understanding of the cause and natural course of gastroparesis and to advance the diagnosis and treatment of this disorder. www.jhucct.com/gpcrc

Chapter 8
Cancer

Lara Traeger, Jamie M. Jacobs, Giselle Perez-Lougee, Joseph A. Greer, and Elyse R. Park

8.1 Cancer

Cancer involves the uncontrolled growth of abnormal cells in the body. Internal factors (e.g., genetic mutations) and external factors (e.g., tobacco use, sun exposure, or infectious agents such as hepatitis C virus) increase risk for developing specific cancer types. In many cases, cancer may develop over several years before available tests can detect it. Physicians stage cancers at the time of diagnosis and use this information to plan treatment and evaluate prognosis. Solid tumors typically are staged according to the size of the primary tumor, involvement of regional lymph nodes, and spread to distal parts of the body. Hematologic cancers including leukemia and lymphoma are identified and staged based on different cellular classification systems.

L. Traeger, Ph.D. (✉) • E.R. Park, Ph.D., M.P.H.
Behavioral Medicine Service, Department of Psychiatry, Massachusetts General Hospital, Harvard Medical School, Boston, MA, USA
e-mail: ltraeger@mgh.harvard.edu; epark@mgh.harvard.edu

J.M. Jacobs, Ph.D. • G. Perez-Lougee, Ph.D.
Massachusetts General Hospital, 55 Fruit Street, Boston, MA 02114, USA
e-mail: jjacobs@mgh.harvard.edu; gperez@mgh.harvard.edu

J.A. Greer, Ph.D.
Center for Psychiatric Oncology & Behavioral Sciences, Massachusetts General Hospital Cancer Center, Yawkey Suite 10B, 55 Fruit Street, Boston, MA 02114, USA
e-mail: jgreer2@mgh.harvard.edu

© Springer Science+Business Media New York 2017
A.-M. Vranceanu et al. (eds.), *The Massachusetts General Hospital Handbook of Behavioral Medicine*, Current Clinical Psychiatry,
DOI 10.1007/978-3-319-29294-6_8

8.1.1 Demographics

Cancer represents a worldwide burden, affecting both more and less economically developed countries [1]. As of 2014 approximately 14.5 million people in the USA were living with a history of cancer, ranging from a recent diagnosis to long-term survivorship [2]. Prostate and breast cancers are the most commonly diagnosed cancers in US men and women, respectively, with lung and colorectal cancers representing the second and third most common cancers for both sexes. Across all cancers, the US 5-year relative survival rate is 68 %, representing an increase over the past several decades due to improvements in early screening and treatment [2].

Cancer survival rates vary by cancer type and stage, individual differences (e.g., biobehavioral factors and comorbid health issues), and disparities in access to care, among other factors. For instance, the current US 5-year relative survival rates for colorectal cancer versus lung cancer are 90 % versus 54 % (local disease), 71 % versus 17 % (regional disease), and 13 % versus 4 % (distal disease). Most lung cancers are diagnosed at an advanced stage, and this cancer type accounts for the highest estimated proportion of US cancer-related deaths in men and women for 2015 [2]. Patients in poverty face significant barriers to early cancer screening, detection and optimal treatment. Poverty and social inequities contribute to poorer cancer outcomes for many US racial/ethnic minority patients [3]; across all cancer types, non-Hispanic black adults face greater risk of cancer-related death than any other racial/ethnic group [2].

For simplicity, this chapter will use the term "patient" when referring to individuals with cancer. However, many practitioners, advocates, and individuals affected by cancer consider survivorship to start at diagnosis, given that the need to focus on health and well-being begins at diagnosis and continues to evolve over time.

8.2 Patient Experiences

When patients engage in cancer care, they enter a complex system of medical, nursing, pharmacy, and allied health professionals. Treatments are multidisciplinary and may involve surgery, chemotherapy, and/or radiation, depending on the type and stage of cancer and other clinical factors. Other treatments include stem cell or bone marrow transplant, hormone therapy, immunotherapy, and targeted therapies. These systemic therapies can be administered alone or in combination, which requires a high level of coordination among providers.

Patients often experience greater symptom burden from treatment than from the cancer itself. For patients receiving active therapy, symptoms such as fatigue, nausea/vomiting, constipation, diarrhea, and neuropathic pain can negatively impact daily functioning and quality of life (QOL; [4–6]). Since active therapies primarily are administered in outpatient settings, patients must triage and manage complications while at home. Self-care routines involve adhering to adjuvant medications (e.g., antiemetics), altering diet and activity levels, and maintaining communication with oncology providers. The high prevalence of poorly controlled symptoms [6] underscores the importance of self-care and collaboration with the oncology team. Moreover, some problems such as fatigue respond minimally to available medical treatments [7, 8]. This gap further highlights the importance of behavioral strategies to help patients manage symptoms and their impact on QOL. Survivorship care guidelines also emphasize the importance of health behaviors (e.g., smoking cessation, nutrition, physical activity) well after treatment completion, in order to minimize chronic and late-onset complications and reduce risk of recurrence, new cancer, or comorbid disease [9].

Following completion of active treatment, patients attend regular follow-up oncology visits for surveillance; a portion of patients may receive additional treatment (e.g., endocrine therapy) to reduce risk of progression or recurrence. Patients may continue to experience fears of suffering, disease recurrence, disease progression, mortality, or the impact of cancer on loved ones. Some treatments will lead to disfigurement (e.g., mastectomy, rectal excision, or ostomy placement) and/or changes in sexual and reproductive health [10]. Patients may struggle with concerns about body image and identity (see more information in section, *Specific Populations: Long-Term Survivorship*). Moreover, cognitive changes and other health factors may delay or impede return to work, exacerbating the economic strain of cancer. Patients with metastatic disease may continue with active treatment to help control cancer progression and/or palliate pain symptoms; complex factors influence the decision to discontinue treatment in these cases [11].

8.2.1   Depression

Adults with cancer face higher risk of major depression relative to those in the general population [12]. In hematology/oncology settings, the prevalence of major depressive disorder is approximately 15 %, and the prevalence of major and minor depression and dysthymia combined is approximately 21 %. Low engagement in medical care has been identified as a marker of depression in cancer [13]. Depression symptoms increase patient risk for misunderstanding provider recommendations, fearing cancer treatment complications, and perceiving practical barriers to treatment [14], with some evidence that depressed patients are less likely to accept and complete optimal treatment regimens [15]. Among patients with end-stage cancer, depression symptoms also may interfere with acceptance of prognosis [16], which can complicate decision-making about end-of-life care [17].

8.2.2 Anxiety

For many patients, anxiety can fluctuate at specific points such as before receipt of test results or at the start or completion of treatment. Worried thoughts are commonly marked by fears of cancer recurrence and progression. However, a minority of patients will experience clinically significant anxiety symptoms [18] and approximately 10 % of adult patients will meet criteria for an anxiety disorder [19]. Post-traumatic stress symptoms also have been reported secondary to cancer-related events [20]. Moderate-to-severe anxiety affects a patient's ability to differentiate real versus imagined threat. Patients with anxiety experience more severe symptom burden, engage in less effective medical decision-making, and are more likely to experience chemotherapy dose delays/reductions [21–23]. Social anxiety may limit critical communication with oncology providers. Needle phobia interferes with critical tests and treatments. Even subclinical anxiety may cause patients to either avoid or compulsively seek prognostic information [24].

8.2.3 Cognitive-Behavioral Cycle of Psychological Distress and Disability

Psychological distress can exacerbate general medical symptoms through a reinforcing cycle [25, 26]. For instance, patients who are anxious about their existing dyspnea (breathlessness) may attempt to avoid worsening this problem by decreasing physical activity. Paradoxically, this strategy can lead patients to heighten their attention to even slight or transient respiratory sensations. This path can evolve into a cycle in which distress and avoidance further heighten sensitivity, anxiety, and avoidance of physical activity, increasing risk of physical deconditioning.

8.2.4 Resiliency and Growth

In some cases, patients with cancer may be able to protect themselves from decrements in QOL by maintaining flexibility and recalibrating/reprioritizing expectations and goals in their life [27]. A growing literature also highlights that patients may channel emotionally disruptive cancer experiences into positive life changes [28]. Across both health and non-health-related traumas, younger age and severity of the traumatic event have been associated with more personal growth [28]. Moreover, in cancer, younger patients report higher rates of psychological distress relative to older patients [29]. Taken together, these findings support that psychological responses to cancer may evolve with increasing age, and that those who experience cancer as more disruptive also may be more likely to report personal growth from their cancer experiences [30].

8.3   Behavioral Medicine in Cancer

8.3.1   Background and Rationale

Behavioral medicine for patients with cancer targets the following aims: (1) reduce psychological distress, (2) improve quality of life (QOL) and functional status, (3) increase adherence to medical regimens or specific health behaviors, and/or (4) manage side effects related to cancer or its treatment. Practitioners also may assist patients and families in coping with anticipatory grief, bereavement, loss of dignity, or other existential or end-of-life concerns. Behavioral medicine interventions commonly are multi-modal and target multiple outcomes. Trained providers may deliver interventions in individual or group settings, or in a clinical setting such as a chemotherapy or radiotherapy unit. Common intervention strategies include cognitive-behavioral, supportive-expressive, and relaxation- or mindfulness-based techniques, as described in this chapter. When possible, practitioners should collaborate with the oncology team and other specialists involved in the patient's care.

8.3.2   Assessment

Behavioral medicine assessments in cancer focus on presenting concerns. Current quality cancer care guidelines identify screening for psychological distress, pain, and fatigue as part of the standard of care [31]. See Table 8.1 for a brief list of example self-report instruments. With respect to psychological distress, single items (e.g., depression or anxiety rating in the past week) provide rapid screens whereas unidimensional instruments offer more robust scores that can be evaluated against established cut-offs [48]. For instance, the 14-item Hospital Anxiety and Depression Scale (HADS; [35]) is an efficient measure of anxiety and depression symptoms that has shown good psychometric properties in psychosocial intervention trials in cancer [49]. The nine-item Patient Health Questionnaire (PHQ-9; [36]) is a validated and recommended screen for clinical depression in longitudinal cancer studies [50]. Patients who screen positive for psychological distress should be referred for more in-depth practitioner assessment when available [51].

Identification of pain and fatigue depends on patient self-report [52]. While there are no gold standard measures, simple one-item screens can facilitate symptom tracking over time. Unidimensional instruments such as the Brief Pain Inventory [37] and Brief Fatigue Inventory [38] evaluate symptom severity and impact on functioning. Longer, multidimensional instruments (e.g., Multidimensional Fatigue Inventory [42]) evaluate symptoms across somatic, cognitive, affective, and behavioral dimensions. Practitioners should explore the effects of symptoms on sleep, relationships, and other QOL domains. This information may be part of, or a trigger for, a multidisciplinary evaluation to develop an appropriate care plan.

Table 8.1 Behavioral medicine assessment in cancer: example self-report instruments

Types	Domains	Example instruments	Citations
Rapid screens	Pain, fatigue, various	Visual analog scale	See reviews, [32, 33]
	Pain, fatigue, various	Numeric rating scale	
	Pain, fatigue, various	Verbal rating scale	
	Anxiety, depression	Patient Health Questionnaire-4	[34]
Unidimensional instruments	Anxiety, depression	Hospital Anxiety and Depression Scale	[35]
	Depression	Patient Health Questionnaire-9	[36]
	Pain	Brief Pain Inventory	[37]
	Fatigue	Brief Fatigue Inventory	[38]
	Medication adherence	Modified Morisky Medication Adherence Scale	[39]
	Physical activity	Physical Activity Questionnaire	[40]
Multidimensional instruments	Quality of life	Functional Assessment of Cancer Therapy	[41]
	Fatigue	Multidimensional Fatigue Inventory	[42]
	Social support	Multidimensional Scale of Perceived Social Support	[43]
	Social support	Medical Outcomes Social Support Survey	[44]
Multi-symptom inventories	Multiple relevant symptoms	Edmonton Symptom Assessment Scale	[128]
		MD Anderson Symptom Inventory	[45]
		Memorial Symptom Assessment Scale	[46]
		Rotterdam Symptom Checklist	[47]

A number of factors affect behavioral medicine assessment in patients with cancer. For one, symptoms frequently cluster together. Depression and anxiety can co-occur with cancer- or treatment-related fatigue, pain, poor appetite, cognitive changes, and respiratory difficulties [53–55]. Anxiety symptoms also can indicate the presence of a metabolic disorder, cardiac symptoms, adverse medication effects, or abrupt withdrawal from medications such as opioids. When conducting a differential diagnosis of new onset psychiatric symptoms, practitioners must include cancer-related complications.

A second factor is that, as mentioned earlier, psychiatric symptoms fluctuate during active cancer therapies and points of transition (e.g., initiating or completing treatment). This factor complicates the differentiation of problems such as major depressive disorder, adjustment disorder, and normative emotional responses to cancer [56]. Fluctuations highlight the need to evaluate patients regularly throughout their cancer trajectory.

Finally, we suggest adapting assessments for patients who are experiencing cognitive changes due to cancer, treatment complications, or other factors. Practitioners may supplement symptom inventories by eliciting qualitative information about functioning throughout a typical day, without requiring 1- or 2-week recall. Family and close friends may provide corroborative information about symptom patterns over time. These strategies also may assist practitioners in assessing patients who minimize somatic symptoms because they consider them to be an expected part of cancer or normal aging; want to be perceived as a good patient; or fear that symptom disclosure might delay their current anticancer treatment.

8.3.3 Psychoeducation

Psychoeducation incorporates health information with psychological support and stress management elements. Practitioners may use psychoeducation to help patients reduce emotional distress or confusion around their cancer diagnosis [57]; prepare for anticancer treatments and potential side effects [48]; and improve stress management, pain management, and QOL [48, 58, 59]. Psychoeducation also may be instrumental in reinforcing adherence to self-administered treatments such as oral chemotherapies or supportive care regimens [60]. For instance, patients who are prescribed opioids for pain may benefit from reviewing information about pain, the role of long-acting versus short-acting medications, and strategies for managing opioid side effects such as constipation. Practitioners may facilitate opportunities for the patient to clarify clinical misconceptions with the oncology team in a supportive environment.

8.3.4 Motivational Interviewing

Motivational interviewing (MI) is a counseling style in which open-ended questions are used to help patients elicit intrinsic motivation to work toward stated goals [61]. Brief MI may set the stage for a behavioral medicine intervention and then may be used over the course of the intervention to explore ambivalence and revisit goals. For patients with cancer, MI may help them to change behaviors that are relevant to health, QOL, and cancer prevention, such as smoking cessation [62]. MI also may elicit motivation for adherence to active cancer treatments, long-term endocrine therapies, and supportive care regimens. The practitioner should monitor motivation given that patients may experience decreased self-efficacy or sense of control in the context of intensive treatments and uncertain disease course. MI also may facilitate motivation for increasing or maintaining health behaviors after patients have completed active treatments, in order to reduce risk of residual and late-onset complications.

8.3.5 Cognitive Behavioral Therapy

Cognitive behavioral therapy (CBT) reflects a time-limited and skills-based approach, with a focus on reducing symptoms. CBT is rooted in the theory that a person's interpretation of a stressor influences the persons' emotional response and the ability to problem-solve the stressful situation. A CBT intervention may begin with an explanation of the theoretical model of CBT and rationale for the proposed strategies. The practitioner and patient may optimize therapeutic gains by discussing upfront the roles of session attendance and practice exercises between sessions.

CBT in cancer can be used to empower patients with skills for optimal self-care. CBT interventions have been shown to reduce depression, anxiety, and sleep disturbances and improve symptom management and QOL in cancer [63–68]. Depression and anxiety are related to problems with completion of treatment regimens [69]. CBT interventions can be formulated to co-target patient skills for improving mood, adherence, and self-care behaviors [70]. Below, we describe common CBT strategies and other interventions that may be paired with CBT (e.g., relaxation training), with attention to adapting them for patients with cancer. Each technique can be used as a stand-alone intervention or combined into a larger protocol, as described in this chapter's case illustration and as shown in a structured protocol that Greer and colleagues developed to treat anxiety in patients with advanced cancer (see Table 8.2; [64, 71]).

Behavioral Activation. Behavioral activation (BA) is an empirically validated treatment which helps patients to increase or reengage in pleasurable and meaningful activities, and therefore increase exposure to natural reinforcements [72]. BA may help patients with cancer to improve depression, anxiety, QOL and functional status [72, 73]. Importantly, factors such as fatigue or compromised immune function can impede engagement in activities that are important to a patient's QOL and identity. Practitioners and patients may work on (1) finding new ways in which the patient can stay engaged in areas of life that bolster QOL and identity, and (2) communicating with the oncology team about modifiable symptoms. Since patients may find cancer to be a socially isolating experience, practitioners and patients may problem-solve ways for the patient to maintain connections with loved ones and/or forge new connections with other patients. Finally, practitioners and patients can pair BA with health behavior goals (e.g., physical activity) that target both health and QOL.

Cognitive Restructuring. Cognitive restructuring, a core CBT element, involves increasing awareness of severe, irrational and unhelpful thoughts about a stressful situation ("*My test results are going to show that my cancer has returned*") and then replacing these thoughts with more accurate and helpful ones ("*While I don't know what the test results will show, I have a good team supporting me*"). The practitioner may use Socratic questioning to help patients challenge their severe thoughts and

Table 8.2 Brief structured intervention for treating anxiety in advanced cancer

Module	No. of sessions	Techniques	Description
1	1	Psychoeducation goal setting	– Explore patient's cancer-related experiences
			– Discuss patient's understanding of current anxiety in relation to advanced cancer and other factors
			– Introduce and develop cognitive-behavioral model of anxiety in context of patient's concerns
			– Collaborate with patient to set treatment goals
			– Explore motivation for working toward goals
2	1	Relaxation training	– Provide information about physiologic stress response and how it may impact other cancer-related symptoms
			– Assist patient in recognizing own stress symptoms
			– Introduce exercises to elicit the relaxation response
			– Audio record exercises during session and explore ways to develop a regular practice
3	2–3	Coping with cancer fears	– Introduce concept of automatic worried thoughts
			– Identify patient's worries and how they may interfere with functioning and QOL
			– Introduce and practice strategies for differentiating realistic versus unrealistic worries
			– Practice applying strategies for coping with worries that are realistic, unrealistic, or unclear (see Fig. 8.1)
4	1	Activity planning and pacing	– Explore daily activities and priorities, and daily fluctuations in energy/well-being
			– Practice evaluating current level of energy/well-being per day and throughout each day
			– Plan and pace daily activities by feasible blocks of time
			– Modify activities and utilize social support as needed to stay engaged with activities without over-exertion
5	1	Skill review and maintenance	– Review skills covered during prior sessions
			– Problem-solve strategies for maintaining skills

Based on intervention protocol by Greer et al. [71]

practice generating new interpretations. For patients with cancer, a common CBT goal is to foster adaptive appraisals of cancer diagnosis, treatment, and related stressors [48]. However, some patients may experience realistic concerns about feared events such as cancer progression, and in other cases, a patient's risk of progression may not be clear. Greer et al. [74] adapted a decisional model that practitioners may use to help patients assess negative thoughts for realistic and unrealistic components (see Fig. 8.1). When a patient ruminates about realistic risks, acceptance-oriented strategies such as mindfulness (as described later in this chapter) may be warranted. When risk is not clear, practitioners and patients may focus on obtaining more information (e.g., communicating with the oncology team about clinical concerns).

Problem-Solving Therapy. Problem-solving therapy introduces a decision-making framework to help patients identify and resolve current problems while increasing self-efficacy, confidence, and perceived control [75]. For instance, a patient who feels hopeless about managing severe cancer-related gastrointestinal

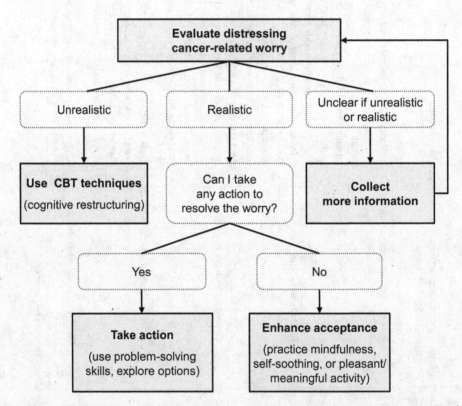

Fig. 8.1 Decisional model for coping with cancer-related worry. Adapted from Greer JA, Graham JS, Safren SA. Resolving treatment complications associated with comorbid medical conditions. In M. Otto & S. Hofmann. (Eds). Avoiding treatment failure in anxiety disorders. New York: Springer, 2009

symptoms might practice: (a) defining the problem ("*I can't enjoy time with friends and family due to my symptoms*"); (b) generating possible solutions (*using daily reminders to take prophylactic medications; practicing mind–body techniques; adjusting daytime activity schedule; communicating with family and oncology team*); (c) selecting optimal solutions; and (d) implementing the chosen solution and monitoring the outcome. Problem-solving therapy has been shown to reduce psychological distress and improve symptom management in patients with cancer [66, 76, 77]. Practitioners and patients should consider how social workers, case managers, and family caregivers, when available, may assist the patient in brainstorming and accessing possible solutions to practical problems (e.g., financial or transportation barriers to treatment).

Exposure. Exposure-based interventions, such as prolonged exposure or systematic desensitization, may be used to reduce anticipatory nausea/vomiting, needle phobia, or anxious avoidance of objects, individuals, or events that patients associate with their cancer and treatment [78, 79]. Generally, the practitioner guides the patient through graded exposure to cues that trigger increasing levels of anxiety, while assisting the patient in utilizing counter-conditioning or other new coping strategies to reduce the anxiety. For instance, during systematic desensitization for a patient with anticipatory nausea/vomiting, the patient may learn to pair a relaxation response with identified stimuli (e.g., sights and sounds that the patient associates with chemotherapy) in order to decondition the unwanted behavioral response (nausea) that has been paired with these stimuli. While exposure requires patients to experience anxiety-provoking stimuli in order to habituate to them, oncology settings commonly use short-acting anxiety medications including benzodiazepines to provide immediate relief from panic symptoms and nausea [80]. The practitioner and oncology team should prioritize strategies for facilitating patient access to feared but time-sensitive procedures and treatments, while also increasing patient skills for reducing their anxiety in the long term.

8.3.6 Relaxation Training and Hypnotherapy

Practitioners may administer relaxation training within the context of CBT or as a stand-alone stress management intervention. A variety of techniques (e.g., progressive muscle relaxation, guided visual imagery, and diaphragmatic breathing) can help patients to activate a hypometabolic physiologic state and reduce physical and emotional tension [81]. Relaxation training has been used to help patients with cancer manage pain, nausea, and fatigue; reduce depression and anxiety symptoms; and improve functional status and QOL [58, 59, 82, 83]. Moreover, relaxation exercises represent a portable strategy that patients can use in oncology settings. For instance, patients can practice relaxation to reduce tension and distress in the moment, while they await or undergo procedures (e.g., breast biopsies), chemotherapy, or radiation treatments [84, 85]. Prior to introducing relaxation, practitioners may provide information about the evolutionary function of stress symptoms and the rationale for eliciting the relaxation response. Practitioners and patients also should account for current symptoms (dyspnea, pain, etc.) when exploring which relaxation techniques will best fit patients' preferences and needs.

Hypnosis in health care settings is a psychotherapeutic technique in which the practitioner helps the patient generate a relaxed state of focused attention and then provides "suggestions for changes in sensation, perception, cognition, affect, mood or behavior" [86, p 81]. For patients with cancer, hypnosis either alone or in combination with CBT has reduced psychological distress, nausea, pain, and fatigue in the context of surgery, active treatments, and terminal disease [87–89], with evidence that hypnosis may reduce the amount of analgesic and sedative medication used during surgery [88]. Practitioners can teach self-hypnosis to patients, for symptom management as needed.

8.3.7 Supportive-Expressive Psychotherapy

Supportive-expressive psychotherapy is one of the most commonly used therapies in practice. In group settings, supportive-expressive psychotherapy fosters a validating environment in which patients can process their experiences with cancer and treatment and receive support from other group members and the facilitator. Components may include validation, supportive/empathic listening, expressive writing, stress management, problem-solving, and education [90]. Patients also may explore ways to improve communication with friends, family, and their oncology team. Supportive-expressive psychotherapy has reduced fatigue, depression, and anxiety symptoms in cancer [65, 91]. Supportive group therapy also may help patients with advanced cancer to process spiritual or existential end-of-life concerns [92].

8.3.8 Mindfulness

Mindfulness-based therapies involve establishing an intentional practice of non-judgmental awareness of present-moment feelings, thoughts, and bodily sensations. Practitioners may introduce mindfulness to help patients cultivate attention, acceptance, and emotional tolerance of current stressors that appear uncontrollable. This type of practice may assist patients in reducing persistent stressful rumination about what caused their disease (a focus on the past), or whether their disease will progress (a focus on the future). Practitioners may guide patients in fostering mindfulness through daily practice of body scans, yoga, or walking and sitting mediations. Mindfulness-based protocols may reduce depression and anxiety symptoms and facilitate personal growth in patients and survivors [93, 94]. Mindfulness in combination with CBT also has shown evidence for improving sexual function in women with gynecologic cancers [95].

8.3.9 Case Illustration

Andre is a 70-year-old contractor, husband, and father of two adult sons who was diagnosed with advanced colon cancer 6 months ago. He attends an oncology clinic every 2 weeks to receive intravenous chemotherapy and meet with his oncology team. While Andre does not always take antiemetic and antidiarrheal medications as his team recommends, he feels proud that he can tolerate chemotherapy side effects that intensify during the few days after each chemotherapy infusion. However, fatigue is the one symptom that Andre can't seem to control. He stopped taking on new contracting jobs and is struggling to complete chores around the house or finish the remodeling work that he started in his own kitchen. Instead, Andre increasingly takes daytime naps—something he can't remember doing since childhood. He is frustrated, irritable, and ashamed. Fatigue is a persistent reminder that he is a weakened version of himself. He believes that his wife is beginning to resent him for lagging on responsibilities at home. When Andre cannot be productive, he views himself as a fraud. He often struggles to get out of bed and face his family and friends, and now prefers to spend more time alone.

Andre's wife has noticed his depressed and irritable moods, despite his efforts to hide them. She mentions them during his next oncology visit. The oncology team nurse suggests a referral for psychosocial services. The nurse normalizes the referral, noting that the team recommends an introductory visit for each patient. Andre does not think his problems warrant attention, but he agrees to meet with a CBT practitioner for evaluation.

At Andre's initial CBT evaluation, the practitioner encourages Andre to tell his story about his cancer experiences. As he explains, she notes his thoughts, feelings, and coping behaviors, and causal relationships among them. She then provides brief psychoeducation about the purpose and rationale for CBT in the context of Andre's presenting concerns. The practitioner also addresses Andre's ambivalence about engaging in CBT. He notes that at this time, he is motivated in part by his wife's concern (*"It makes her happy that I'm seeing you."*). The practitioner normalizes Andre's belief that needing support is a sign of weakness, by providing information about common physical and emotional distress symptoms experienced by individuals in his situation. She uses MI to help Andre identify his intrinsic motivation for enhancing strategies to improve his coping and QOL. Andre agrees to initiate CBT. The practitioner and Andre agree to schedule sessions in tandem with Andre's chemotherapy visits when possible and to avoid scheduling on days immediately following chemotherapy when side effects are most severe.

The first session focuses on Andre's current concerns. The practitioner creates a CBT model to illustrate causal relationships among Andre's physical experiences (*fatigue*), thoughts (*I am a weakened version of myself*), feelings (*despondence, shame*), and coping behaviors (*social isolation*). She uses Socratic questioning to assist Andre in identifying these relationships and further developing the model. The practitioner and Andre then work to identify his treatment goals (*to increase my energy; reduce my depressed mood and irritability; and be productive at home*).

The practitioner introduces specific CBT techniques to address Andre's goals and conveys optimism in his ability to achieve them. They formulate a treatment plan that targets his concerns about fatigue, mood, and productivity. Andre's elevated score on a self-report measure of depression supports that depression impacts his QOL and highlights specific depression symptoms that may be amenable to change. At each subsequent session, Andre completes the self-report measure to monitor goal progress. The practitioner uses MI as needed to help Andre elicit personal autonomy and motivation to work toward his goals.

The practitioner first provides psychoeducation about cancer-related symptoms and mood, and their influences on QOL. During this discussion, Andre considers how his belief that fatigue is a sign of weakness could worsen his overall experience of fatigue. He also realizes that while he avoids taking adjuvant medications whenever possible, his gastrointestinal symptoms further limit him from leaving the house and making plans with family and friends. Overall, Andre reflects that by enhancing his self-care and adherence to medication targeting his symptoms, he might improve his current QOL.

The practitioner introduces BA to help Andre reengage in meaningful and enjoyable activities. They spend time brainstorming activities that would help Andre connect with his identity as a contractor and productive person, while also accounting for times in which his energy level is low. To this end, the practitioner introduces time-based pacing, in which activities are limited to specific amounts of time based on current energy capacity. The practitioner and Andre also problem-solve strategies for improving adherence to adjuvant medications that will reduce interference of nausea and gastrointestinal distress on Andre's target activities. Andre commits to logging daily activities, along with fatigue and mood severity.

Andre's daily logs show that his target activities frequently do not improve mood. On the self-report measure of depression, Andre continues to score high on items such as guilty thoughts. Through Socratic questioning, the practitioner helps Andre to identify severe negative self-talk that interfered with his target activities. Andre also pinpoints longstanding beliefs ("*A man's worth is measured by his work*," "*If you live a moral life, you will be rewarded.*") that cause him to devalue his target activities, criticize himself for not working, and blame himself for developing cancer. He is able to connect these thoughts with his irritability and shame and with his attempts to forgo naps and work beyond his physical limit.

Over the next two sessions, Andre begins to apply cognitive restructuring to challenge his negative thoughts and generate more helpful self-talk. He finds it particularly helpful to consider evidence that supports versus contradicts the thoughts and to consider what he might choose to say to a close friend in a similar situation. Andre expresses to the practitioner that while this strategy does not eliminate his sadness and shame, it has begun to reduce them. Moreover, he utilized communication skills discussed during sessions to address his painful belief that his wife thought of him as a burden, by "gathering more information" through a conversation with her. He notes that they still have much to work through, but he has been buoyed by renewed warmth and communication between them.

Andre increasingly recognizes when he is relying on unhelpful thoughts and behavioral reactions to his fatigue. He continues to work with the practitioner on reframing his perceptions of daytime naps in a more helpful light and to redefine what it means to be a productive person. Andre also begins to practice mindfulness, in order to calm his racing thoughts and work on accepting aspects of fatigue that he cannot change. As Andre focuses on helpful self-talk, his thoughts and behaviors reflect more commitment to staying engaged with family and friends and to remaining vigilant against old beliefs that he is not worthy of their respect.

By the tenth CBT session, Andre is regularly using his CBT strategies to good effect. He and the practitioner discuss therapy termination. The practitioner validates his efforts and works with him to brainstorm strategies for maintaining his skills. Following their last session, the practitioner stays in contact with Andre and his oncology team. Andre continues to meet with the practitioner from time to time for booster sessions or general support in coping with his advanced disease.

8.4   Specific Populations

8.4.1   Aging and Cancer

Among patients with cancer, older age increases the likelihood of treatment complications and pain [96, 97]. As patients age, they also may face increasingly restricted social and financial resources. Patients therefore may benefit from support in problem-solving ways to pay for and adhere to complex supportive care regimens. Some patients also may need assistance in accessing transportation to oncology visits and managing responsibilities at home. Practitioners and patients may call upon case managers and family members to help mobilize support. For some patients, dementia-related cognitive impairment can impede both problem-solving and informed decision-making. Practitioners may help to ensure ethical treatment planning by coordinating with existing health care proxies or facilitating the establishment of a guardian.

Despite their risk for cancer-related burden, elderly patients commonly report lower rates of psychological distress relative to younger adult patients [29]. This paradox may reflect age-related changes in psychological responses to cancer, expressions of distress, and/or ways of coping with health threats and loss. Practitioners may supplement commonly used depression screening instruments with items (such as daily mood variation or diffuse physical complaints) that have been suggested to enhance depression identification in elderly patients [98]. Practitioners also may assess symptoms in the context of coping behaviors (e.g., minimization or reframing of symptoms) that influence self-report [129]. Behavioral medicine intervention strategies can be adapted to help patients cope with changes in health status that co-occur with life role transitions such as shifting from caregiver to care recipient or from active wage earner to retiree.

8.4.2 Long-Term Survivorship

Over the past several decades, the increase in cancer incidence coupled with improvements in cancer screening and treatment have led to a growing number of cancer survivors [99]. Approximately 40 % of US survivors are at least 10 years post-diagnosis [100]. Cancer survivorship can involve complex health care needs— highlighting the importance of ongoing health behaviors and self-care. For instance, fatigue may persist well after treatment completion [101]. Survivors also face elevated risk of secondary cancers, cardiac complications, osteoporosis, sexual and reproductive health problems, and neurocognitive changes [102–105]. More than half of survivors of childhood cancer may experience at least one moderate-to-severe late-onset complication [106].

The psychosocial sequelae of survivorship suggest additional targets for intervention. Many survivors experience ongoing fear of cancer recurrence and other health problems. While survivors may struggle to reconcile their cancer experiences with their premorbid identity or their vision for the future, they may feel socially isolated or pressured by others to move on. Survivors of childhood and adolescent cancers may feel that they missed significant life milestones [107]. Body changes and disfigurement [108] can further impact normative social and identity development. Transition into adulthood may evoke worries about being able to start a family [109]. Residual treatment complications also increase risk for subsequent underemployment and underinsurance [110, 111].

Survivors may pursue formal psychosocial support at specific times such as the anniversary of their diagnosis or treatment completion, or at points when follow-up oncology visits decrease in frequency. Behavioral medicine interventions for survivors commonly incorporate CBT, psychoeducation, stress management, and emotional expression strategies [112]. Practitioners should conduct a detailed assessment, including the time and circumstances of cancer diagnosis and treatment, and tailor interventions to individual needs, developmental stage (both current and at time of diagnosis) and cancer history. Relevant intervention targets include psychological adjustment to survivorship, health promotion and prevention (e.g., smoking cessation, substance use reduction, healthy eating, and physical activity) and specific symptoms and concerns (e.g., fatigue, insomnia, psychological distress, and fear of recurrence) [112, 113, 130]. Survivors of early childhood cancer also may benefit from social skills training and assistance with reintegrating into school, whereas survivors of adult cancer many benefit from strategies to process changes in identity, adjust to functional losses, cope with uncertainty, and evaluate life goals and values. Survivors who are coping with disfigurement or disability may need support around change in body image and function. Interventions also may assist family members in addressing their needs and concerns.

8.5 Behavioral Medicine in Practice: Challenges and Opportunities

Recommended resources for practice settings are provided in Table 8.3. Current clinical guidelines include psychosocial care as a component of quality cancer care (e.g., [31]). However, while monitoring multiple health priorities, oncology clinicians have limited time to evaluate patient distress, coping and health behaviors that may be key targets for behavioral medicine intervention. In a survey of US oncologists, almost two-thirds endorsed screening patients routinely for distress whereas only 14 % used validated screening instruments. Moreover, oncologists were less likely to screen if they perceived time constraints and concerns about their ability to detect distress [114]. Among US National Cancer Institute-designated cancer centers, case managers and clinical social workers represent the most common psychosocial care providers (67 %). Most of the institutions provide primary funding for these services, with additional support from fee-for-service structures and grants [115]. Across geographic regions and cancer care settings, patient access to psychosocial services varies widely. Cancer centers commonly face challenges to psychosocial staffing and limited options for community referral.

Both clinical researchers and oncology practices have been expanding behavioral medicine intervention delivery in order to reduce barriers to care related to advanced disease, debilitating side effects, or limited access to specialty mental health providers. Phone-based and mobile (mHealth) interventions may help to reduce symptoms in patients with cancer and represent critical strategies for providing information and self-management support over time [116, 117]. Several trials have tested nursing-led interventions, with some support for improving patient-reported symptoms and QOL [118–120]. Palliative care nurses also may be trained to use basic CBT during home hospice visits although patient health status may limit participation [121, 122]. Interventions also can be adapted for delivery to couples, families, and family caregivers [123, 124]. Interventions that reduce caregiver burden and increase caregiver support may in turn allow caregivers to help improve patient medical adherence and management of side effects [125].

Research also is ongoing to increase our understanding of the pathogenesis of treatment complications, including biobehavioral factors that may underlie individual differences in risk for complications. For instance, depression may share biological mechanisms with cancer-related fatigue and pain for some patients [126, 127]. Advances in our understanding of symptom pathways will help researchers to develop novel strategies for identifying, treating, and/or preventing treatment complications that impact health and QOL.

Table 8.3 Resources

American Cancer Society
Internet address: www.cancer.org
National Cancer Information Center: 1-800-227-2345

American Psychosocial Oncology Society
Internet address: http://www.apos-society.org
Helpline: 1-866-276-7443

Cancer Support Community
Internet address: http://www.cancersupportcommunity.org
Cancer Support Helpline: 1-888-793-9355

National Cancer Institute at the U.S. National Institutes of Health
Internet address: www.cancer.gov
National Cancer Institute Contact Center: 1-800-422-6237

Suggested readings

Books

Holland JC, Breitbart WS, Jacobsen PB, Loscalzo MJ, McCorkle R, Butow PN, editors. Psycho-oncology. 3rd ed. New York: Oxford University Press; 2015

Holland JC, Hughes MK, Greenberg DB, editors. Psycho-oncology: a quick reference on the psychosocial dimensions of cancer symptom management. 2nd ed. Charlottesville, VA: American Psychosocial Oncology Society; 2015

Guidelines and reports

Adler NE, Page A. National Institute of Medicine (US) Committee on Psychosocial Services to cancer patients/families in a community setting: Cancer care for the whole patient: meeting psychosocial health needs. Washington, DC: National Academies Press; 2008

American Society of Clinical Oncology. ASCO clinical practice survivorship guidelines and adaptations: summary of recommendations tables. American Society of Clinical Oncology; 2014. http://www.instituteforquality.org/practice-guidelines

National Comprehensive Cancer Network. NCCN clinical practice guidelines in oncology: supportive care, version 1.2015. Fort Washington, PA: National Comprehensive Cancer Network; 2015. http://www.nccn.org/professionals/physician_gls/f_guidelines.asp

References

1. Torre LA, Bray F, Siegel RL, Ferlay J, Lortet-Tieulent J, Jemal A. Global cancer statistics, 2012. CA Cancer J Clin. 2015;65(2):87–108.
2. American Cancer Society. Cancer facts & figures 2015. Atlanta: American Cancer Society; 2015.
3. Polite BN, Dignam JJ, Olopade OI. Colorectal cancer model of health disparities: understanding mortality differences in minority populations. J Clin Oncol. 2006;24(14):2179–87.
4. Esther Kim JE, Dodd MJ, Aouizerat BE, Jahan T, Miaskowski C. A review of the prevalence and impact of multiple symptoms in oncology patients. J Pain Symptom Manage. 2009;37:715–36.
5. Henry DH, Viswanathan HN, Elkin EP, Traina S, Wade S, Cella D. Symptoms and treatment burden associated with cancer treatment: results from a cross-sectional national survey in the U.S. Support Care. Cancer. 2008;16:791–801.
6. McKenzie H, Hayes L, White K, Cox K, Fethney J, Boughton M, et al. Chemotherapy outpatients' unplanned presentations to hospital: a retrospective study. Support Care Cancer. 2011;19:963–9.

7. Bruera E, Valero V, Driver L, Shen L, Willey J, Zhang T, et al. Patient-controlled methylphenidate for cancer fatigue: a double-blind, randomized, placebo-controlled trial. J Clin Oncol. 2006;24:2073–8.
8. Spathis A, Fife K, Blackhall F, et al. Modafinil for the treatment of fatigue in lung cancer: results of a placebo-controlled, double-blind, randomized trial. J Clin Oncol. 2014;32:1882–8.
9. Ligibel JA, Denlinger CS. New NCCN guidelines for survivorship care. J Natl Compr Canc Netw. 2013;11(5S):640–4.
10. Dizon DS, Suzin D, McIlvenna S. Sexual health as a survivorship issue for female cancer survivors. Oncologist. 2014;19(2):202–10.
11. Pirl WF, Greer JA, Irwin K, Lennes IT, Jackson VA, Park ER, et al. Processes of discontinuing chemotherapy for metastatic non-small-cell lung cancer at the end of life. J Oncol Pract. 2015;11(3):e405–12.
12. Honda K, Goodwin RD. Cancer and mental disorders in a national community sample: findings from the National Comorbidity Survey. Psychother Psychosom. 2004;73(4):235–42.
13. Akechi T, Ietsugu T, Sukigara M, Okamura H, Nakano T, Akizuki N, et al. Symptom indicator of severity of depression in cancer patients: a comparison of the DSM-IV criteria with alternative diagnostic criteria. Gen Hosp Psychiatry. 2009;31(3):225–32.
14. Ell K, Sanchez K, Vourlekis B, Lee PJ, Dwight-Johnson M, Lagomasino I, et al. Depression, correlates of depression, and receipt of depression care among low-income women with breast or gynecologic cancer. J Clin Oncol. 2005;23(13):3052–60.
15. Colleoni M, Mandala M, Peruzzotti G, Robertson C, Bredart A, Goldhirsch A. Depression and degree of acceptance of adjuvant cytotoxic drugs. Lancet. 2000;356(9238):1326–7.
16. Thompson GN, Chochinov HM, Wilson KG, McPherson CJ, Chary S, O'Shea FM, et al. Prognostic acceptance and the well-being of patients receiving palliative care for cancer. J Clin Oncol. 2009;27(34):5757–62.
17. Brink P, Smith TF, Kitson M. Determinants of do-not-resuscitate orders in palliative home care. J Palliat Med. 2008;11(2):226–32.
18. Brintzenhofe-Szoc KM, Levin TT, Li Y, Kissane DW, Zabora JR. Mixed anxiety/depression symptoms in a large cancer cohort: prevalence by cancer type. Psychosomatics. 2009;50:383–91.
19. Mitchell AJ, Chan M, Bhatti H, Halton M, Grassi L, Johansen C, et al. Prevalence of depression, anxiety, and adjustment disorder in oncological, haematological, and palliative-care settings: a meta-analysis of 94 interview-based studies. Lancet Oncol. 2011;12:160–74.
20. Gurevich M, Devins GM, Rodin GM. Stress response syndromes and cancer: conceptual and assessment issues. Psychosomatics. 2002;43:259–81.
21. Andrykowski MA. The role of anxiety in the development of anticipatory nausea in cancer chemotherapy: a review and synthesis. Psychosom Med. 1990;52:458–75.
22. Greer JA, Pirl WF, Park ER, Lynch TJ, Temel JS. Behavioral and psychological predictors of chemotherapy adherence in patients with advanced non-small cell lung cancer. J Psychosom Res. 2008;65:549–52.
23. Latini DM, Hart SL, Knight SJ, Cowan JE, Ross PL, Duchane J, et al. The relationship between anxiety and time to treatment for patients with prostate cancer on surveillance. J Urol. 2007;178:826–31.
24. Traeger L, Greer JA, Fernandez-Robles C, Temel JS, Pirl WF. Evidence-based treatment of anxiety in patients with cancer. J Clin Oncol. 2012;30(11):1197–205.
25. den Hollander M, de Jong JR, Volders S, Goossens ME, Smeets RJ, Vlaeyen JW. Fear reduction in patients with chronic pain: a learning theory perspective. Expert Rev Neurother. 2010;10:1733–45.
26. Vlaeyen JW, Linton SJ. Fear-avoidance and its consequences in chronic musculoskeletal pain: a state of the art. Pain. 2000;85:317–32.
27. Lepore SJ, Eton DT. Response shifts in prostate cancer patients: an evaluation of suppressor and buffer models. In: Schwartz CE, Sprangers MAG, editors. Adaptation to changing health: response shift in quality-of-life research. Washington, DC: American Psychological Association; 2000. p. 37–51.

28. Helgeson VS, Reynolds KA, Tomich PL. A meta-analytic review of benefit finding and growth. J Consult Clin Psychol. 2006;74(5):797–816.
29. Wilson KG, Chochinov HM, Skirko MG, Allard P, Chary S, Gagnon PR. Depression and anxiety disorders in palliative cancer care. J Pain Symptom Manage. 2007;33(2):118–29.
30. Blank TO, Bellizzi KM. A gerontologic perspective on cancer and aging. Cancer. 2008;112(11S):2569–76.
31. National Comprehensive Cancer Network. NCCN clinical practice guidelines in oncology: distress management, version 1.2015. Fort Washington: National Comprehensive Cancer Network; 2015.
32. Caraceni A, Brunelli C, Martini C, Zecca E, De Conno F. Cancer pain assessment in clinical trials. A review of the literature (1999–2002). J Pain Symptom Manage. 2005;29(5):507–19.
33. Hjermstad MJ, Fayers PM, Haugen DF, Caraceni A, Hanks GW, Loge JH. Studies comparing Numerical Rating Scales, Verbal Rating Scales, and Visual Analogue Scales for assessment of pain intensity in adults: a systematic literature review. J Pain Symptom Manage. 2011;41(6):1073–93.
34. Kroenke K, Spitzer RL, Williams JB, Löwe B. An ultra-brief screening scale for anxiety and depression: the PHQ-4. Psychosomatics. 2009;50(6):613–21.
35. Zigmond AS, Snaith RP. The hospital anxiety and depression scale. Acta Psychiatr Scand. 1983;67:361–70.
36. Kroenke K, Spitzer RL, Williams JB. The PHQ-9: validity of a brief depression severity measure. J Gen Intern Med. 2001;16(9):606–13.
37. Cleeland CS, Ryan KM. Pain assessment: global use of the Brief Pain Inventory. Ann Acad Med Singapore. 1994;23(2):129–38.
38. Mendoza TR, Wang XS, Kugaya A, et al. The rapid assessment of fatigue severity in cancer patients; use of the brief fatigue inventory. Cancer. 1999;85(5):1186–96.
39. Morisky DE, Green LW, Levine DM. Concurrent and predictive validity of a self-reported measure of medication adherence. Med Care. 1986;24(1):67–74.
40. Meyerhardt JA, Heseltine D, Niedzwiecki D, et al. Impact of physical activity on cancer recurrence and survival in patients with stage III colon cancer: findings from CALGB 89803. J Clin Oncol. 2006;24:3535–41.
41. Cella DF, Tulsky DS, Gray G, Sarafian B, Linn E, Bonomi A, et al. The Functional Assessment of Cancer Therapy Scale: development and validation of the general measure. J Clin Oncol. 1993;11:570–9.
42. Smets EMA, Garssen B, Bonke B, De Haes JC. The multidimensional fatigue inventory (MFI) psychometric qualities of an instrument to assess fatigue. J Psychom Res. 1995;39(5):315–25.
43. Zimet GD, Dahlem NW, Zimet SG, Farley GK. The multidimensional scale of perceived social support. J Pers Assess. 1988;52(1):30–41.
44. Sherbourne CD, Stewart AL. The MOS social support survey. Soc Sci Med. 1991;32(6):705–14.
45. Cleeland CS, Mendoza TR, Wang XS, Chou C, Harle MT, Morrissey M, et al. Assessing symptom distress in cancer patients: the M.D. Anderson Symptom Inventory. Cancer. 2000;89:1634–46.
46. Portenoy RK, Thaler HT, Kornblith AB, Lepore JM, Friedlander-Klar H, Kiyasu E, et al. The Memorial Symptom Assessment Scale: an instrument for the evaluation of symptom prevalence, characteristics and distress. Eur J Cancer. 1994;30A(9):1326–36.
47. de Haes JC, van Knippenberg FC, Neijt JP. Measuring psychological and physical distress in cancer patients: structure and application of the Rotterdam Symptom Checklist. Br J Cancer. 1990;62(6):1034–8.
48. Jacobsen PB, Jim HS. Psychosocial interventions for anxiety and depression in adult cancer patients: achievements and challenges. CA Cancer J Clin. 2008;58(4):214–30.

49. Luckett T, Butow PN, King MT, Oguchi M, Heading G, Hackl NA, et al. A review and recommendations for optimal outcome measures of anxiety, depression and general distress in studies evaluating psychosocial interventions for English-speaking adults with heterogeneous cancer diagnoses. Support Care Cancer. 2010;18(10):1241–62.

50. Johns SA, Kroenke K, Krebs EE, Theobald DE, Wu J, Tu W. Longitudinal comparison of three depression measures in adult cancer patients. J Pain Symptom Manage. 2013;45(1):71–82.

51. Pirl WF, Fann JR, Greer JA, Braun I, Deshields T, Fulcher C, Harvey E, Holland J, Kennedy V, Lazenby M, Wagner L, Underhill M, Walker DK, Zabora J, Zebrack B, Bardwell WA. Recommendations for the implementation of distress screening programs in cancer centers: report from the American Psychosocial Oncology Society (APOS), Association of Oncology Social Work (AOSW), and Oncology Nursing Society (ONS) joint task force. Cancer. 2014;120(19):2946–54.

52. Jean-Pierre P, Figueroa-Moseley CD, Kohli S, Fiscella K, Palesh OG, Morrow GR. Assessment of cancer-related fatigue: implications for clinical diagnosis and treatment. Oncologist. 2007;12(S1):11–21.

53. Brown LF, Kroenke K. Cancer-related fatigue and its associations with depression and anxiety: a systematic review. Psychosomatics. 2009;50:440–7.

54. Delgado-Guay M, Parsons HA, Li Z, Palmer JL, Bruera E. Symptom distress in advanced cancer patients with anxiety and depression in the palliative care setting. Support Care Cancer. 2009;17:573–9.

55. So WK, Marsh G, Ling WM, Leung FY, Lo JC, Yeung M, et al. The symptom cluster of fatigue, pain, anxiety, and depression and the effect on the quality of life of women receiving treatment for breast cancer: a multicenter study. Oncol Nurs Forum. 2009;36:E205–14.

56. Winell J, Roth AJ. Depression in cancer patients. Oncology (Williston Park). 2004;18(12):1554–60.

57. Galway K, Black A, Cantwell M, Cardwell CR, Mills M, Donnelly M. Psychosocial interventions to improve quality of life and emotional wellbeing for recently diagnosed cancer patients. Cochrane Database Syst Rev. 2012;11:CD007064.

58. Faller H, Schuler M, Richard M, Heckl U, Weis J, Küffner R. Effects of psycho-oncologic interventions on emotional distress and quality of life in adult patients with cancer: systematic review and meta-analysis. J Clin Oncol. 2013;31(6):782–93.

59. Sheinfeld Gorin SS, Krebs P, Badr H, Janke EA, Jim HS, Spring B, et al. Meta-analysis of psychosocial interventions to reduce pain in patients with cancer. J Clin Oncol. 2012;30(5):539–47.

60. McCue DA, Lohr LK, Pick AM. Improving adherence to oral cancer therapy in clinical practice. Pharmacotherapy. 2014;34(5):481–94.

61. Emmons KM, Rollnick S. Motivational interviewing in health care settings: opportunities and limitations. Am J Prev Med. 2001;20(1):68–74.

62. Park ER, Japuntich S, Temel J, Lanuti M, Pandiscio J, Hilgenberg J, et al. A smoking cessation intervention for thoracic surgery and oncology clinics: a pilot trial. J Thorac Oncol. 2011;6(6):1059–65.

63. Gielissen MF, Verhagen S, Witjes F, Bleijenberg G. Effects of cognitive behavior therapy in severely fatigued disease-free cancer patients compared with patients waiting for cognitive behavior therapy: a randomized controlled trial. J Clin Oncol. 2006;24(30):4882–7.

64. Greer JA, Traeger L, Bemis H, Solis J, Hendriksen ES, Park ER, et al. A pilot randomized controlled trial of brief cognitive-behavioral therapy for anxiety in patients with terminal cancer. Oncologist. 2012;17(10):1337–45.

65. Kangas M, Bovbjerg DH, Montgomery GH. Cancer-related fatigue: a systematic and meta-analytic review of non-pharmacological therapies for cancer patients. Psychol Bull. 2008;134(5):700–41.

66. Lee Y-H, Chiou P-Y, Chang P-H, Hayter M. A systematic review of the effectiveness of problem-solving approaches towards symptom management in cancer care. J Clin Nurs. 2011;20:73–85.

67. Osborn RL, Demoncada AC, Feuerstein M. Psychosocial interventions for depression, anxiety, and quality of life in cancer survivors: meta-analyses. Int J Psychiatry Med. 2006;36:13–34.
68. Smith MT, Huang MI, Manber R. Cognitive behavior therapy for chronic insomnia occurring within the context of medical and psychiatric disorders. Clin Psychol Rev. 2005;25:559–92.
69. Kissane D. Beyond the psychotherapy and survival debate: the challenge of social disparity, depression and treatment adherence in psychosocial cancer care. Psychooncology. 2009;18:1–5.
70. Safren SA, Gonzalez JS, Soroudi N. Coping with chronic illness: a cognitive-behavioral therapy approach for adherence and depression: therapist guide. New York: Oxford University Press; 2008.
71. Greer JA, Park ER, Prigerson HG, Safren SA. Tailoring cognitive-behavioral therapy to treat anxiety comorbid with advanced cancer. J Cogn Psychother. 2010;24(4):294–313.
72. Hopko DR, Armento ME, Robertson S, Ryba MM, Carvalho JP, Colman LK, et al. Brief behavioral activation and problem-solving therapy for depressed breast cancer patients: randomized trial. J Consult Clin Psychol. 2011;79(6):834–49.
73. Hopko DR, Robertson SMC, Carvalho JP. Sudden gains in depressed cancer patients treated with behavioral activation therapy. Behav Ther. 2009;40(4):346–56.
74. Greer JA, Graham JS, Safren SA. Resolving treatment complications associated with comorbid medical conditions. In: Otto M, Hofmann S, editors. Avoiding treatment failure in anxiety disorders. New York: Springer; 2009. p. 317–46.
75. D'Zurilla TJ, Nezu AM. Problem-solving therapy: a positive approach to clinical intervention. 3rd ed. New York: Springer; 2007.
76. Nezu AM, Nezu CM, Felgoise SH, McClure KS, Houts PS. Project Genesis: assessing the efficacy of problem-solving therapy for distressed adult cancer patients. J Consult Clin Psychol. 2003;71(6):1036–48.
77. Nezu AM, Nezu CM, Friedman SH, Faddis S, Houts PS. Helping cancer patients cope: a problem-solving approach. Washington, DC: American Psychological Association; 1998.
78. Roscoe JA, Morrow GR, Aapro MS, Molassiotis A, Olver I. Anticipatory nausea and vomiting. Support Care Cancer. 2011;19(10):1533–8.
79. Wolitzky-Taylor KB, Horowitz JD, Powers MB, Telch MJ. Psychological approaches in the treatment of specific phobias: a meta-analysis. Clin Psychol Rev. 2008;28(6):1021–37.
80. Holland JC, Hughes MK, Greenberg DB, editors. Quick reference for oncology clinicians: the psychiatric and psychological dimensions of cancer symptom management. Charlottesville: American Psychosocial Oncology Society; 2006.
81. Wallace RK, Benson H, Wilson NF. A wakeful hypometabolic physiologic state. Am J Physiol. 1971;221(3):795–9.
82. Jacobsen PB, Meade CD, Stein KD, Chirikos TN, Small BJ, Ruckdeschel JC. Efficacy and costs of two forms of stress management training for cancer patients undergoing chemotherapy. J Clin Oncol. 2002;20:2851–62.
83. Luebbert K, Dahme B, Hasenbring M. The effectiveness of relaxation training in reducing treatment-related symptoms and improving emotional adjustment in acute non-surgical cancer treatment: a meta-analytical review. Psychooncology. 2001;10(6):490–502.
84. Krischer MM, Xu P, Meade CD, Jacobsen PB. Self-administered stress management training in patients undergoing radiotherapy. J Clin Oncol. 2007;25(29):4657–62.
85. Park ER, Traeger L, Willett J, Gerade B, Webster A, Rastegar S, et al. A relaxation response training for women undergoing breast biopsy: exploring integrated care. Breast. 2013;22(5):799–805.
86. Montgomery GH, Hallquist MN, Schnur JB, David D, Silverstein JH, Bovbjerg DH. Mediators of a brief hypnosis intervention to control side effects in breast surgery patients: response expectancies and emotional distress. J Consult Clin Psychol. 2010;78(1):80–8.
87. Liossi C, White P. Efficacy of clinical hypnosis in the enhancement of quality of life of terminally ill cancer patients. Contemp Hypn. 2001;18(3):145–60.

88. Montgomery GH, Bovbjerg DH, Schnur JB, David D, Goldfarb A, Weltz CR, et al. A randomized clinical trial of a brief hypnosis intervention to control side effects in breast surgery patients. J Natl Cancer Inst. 2007;99(17):1304–12.

89. Montgomery GH, David D, Kangas M, Green S, Sucala M, Bovbjerg DH, et al. Randomized controlled trial of a cognitive-behavioral therapy plus hypnosis intervention to control fatigue in patients undergoing radiotherapy for breast cancer. J Clin Oncol. 2014;32(6):557–63.

90. Raingruber B. The effectiveness of psychosocial interventions with cancer patients: an integrative review of the literature (2006–2011). ISRN Nurs. 2011;2011:638218.

91. Miovic M, Block S. Psychiatric disorders in advanced cancer. Cancer. 2007;110(8):1665–76.

92. Breitbart W. Spirituality and meaning in supportive care: spirituality-and meaning-centered group psychotherapy interventions in advanced cancer. Support Care Cancer. 2002;10(4):272–80.

93. Piet J, Würtzen H, Zachariae R. The effect of mindfulness-based therapy on symptoms of anxiety and depression in adult cancer patients and survivors: a systematic review and meta-analysis. J Consult Clin Psychol. 2012;80(6):1007–20.

94. Rouleau CR, Garland SN, Carlson LE. The impact of mindfulness-based interventions on symptom burden, positive psychological outcomes, and biomarkers in cancer patients. Cancer Manag Res. 2015;7:121–31.

95. Brotto LA, Erskine Y, Carey M, Ehlen T, Finlayson S, Heywood M, et al. A brief mindfulness-based cognitive behavioral intervention improves sexual functioning versus wait-list control in women treated for gynecologic cancer. Gynecol Oncol. 2012;125(2):320–5.

96. Kundu SD, Roehl KA, Eggener SE, Antenor JA, Han M, Catalona WJ. Potency, continence and complications in 3,477 consecutive radical retropubic prostatectomies. J Urol. 2004;172(6 Pt 1):2227–31.

97. McGuire DB. Occurrence of cancer pain. J Natl Cancer Inst Monogr. 2004;32:51–6.

98. Nelson CJ, Cho C, Berk AR, Holland J, Roth AJ. Are gold standard depression measures appropriate for use in geriatric cancer patients? A systematic evaluation of self-report depression instruments used with geriatric, cancer, and geriatric cancer samples. J Clin Oncol. 2010;28(2):348–56.

99. Siegel R, DeSantis C, Virgo K, Stein K, Mariotto A, Smith T, et al. Cancer treatment and survivorship statistics, 2012. CA Cancer J Clin. 2012;62(4):220–41.

100. de Moor JS, Mariotto AB, Parry C, Alfano CM, Padgett L, Kent EE, et al. Cancer survivors in the United States: prevalence across the survivorship trajectory and implications for care. Cancer Epidemiol Biomarkers Prev. 2013;22(4):561–70.

101. Bower JE, Ganz PA, Desmond KA, Rowland JH, Meyerowitz BE, Belin TR. Fatigue in breast cancer survivors: occurrence, correlates, and impact on quality of life. J Clin Oncol. 2000;18(4):743–53.

102. Armstrong GT, Liu Q, Yasul Y, Huang S, Ness KK, Leisenring Q, et al. Long-term outcomes among adult survivors of childhood central nervous system malignancies in the Childhood Cancer Survivor Study. J Natl Cancer Inst. 2009;101(13):946–58.

103. Ford JS, Kawashima T, Whitton J, Leisenring W, Laverdière C, Stovall M, et al. Psychosexual functioning among adult female survivors of childhood cancer: a report from the childhood cancer survivor study. J Clin Oncol. 2014;32(28):3126–36.

104. Meirow D, Nugent D. The effects of radiotherapy and chemotherapy on female reproduction. Hum Reprod Update. 2001;7(6):535–43.

105. Mueller S, Fullerton HJ, Stratton K, Leisenring W, Weathers RE, Stovall M, et al. Radiation, atherosclerotic risk factors, and stroke risk in survivors of pediatric cancer: a report from the childhood cancer survivor study. Int J Radiat Oncol Biol Phys. 2013;86(4):649–55.

106. Michel G, Greenfield DM, Absolom K, Ross RJ, Davies H, Eiser C. Follow-up care after childhood cancer: survivors' expectations and preferences for care. Eur J Cancer. 2009;45(9):1616–23.

107. Jones BLJ. Promoting healthy development among survivors of adolescent cancer. Fam Community Health. 2008;31:S61–70.
108. Kinahan KE, Sharp LK, Seidel K, Leisenring W, Didwania A, Lacouture ME, et al. Scarring, disfigurement, and quality of life in long-term survivors of childhood cancer: a report from the childhood cancer survivor study. J Clin Oncol. 2012;30(20):2466–74.
109. Schover LR, Rybicki LA, Martin BA, Bringelsen KA. Having children after cancer: a pilot survey of survivors' attitudes and experiences. Cancer. 1999;86(4):697–709.
110. Kirchhoff AC, Krull KR, Ness KK, Armstrong GT, Park ER, Stovall M, et al. Physical, mental and neurocognitive status and employment outcomes in the childhood cancer survivor study cohort. Cancer Epidemiol Biomarkers Prev. 2011;20(9):1838–49.
111. Kirchhoff AC, Leisenring W, Krull KR, Ness KK, Friedman DL, Armstrong GT, et al. Unemployment among adult survivors of childhood cancer: a report from the childhood cancer survivor study. Med Care. 2010;48(11):1015–25.
112. Stanton AL, Rowland JH, Ganz PA. Life after diagnosis and treatment of cancer in adulthood: contributions from psychosocial oncology research. Am Psychol. 2015;70(2):159–74.
113. Brier MJ, Schwartz LA, Kazak AE. Psychosocial, health-promotion, and neurocognitive interventions for survivors of childhood cancer: a systematic review. Health Psychol. 2015;34(2):130–48.
114. Pirl WF, Muriel A, Hwang V, Kornblith A, Greer J, Donelan K, et al. Screening for psychosocial distress: a national survey of oncologists. J Support Oncol. 2007;5(10):499–504.
115. Deshields T, Kracen A, Nanna S, Kimbro L. Psychosocial staffing at National Comprehensive Cancer Network member institutions: data from leading cancer centers. Psychooncology. 2016;25(2):164–9.
116. Gustafson DH, Hawkins R, McTavish F, Pingree S, Chen WC, Volrathongchai K, et al. Internet-based interactive support for cancer patients: are integrated systems better? J Commun. 2008;58(2):238–57.
117. Park ER, Puleo E, Butterfield RM, Zorn M, Mertens AC, Gritz ER, et al. A process evaluation of a telephone-based peer-delivered smoking cessation intervention for adult survivors of childhood cancer: the partnership for health study. Prev Med. 2006;42(6):435–42.
118. McCorkle R, Dowd M, Ercolano E, Schulman-Gree D, Williams AL, Siefert ML, et al. Effects of a nursing intervention on quality of life outcomes in post-surgical women with gynecological cancers. Psychooncology. 2009;18(1):62–70.
119. Wagner EH, Ludman EJ, Aiello Bowles EJ, Penfold R, Reid RJ, Rutter CM, et al. Nurse navigators in early cancer care: a randomized, controlled trial. J Clin Oncol. 2014;32:12–8.
120. Young JM, Butow PN, Walsh J, Durcinoska I, Dobbins TA, Rodwell L, et al. Multicenter randomized trial of centralized nurse-led telephone-based care coordination to improve outcomes after surgical resection for colorectal cancer: the CONNECT intervention. J Clin Oncol. 2013;31:3585–91.
121. Mannix KA, Blackburn IM, Garland A, Gracie J, Moorey S, Reid B, et al. Effectiveness of brief training in cognitive behaviour therapy techniques for palliative care practitioners. Palliat Med. 2006;20(6):579–84.
122. Moorey S, Cort E, Kapari M, Monroe B, Hansford P, Mannix K, et al. A cluster randomized controlled trial of cognitive behaviour therapy for common mental disorders in patients with advanced cancer. Psychol Med. 2009;39(5):713–23.
123. Badr H, Krebs P. A systematic review and meta-analysis of psychosocial interventions for couples coping with cancer. Psychooncology. 2013;22(8):1688–704.
124. Northouse LL, Katapodi MC, Song L, Zhang L, Mood DW. Interventions with family caregivers of cancer patients: meta-analysis of randomized trials. CA Cancer J Clin. 2010;60(5):317–39.
125. Northouse L, Williams AL, Given B, McCorkle R. Psychosocial care for family caregivers of patients with cancer. J Clin Oncol. 2012;30(11):1227–34.
126. Reyes-Gibby CC, Swartz MD, Yu X, Wu X, Yennurajalingam S, Anderson KO, et al. Symptom clusters of pain, depressed mood, and fatigue in lung cancer: assessing the role of cytokine genes. Support Care Cancer. 2013;21(11):3117–25.

127. Thornton LM, Andersen BL, Blakely WP. The pain, depression, and fatigue symptom cluster in advanced breast cancer: covariation with the hypothalamic-pituitary-adrenal axis and the sympathetic nervous system. Health Psychol. 2010;29(3):333–7.

128. Bruera E, Kuehn N, Miller MJ, Selmser P, Macmillan K. The Edmonton Symptom Assessment System (ESAS): a simple method of the assessment of palliative care patients. J Palliat Care. 1991;7:6–9.

129. Leventhal EA, Crouch M. Are there differences in perceptions of illness across the lifespan? In KJ Petrie, JA. Weinman (Eds.). Perceptions of health and illness: Current research and applications (pp. 77–102). Netherlands: Harwood Academic Publishers; 1997.

130. Demark-Wahnefried W, Pinto BM, Gritz ER. Promoting health and physical function among cancer survivors: potential for prevention and questions that remain. J Clin Oncol. 2006;24(32):5125–31.

Abbreviations

ACS	American Cancer Society
BA	Behavioral activation
CBT	Cognitive behavioral therapy
MI	Motivational interviewing
NCCN	National Comprehensive Cancer Network
QOL	Quality of life

Chapter 9
Neurological Conditions

Jennifer A. Burbridge and Catherine L. Leveroni

9.1 Introduction

9.1.1 Prevalence of Psychological and Psychiatric Comorbidities

Neurological disorders are diseases of the brain, spine, and nerves. These conditions are often associated with decline in physical and/or cognitive function, and represent a huge stressor to patients and their caregivers. Depression and anxiety are common in patients with chronic neurological disease. Although not the case for all, patients with neurological conditions are more likely to experience depression during their lifetimes than the general public or patients with many other chronic medical conditions [1]. For example, the incidence rates of depression range from 36 to 65 % in patients with multiple sclerosis (e.g., [2–4]), from 25 to 79 % following cerebrovascular accident [5], from 30 to 50 % in patients with Parkinson's disease [6, 7], and around 66 % in patients with medically intractable epilepsy [8]. Anxiety is also fairly common. Approximately 29 % of individuals experience anxiety following stroke or a transient ischemic attack [9]. The incidence rate of anxiety following acquired brain injury ranges from 11 to 70 % depending on the study [10]. In patients with chronic epilepsy, the incidence of anxiety disorder is 22.8 % and the incidence of anxiety symptoms is 34.2 % [11].

J.A. Burbridge, Ph.D. (✉) • C.L. Leveroni, Ph.D.
Behavioral Medicine Service, Department of Psychiatry, Massachusetts General Hospital, Harvard Medical School, Boston, MA, USA
e-mail: jburbridge@mgh.harvard.edu

© Springer Science+Business Media New York 2017
A.-M. Vranceanu et al. (eds.), *The Massachusetts General Hospital Handbook of Behavioral Medicine*, Current Clinical Psychiatry, DOI 10.1007/978-3-319-29294-6_9

The presence of psychiatric comorbidities is associated with poorer outcomes in neurological populations. Depression has been associated with poorer quality of life, reduced medication adherence, relationship and vocational issues, increased cognitive impairment, and increased risk of suicide [6, 12–14]. Depression is also associated with a negative response to treatments, a prolonged course of illness, and slower rate of recovery [14]. In light of these factors, treatments including psychotherapy are crucial in the medical management of patients with neurological conditions [14]. Anxiety conditions, including panic attacks, generalized anxiety, obsessive compulsive behaviors, and social phobia, can complicate neurology patient's daily functioning, adherence with treatment, and ability to participate in rehabilitation [15].

9.1.2 The Biopsychosocial Mode in Neurological Populations

While there have been numerous etiologies proposed to account for the high rates of psychiatric comorbidities in neurological disease, most favor a model that accounts for psychological, social-level, and biological variables, as well as their complex interrelationships. From a psychological standpoint patients with neurological disorders are at increased risk for stress and distress by virtue of having a chronic illness over which they have little control. Furthermore, the course of neurological conditions can be unpredictable: some patients struggle with recurrent or intermittent symptoms while others are faced with an incurable illness that has variable rates of progression. This uncertainty can foster increased symptoms of depression and anxiety (e.g., [16]). Discomfort related to somatic symptoms (e.g., pain, fatigue, insomnia, dizziness, weakness), cognitive symptoms (e.g., memory loss, aphasia, perceptual distortions, executive dysfunction), and motor symptoms (e.g., hemiparesis, ataxia, tremor, rigidity, dsykinesias, gait dysfunction) compound distress. Patients with neurological conditions can experience significant restrictions in their ability to live normal lives due to the illness itself or the side effects of the medications. Patients frequently report that their condition has an adverse impact on their quality of life, even with treatment [17]. Many patients are unable to drive, work, or care for themselves or others. This loss of functional independence can be a source of frustration, despondency, and anxiety. Finally, chronic neurological disease and its associated functional disability can exert a negative impact on a patient's self-concept and self-esteem. The resultant loss of confidence can foster feelings of despondency and loss of hope. It also can alter the dynamics of close relationships as often partners or family members have to care for the patient, leading to interpersonal discord and further increasing symptoms of depression and anxiety.

Individuals with neurological conditions are also vulnerable to psychiatric symptoms and disorders due to the direct impact of the disease process on the neural systems involved in the experience and expression of emotion. Emotions and behaviors are regulated by a complex system of distributed and interconnected brain regions; therefore, it is not surprising that diverse neuropathologies can induce alterations in mood and behavior. Indeed, psychiatric symptoms can represent the direct manifestation of brain disease affecting distributed neural systems in neurological populations. Disease or injury that disrupts the structural and functional integrity of the limbic system can lead to anxiety and depression. For example, in patients with temporal lobe epilepsy, depression and anxiety can be linked to pathology and abnormal epileptiform activity in limbic systems structures [18]. Moreover, the incidence varies depending on the laterality of the seizure focus. Depression is more common in patients with left than right temporal lobe epilepsy [19]. This observation further strengthens the argument that depression can be driven by altered limbic system functioning. Depression has also been associated with abnormal connectivity within limbic systems structures in individuals with multiple sclerosis and Parkinson's disease [20, 21].

Psychiatric disorders are also common in patients with disease that primarily affect the basal ganglia. For example, the neuropsychiatric syndromes that accompany Huntington's disease, which can include tics, obsessions, and compulsions, are believed the direct manifestation of altered fronto-striatal functioning [22]. Patients with diseases that are circumscribed to the cerebellum additionally can present with a primary affective and behavioral syndrome [23]. Depression and anxiety can result from damage to the frontal cortex. In Traumatic Brain Injury survivors, depression has been predicted by presence of intracranial lesions or reduced gray matter volume, especially in the left frontal area [24, 25]. In these patients, depression is hypothesized to be mediated by deactivation of lateral and dorsolateral prefrontal cortex and increased activation of limbic regions including the amygdala [24].

9.2 Evidence Base for CBT Interventions in Neurological Populations

Managing psychiatric illness in patients with neurological conditions has been the focus of much research. However, across neurological populations, investigations on the effectiveness of CBT have yielded mixed results. This is because the literature is fraught with methodological issues that reduce the generalizability of the findings, including small sample sizes, uncontrolled studies, patient heterogeneity, and variability in focus of treatment and strategies. Despite these limitations, there is mounting evidence that cognitive-behavioral interventions are clinically meaningful to patient groups. CBT has been found to enhance quality of life, adjustment to chronic illness, and overall coping in patients with epilepsy [26]. It was also noted to improve quality of life and performance of activities of daily living (ADLs) in patients with mild cognitive impairment (MCI) and dementia [27]. CBT has also been found to improve quality of life in patients with multiple sclerosis; the improvement was mediated by increased positive affect and reduced depression, but not by changes in subject's level of fatigue [28].

Cognitive-behavioral interventions also have shown promise as a treatment for depression and anxiety in patients with epilepsy [29], multiple sclerosis [13], mild cognitive impairment and dementia [27], Parkinson's disease [6], and acquired brain injuries of varied etiology [30–32]. Thus, taken together, investigations suggest that CBT is not a "panacea" in neurological populations [32]. Reductions are generally observed in symptoms and behaviors that were specifically targeted by the intervention. The benefits do not generalize to symptoms and behaviors that were not specifically addressed. For example, in review of studies of CBT for traumatic brain injury (TBI) survivors, Waldron et al. [32] note that successful intervention aimed at anger management in TBI did not also reduce depression and anxiety in the sample. In a recent review of the impact of CBT interventions on depressive symptoms in patients with epilepsy, Gandy et al. [29] determined that the most effective interventions were tailored to ameliorate depressive symptoms. Depression was less likely reduced if the intervention was targeted toward disease variables such as seizure reduction. In addition, the group investigated the efficacy of a CBT intervention targeting depression in a randomized controlled trial. They found that the intervention reduced the likelihood of depression and suicidal ideation but did not have a significant impact on quality of life [33]. The take-home message for therapists working with patients with neurological conditions seems clear: the most effective interventions for patients should be tailored to target the individual patient's specific symptoms.

9.2.1 Special Considerations: CBT in Patients with Cognitive Impairments

One of the most significant challenges therapists face when treating patients with neurological conditions can be cognitive impairment. Studies have shown an association between increased cognitive impairment and psychiatric symptomatology in neurological groups demonstrating the need for empirically supported treatments for these patients. In particular, depression has been found to be increased in patients with executive dysfunction. This has been observed across numerous populations including TBI, epilepsy, multiple sclerosis, and Parkinson's disease [16, 24, 34]. Patients with executive dysfunction are at risk for depression and anxiety because the frontal-subcortical networks involved in emotion regulation also subserve executive aspects of cognition. In addition, executive cognitive deficits can interfere with a person's ability to cope with psychiatric symptoms as well as everyday life stressors. Executive dysfunction can limit a patient's ability to think flexibly, generate solutions to everyday problems, and guide behavior toward effective solutions. In addition, patients with executive deficits can experience difficulty regulating emotion and affect. This can have a negative impact on interpersonal functioning and reduce the quality of relationships, leading to decreased social support and increased symptomatology. However, despite the need for therapeutic interventions, cognitive impairment can interfere with a patient's ability to acquire cognitive-behavioral concepts, implement and monitor goal-directed strategies in a consistent manner, and follow through on homework, despite good intentions. In light of these factors, CBT outcomes can be complicated and less favorable in patients with cognitive deficits [58].

On the other hand, cognitive-behavioral interventions can be particularly well suited for patients with cognitive deficits. The interventions are directive, flexible, and they can be adjusted for patients with memory impairment. Therapists can use aids such as planners, handouts, digital voice recorders, and reinforcement of strategies with caregivers, thereby focusing a patient's behavior and boosting his or her ability to retain what was learned in session [6]. There is reason to believe that such strategies will enhance a patient's ability to benefit from a CBT intervention. For example, Mohlman and colleagues ([35], 2005) examined the effectiveness of two CBT interventions in older adults with late life onset GAD and variable deficits in executive functioning (e.g., hypothesis generation, allocation of attention, self-monitoring). One intervention was traditional and the other was "enhanced" by learning and memory aids, reminders of homework, trouble shooting phone calls, and a weekly review of all of the concepts and strategies learned to date. They found that both interventions reduced anxiety in their sample, but the effect size was greater for the enhanced CBT group. Further, they observed concomitant improvement in aspects of executive functions in the responders from both groups.

Modular CBT also can target aspects of executive functioning as a primary aim of the intervention. When thinking about interventions for neurological populations, one can conceptualize executive functioning according to anatomically and behaviorally distinct functional "circuits" and executive subsystems, and devise strategies to intervene at each level of the system [59]. For example, structured activity scheduling, exercises to generate ideas and solutions in everyday life, and monitoring of goal-directed activities may help patients struggling with apathy, loss of spontaneity, and reduced initiative/drive. Training in techniques to monitor behavior, regulate anger and emotion, and enhance understanding of the impact of behavior on others is appropriate for patients with primary disinhibition. Techniques such as mindfulness and "distractibility delay" [36, 37] may help patients better modulate attentional functions.

Many cognitive-behavioral techniques target metacognitive skills, such as organization, planning, prioritization, and awareness. For example, Safren [38] developed a modular CBT for the treatment of depression and management of dysexecutive behaviors in adults with Attention Deficit Hyperactivity Disorder. With strategies to enhance organization, planning, prioritization, task monitoring, attentional allocation, and task completion, the intervention is appealing for use in neurological populations. CBT also can enhance cognitive rehabilitation in patients with cognitive deficits. For example, executive cognitive rehabilitation (i.e., Goal Management Therapy) has been found to have a greater impact on a patient's functioning if it is combined with cognitive-behavioral strategies such as problem solving and homework [39]. The strategies learned in CBT can help move patients with executive functioning deficits toward active, adaptive coping. In this way, CBT can help neurology patients manage despite their cognitive functions. This improvement in functioning has the potential to relieve stress, depression, and anxiety. In this chapter, we will discuss more specific ways in which cognitive-behavioral techniques can help patients with neurological conditions minimize the impact of cognitive deficits in their day-to-day lives.

9.3   Specific CBT Approach/Goals/Skills

CBT is a particularly appealing intervention for individuals with neurological conditions. It is collaborative and by using modules, allows for clinical flexibility which is an integral part of working with this population. It is structured but can also be adapted to accommodate patients with cognitive problems. The goals are concrete. It teaches alternative coping strategies: stress management, problem solving, and increased self-efficacy. Furthermore, it can help patients set and reach appropriate goals and evaluate their achievements in post-illness as opposed to pre-illness terms [40, 41].

CBT for neurological conditions can best be conceptualized as drawing skills and strategies from multiple treatment modules, and applying them as needed to an individual patient's symptoms and circumstances. Because there are key features that cut across many neurological conditions, we have created four modules that can be widely applicable. Within and across modules, the treatment plan and skills can be tailored to a patient's individual needs. The first module includes CBT skills for managing the day-to-day stress of having a neurological condition and its impact on current functioning. The second module includes skills to help with current mood and mood regulation issues. The third module includes skills to help patients cope with the long-term emotional effects of how their lives changed, such as uncertainty about the future and progression of their condition. Finally, the fourth module includes skills to help patients cope with neurocognitive and neurobehavioral impairments that can accompany neurological disorders. For each module, we will also address how to manage challenging symptoms and their impact on the session itself.

9.3.1   Assessment

Perhaps more so than with other populations, assessment is an essential component of successful CBT treatment. Determining a patient's psychiatric and physical symptoms, current stressors and neurocognitive deficits will inform what the treatment will be and how it will be done. Many times, patients are referred by their neurologists because they or the patient's family members have noticed symptoms, but often the patients themselves may not be able to articulate them. While patients may be in distress, they may not be able to connect that distress to psychological issues or realize there is a way to target and work on psychological phenomena. Ascertaining patients' goals for CBT requires structure and education from the therapist, as well as input from the patient and his or her family caregivers. Neurology patients often see multiple providers each week for "checkup" visits, and they don't always understand that CBT is a psychological treatment in which therapist and patient do ongoing work together over the course of a number of sessions. They might not understand why they were referred, only that their physician asked them to make an appointment. Thus, it is important to educate patients about exactly what CBT entails and assess whether this type of therapy is the right fit for the patient's needs. Another reason to conduct a thorough assessment is that patients often have complex medical histories and aren't always the most reliable reporters, especially within a 50-min session. It can be very useful to get collateral information from family during the assessment, as they may be able to better describe pre-illness functioning as well as current symptoms and stressors. Finally, as part of the assessment, it can be incredibly helpful to review neuropsychological test findings, if they have been done. These results can inform the therapist about any cognitive deficits that might affect treatment, as well as the patient's strengths and weaknesses from a neuropsychological perspective. The therapist can then tailor therapy to the patient's optimal learning style and modify the skills themselves or how they should be taught (e.g., slow processing speed, short-term memory deficits, strengths in verbal learning, executive dysfunction, etc.) as part of the treatment. The therapist will want to be aware of symptoms that are specific to the patient's neurological condition versus related to a psychiatric comorbidity. For example, before coming up with a plan for an exposure exercise, it would be important to discriminate panic attacks from complex partial seizures for the patient who experiences both. Ideally, a therapist would also collaborate with the patient's neurology team to acquire accurate medical and diagnostic information as well as identify potential limitations that could affect CBT treatment. For example, if a patient wants to increase the amount of time she spends with friends for emotional support, but the patient is unable to drive herself for visits (and isn't happy with this restriction), the therapist will need to be aware of these limitations and problem solve alternative transportation possibilities. Finally, if the patient has not had neurological testing, this may be the time to make a referral.

When discussing the treatment plan, it is critical to set concrete goals for therapy and how the therapist is going to help the patient achieve these goals. Often patients are overwhelmed by their life circumstances and also have some degree of cognitive deficits. Thus, the therapist's role in the intake assessment is to help the patient identify and prioritize his or her stressors and symptoms. In other words, the therapist helps translate the patient's feelings of stress and unmanageable life circumstances into a succinct and relevant treatment plan. After the assessment, the therapist's next task is to help the patient articulate clear, observable, measurable therapy goals with an emphasis on how each skill is intended to improve a symptom and/or their quality of life. This also involves explaining the rationale for each skill in a way that makes sense to the patient. CBT with patients who have neurological conditions should be conceptualized as a short-term treatment, with an emphasis on building skills; however, the precise number of sessions is determined on an individual basis. Somewhere between 8 and 12 sessions appears to be a good range. The therapist should revisit goals on a regular basis to help the patient to identify and label the strategies (so patients know when they are using them and when they are not), as well as facilitate their understanding of how strategies map on to real-life circumstances.

9.3.2   MODULE 1: Managing Disease-Specific Stress and Impact on Daily life

The skills in the first module address the immediate stress associated with having a neurological condition and the impact of their condition on aspects of daily functioning (e.g., driving, working, ambulating, etc.). Common stressors reported by patients include loss of independence/needing to rely heavily on others, changes in ability to work, coping with pain, having to stop driving, medication side effects, and physical limitations. For example, at times patients with a seizure disorders may be unable to drive unless they have been seizure free for 6 months to 1 year (depending on specific regulations in their state). Other patients with medically intractable daytime seizures may not be able to drive indefinitely. Depending on where a person lives, this could have a dramatic effect on his or her daily life. For other patients, in addition to driving, their ability to ambulate is also affected. Getting around with a wheelchair or a walker makes everything a little bit harder, especially if physical changes are one part of a progressive disease. Patients with neurological conditions are often taking multiple medications with unpleasant side effects such as fatigue, weight gain, and cognitive changes. Many patients must stay on these medications for the rest of their lives. It is the cumulative effect of these numerous daily stressors that contribute to patients' overall distress and level of functioning.

   Relaxation. The first set of skills in this module teaches patients how to decrease physical symptoms of stress via diaphragmatic breathing, progressive muscle relaxation (PMR), and guided imagery [42]. These skills provide a quick way to slow down the stress response, as well as provide strategies that can be used immediately and anywhere. Depending on patients' physical abilities, PMR can be tailored to an individual's situation. For example, patients who have muscle weakness or pain can target other muscle areas or focus more on breath work. These skills are often taught early in the treatment and are an ongoing component of homework practice.

   Problem Solving. The second set of skills in this module involves teaching patients more effective problem-solving skills. The strategies discussed are based on organizing and planning skills developed by Safren et al. [36, 37]. Skills such as breaking tasks down into smaller parts and examining the pros/cons of a situation help patients find practical solutions to stressors that interfere with daily activities such as transportation, medication adherence, sleep problems, and exercise. Furthermore, teaching patients better organizational skills such as how to effectively use a daily task list and how to use a calendar to track appointments also help reduce stress and anxiety.

Self-Monitoring. Finally, teaching patients to monitor and track symptoms and triggers for stress are taught within this module. By teaching patients how to use self-monitoring, they can better understand their feelings and behaviors (e.g., fatigue, pain, seizure frequency, medication side effects, etc.) as well as factors that make them more vulnerable to distress.

Because of the situational obstacles that patients with neurological conditions face as well as fluctuating pain levels and potential cognitive impairments, meeting for regular, weekly CBT sessions can be challenging at times. These factors can contribute to a high cancellation rate in this population. Telepsychiatry CBT and, in particular, video CBT can be helpful in situations when the patient can't come to the office, in order to ensure continuity of treatment. Even with less than perfect adherence, CBT skills can benefit patients as long as the therapist keeps session topics on track and aims to provide continuity between sessions (e.g., "This is what we did last week; how can we apply this skill to what's been going on more recently?" etc.). Each session is an opportunity to get back on track and return to the goals discussed, to assess the skills that are being used and problem solve obstacles in their use of strategies.

9.3.3 MODULE 2: Managing Mood

The skills in this module address specific mood and mood regulation issues that can be both primary (related to brain changes and medications) as well as secondary (emotional reactions to these changes). Common mood symptoms reported by patients are anxiety, depression, and anger. For example, patients can be anxious about medical procedures and surgeries they might need, as well as whether their medications are going to treat their symptoms. Feeling a loss of control is common. For example, a patient with epilepsy may have a seizure at any time, any place, and feels understandably anxious about when or whether this might happen. Patients often restrict their activities, resulting in even more anxiety. Because patients have little control over their symptoms, frustration and anger are commonly experienced. Behavioral and interpersonal consequences of their anger can create additional conflict and make a difficult situation even more challenging.

Activity Scheduling. Patients with neurological conditions often need help adding structure to their lives. While patients may understand the importance of having a daily routine, the process of planning activities can often be stressful if they have physical limitations or pain as a part of their condition. Therefore, it is important for the therapist to understand what medical recommendations have been made in order to help patients develop realistic goals. It is also helpful for the therapist to be creative when brainstorming possible activities. Five or ten minutes of being engaged in a task can yield an enormous emotional benefit. Patients often do not realize the degree to which what they do (or don't do) can affect how they feel. Helping patients create a list of pleasant events is also very useful. Overall, activity scheduling skills include helping patients identify and increase a variety of daily experiences in four key areas: physical activities, interpersonal activities, pleasurable activities, and activities that increase their sense of mastery and self-efficacy.

Cognitive Restructuring. CBT skills aimed at reducing mood symptoms primarily involve cognitive restructuring and identifying unhelpful thoughts that may be contributing to feelings of depression, anger, and frustration [43]. Will my pain ever get better? Will I have another seizure? Will my memory ever go back to how it used to be? How will I be able to get around my community by myself? What if I never go back to work? These are common negative thoughts that patients report and can be examined with cognitive restructuring. While cognitive restructuring requires a capacity for metacognition (thinking about one's thinking), this skill can be modified even for those patients with mild–moderate cognitive deficits. Therapists may choose to use thought records, identification of cognitive distortions, or they may tell patients the negative thought patterns they hear in session, and help generate a list of coping thoughts. Some patients may be better able to "talk out" the process of cognitive restructuring, while others may benefit from writing about their process. The therapist's task is to find a way to teach cognitive restructuring in a way that the patient understands and fits with his or her therapy goals.

Interpersonal Skills. Helping patients understand how their anxiety and depression impact their relationships is another useful CBT strategy. Patients with neurological conditions often have difficulty regulating their feelings, so their emotions will go from 0 to 100 very quickly. This can be confusing and frustrating for patients' friends and family, who may not understand the possible biological etiology of their symptoms or how to help them. Furthermore, patients themselves report feeling overwhelmed and out of control with their feelings, making it even harder for them to effectively problem solve or find the "off" switch. Specific emotion regulation strategies will be discussed in module 4. When patients don't understand their feelings and what causes them, this can lead to interpersonal problems. Furthermore, when there aren't clear medical answers for patients' symptoms, communication problems may develop between patients and their medical providers. Thus, patients can learn more adaptive ways to communicate, such as when to "pause" before reacting, as well as how to build and maintain a strong support system.

9.3.4   MODULE 3: Coping with Chronic and Progressive Stress

The skills in this module are aimed at helping patients cope with the chronic, uncertain, and often progressive nature of their condition as well as the potential for long-term disabilities. In other words, these are skills aimed at coping with chronic and progressive stress. After the initial diagnosis and medical treatment, patients continue to adjust to their situation and what might happen next. Sometimes, they have had months of symptoms without a clear medical diagnosis. Sometimes there isn't a clear medical diagnosis. When patients are told they have a neurological condition, this not only affects their current mood, but it also deeply affects how they view themselves and their future. When you have a brain injury, are you the same person you were before the injury? For most people, our sense of self includes our mind, the way we think, our feelings, how we perceive things—all of which come from a functioning brain. When a neurological condition is identified—a problem with the brain—patients often struggle with their identity and whether their illness or injury requires them to completely start over.

One challenge when working with patients with neurological conditions is that their lives do become different, their disabilities are real, and their frustrations are justified. Sometimes their resources are limited. Entire families are often affected by a patient's neurological condition. For example, a patient who had a stroke may need to depend on her family to help her with basic daily activities. A patient with worsening MS will not be able to continue to live in his third-floor walk-up. If a patient has tremors, an unsteady gait or other ambulatory problems, people are probably going to stare at them. A patient who has a stroke or a brain injury may have long-term cognitive and physical deficits. Patients may not be able to go back to their old jobs and may need to apply for disability benefits. Finances may have changed dramatically. There are parts of their situation that are awful and unpleasant and genuinely unfair. However, it is also likely that there are parts of their lives that can be made better. Skills in this module are aimed at helping patients gain a broader perspective of their life circumstances and learn to think and act in a more acceptance-oriented way. Cognitive restructuring and mindfulness are the two strategies in this module that can help patients make this transition.

Cognitive Restructuring. Cognitive restructuring [43] is a skill that is helpful not only for managing mood, as discussed in module 2, but is also helpful for coping with chronic stress. The reality for patients is that there are many situations that are outside their control. Common themes and thought patterns seen in patients with neurological conditions include loss of independence, feeling judged by others, frustration around life limitations, tolerating uncertainty, managing cognitive deficits, wanting things to be as they were "before," wondering if they will find happiness again, and living with chronic pain. However, patients can learn to control their reactions to these changes by changing maladaptive thinking patterns. They may not be aware of how their thoughts and feelings can make a tough situation even worse. Cognitive techniques in this module are aimed at letting go of the need to make things as they were before, learning acceptance strategies, shifting to a more forward-thinking style, and being receptive to a different kind of future. Acceptance-oriented cognitive restructuring can help patients rethink ineffective thought patterns that are keeping them stuck. First, the therapist needs to have a realistic understanding of a patient's situation including what they can and cannot change. Getting collateral information from a patient's physician and family ensures that the therapist has a realistic understanding of a patient's circumstances. This is important because the adaptive, coping-oriented thoughts generated in therapy need to be grounded in reality. For example, sometimes patients continue to look for medical explanations and treatments when they really need to accept the limits of medical treatments and their symptoms. The therapist does not want to encourage patients to adopt coping thoughts that are not realistic. Identifying realistic goals can be useful in helping patients find a balance between acceptance and change. Cognitive restructuring is a useful strategy for helping patients mourn their losses and find some acceptance, while also living an authentic, meaningful life. Cognitive restructuring can also be aimed at helping patients identify the small victories (e.g., successfully using public transportation, feeling peaceful for a moment, reading a chapter in a book, having a tough but productive discussion with their doctor) and see them as part of the larger process of building themselves up again.

Mindfulness. Mindfulness is an acceptance-based strategy [44]. To be present in the moment means to accept each moment as it unfolds, without judgment. Mindfulness teaches tolerance and acceptance. Mindfulness also involves shifting one's attention, again and again to the present moment. When practicing mindfulness, one can't be focused on the future or stuck in the past. By teaching patients mindfulness, the therapist gives patients a tool that can ground them to the present, whatever the present moment may look like. It is helpful to do in-session practice of mindfulness so patients understand what it is (such as mindfulness of sounds). Mindfulness is a useful way to illustrate acceptance, without judgment, and then relate this back to their personal task of accepting their situation and their symptoms, just as they are. It is important to emphasize that acceptance doesn't mean giving up, but rather, it means tolerating a tough situation just as it is. By not accepting their situation, a patient doesn't make their situation any better, in fact the situation remains exactly the same, but they experience greater distress. Once patients recognize this concept, they can see how ineffective it is for them to wish their situation was different or as it was before they had symptoms, they can find the parts that they can change, and then take real action.

9.3.5 MODULE 4: Managing Neurocognitive and Neurobehavioral Symptoms

The skills in this module involve strategies for managing the neurocognitive and neurobehavioral symptoms that can accompany neurological conditions. The skills here can be tailored to each patient based on information gained in the intake assessment including neurological assessment, as well as information observed directly in the session. Many of the skills in this module have been discussed in previous modules but are applied differently here. The goals of the CBT strategies for the current module are to improve underlying neurocognitive functioning, as well as help patients cope with the direct emotional effects of their neurocognitive symptoms. We have divided this module of skills into two areas: memory loss and executive dysfunction, which are commonly affected in neurological conditions.

9.3.6 Memory Loss

Cognitive-behavioral therapies can be modified to reinforce skill acquisition for patients with memory issues. For patients with memory problems, it is especially important to have a clear written session agenda including goals of session, skills to be discussed, and homework instructions. Patients often become overwhelmed by too many handouts, so we recommend using them judiciously. Keep handouts simple: bullet points, date of session, goals of session, skills to be discussed, and homework instructions. Handouts should be easy to understand and free from extraneous details. Checking patient retention for the main points at the end of the session can help the therapist know if patients are on track and are able to summarize the main point of the session. It is important to review all handouts together with the patient to reinforce session content and its relevance to daily life. Therapists should also encourage patients to share CBT handouts and content from sessions with their family to further reinforce learning and applying skills in everyday life. CBT skills also can be used as an intervention to improve memory and help patients adjust to memory changes. Skills may include having patients keep a notebook to record important information. Other memory aids may include daily monitoring, using a task list/calendar to track appointments, using a timer as a reminder/cue, and relaxation strategies (diaphragmatic breathing, progressive muscle relaxation). Finally, cognitive restructuring is also used to help patients be open to using these aids (versus seeing them as "weakness" and giving up or refusing to use them).

9.3.7 Executive Dysfunction

CBT strategies can also be helpful for remediating some of the neurobehavioral sequelae of neurological processes. Individuals with executive dysfunction are especially vulnerable to experiencing chronic stress of everyday life because executive deficits can profoundly impact patients daily functioning. These deficits often interfere with the ability to initiate goal-directed activities, generate ideas, set priorities and goals, organize complex tasks, and maintain behavioral follow-through. Deficits in executive functioning can also impact emotions. Patients can have difficulty regulating their emotions, as well as their behavior. Thus, CBT strategies for managing executive deficits can have an appreciable impact on quality of life by eliminating barriers to optimal functioning. For the purposes of therapy, it is helpful to conceptualize executive dysfunction as having three dimensions: (1) apathy, (2) disinhibition, and (3) cognitive executive deficits.

Apathy. Many different neurological conditions can result in apathy and reduced behavioral follow-through. These symptoms can be challenging for therapists because they work against the active, change-oriented aspects of CBT. Empathy, validation, and patience are valuable therapist qualities. Because there can be a neurobiological component to these symptoms, motivational interviewing skills

[45] may not be sufficient. Therapists, patients, and their families need to have realistic expectations. Behavioral changes may be subtle but should still be acknowledged and reinforced as positive movement. Patients who are low in initiative may benefit from brainstorming exercises to help them generate ideas and solutions to everyday problems. Patients who have difficulty sustaining behavior can be taught to break down complex tasks into smaller components with a concrete plan for the completion of each step. Some patients initially benefit from reminders and external structure (e.g., from family members) and then work toward increasing independence over time. As mentioned in module 2, activity scheduling and creating a list of pleasant events are helpful strategies for adding structure and meaning to daily life. Using existing lists of pleasant events [46] is useful if the patient is having a hard time generating pleasurable activities. It is important to ask patients to identify positive events, as well as rate how enjoyable or helpful events were. This allows the patient to understand that while he or she may have a limited range of interests, there can still be objective variability within this range. Moreover, the therapist should recognize that while a patient may appear to have limited interests or drive to change based on their affect and behavioral presentation, the patient's subjective experience may be quite different and reveal greater variability.

Disinhibition. Deficits of inhibitory control can significantly contribute to a patient's stress level. Disinhibited patients are impulsive and less likely to think things through. They are also more likely to be emotionally reactive and may easily become irritable, frustrated, and angry. Furthermore, these emotional, behavioral, and cognitive reactions are likely to come up within the session itself and may interfere with rapport. The skills discussed here are principally those developed and used by Linehan [46] for managing emotional distress and dysregulation. These skills help the patient identify common triggers for their emotions and when they are more likely to experience disinhibition and its consequences. For example, therapists can teach patients to take a 10 s pause when they notice the intensity of a situation increasing and then allow for a quick "cool-down" and offer an opportunity for assessment of the situation. During this pause, patients can learn to write down what they are thinking and feeling. These skills can help patients reduce the intensity of their feelings and avoid adding further distress to an already stressful situation. Cognitive restructuring around feelings of anger and frustration can then be added to further identify maladaptive thought patterns and examine the validity of underlying beliefs. Learning when and how to use these skills allows patients to understand the consequences of their behavior/emotional reactions and their effects on relationships.

Cognitive Executive Deficits. The cognitive aspect of executive functioning fits very well with the structure and goals of CBT. These skills are aimed at improving organization, improving prioritization, reducing distractibility, improving attention, as well as overall problem solving. One particular technique called "distractibility delay" [36, 37] helps patients improve their ability to focus on one particular task at a time. This strategy involves having the patient write down distractions as they come up and then return to the task at hand. This is done as many times as the distractions come up, until the task is complete. The idea behind this approach is that by writing down the distraction, patients can note it and mindfully plan to address it later, while still making the original task their priority. Furthermore, organizational and problem-solving skills teach patients how to effectively process information, identify the main point, and how not to get overwhelmed with detail. When creating a task list, patients write down step by step what it is that they need to do. Therapists can educate patients about how stress impacts executive functioning and help identify ways to reduce that stress. To better understand and problem solve stressors, patients can be asked to write down a single sentence about what are feeling stressed about. Helping patients identify one aspect of what they are stressed about teaches patients how to step back, sift through their feelings, and identify a starting point. As with people who have memory deficits, a summary statement at end of session about main points is helpful, as well as making sure patients understand the relevant information from the session. Finally, by asking patients to review their handouts with a support person, they can be accountable for practicing the skills at home. Some patients may need in-between session contact with their therapist (such as a reminder call or voicemail check in) in order to reinforce the information they learned in session.

Interpersonal Skills. The impact of executive dysfunction is stressful not only for the patient but for the people in their lives. Thus, teaching and improving communication skills can help to reduce this stress, particularly when a patient is upset. These skills involve asking a patient to "pause" when they notice they are beginning to get frustrated, and identify what it is that they need from the other person and whether this person can satisfy that need. By defining their goal for themselves first, they can then more clearly state it to someone else. Patients can also be taught to modify their tone and emotional style. Role playing interpersonal situations in session is a very useful technique. Therapists may also want to consider meeting with the patient and their main support person together in order to help identify triggers for miscommunication and also make sure family members are also aware of these skills. Furthermore, it can also be useful for therapists to give feedback to patient directly in the session if they are off track or getting muddled in extraneous details. Extraneous details are often a major trigger for frustration and miscommunication. By giving feedback directly to patients about what it is like to be interacting with them, patients can better identify issues and then make necessary changes. This feedback also provides concrete interpersonal examples to come back to. Finally, in order to manage session time effectively, therapists and patients can negotiate a hand signal or gesture to use when the conversation veers off topic. This allows for in-session learning, circumvents any emotional reactions to being redirected, and provides a gentle way to return to the topic at hand.

Mindfulness. Mindfulness is another strategy that can help improve cognitive executive deficits. This skill involves teaching patients how to slow down, refocus their attention to the present moment, and redirect it when they get distracted [44]. This type of purposeful awareness is challenging when patients have deficits in executive functioning, but with practice, patients can learn to notice sensations, filter out distractions, and bring their attention to one thing at a time. Another component of mindfulness is learning how to be nonjudgmental. The goal of mindfulness

Table 9.1 CBT modules and recommendations for specific patient problems

Module	Strategies	Goals
MODULE 1: Managing disease-specific stress and impact on daily life	Relaxation	Provide education, help patients to elicit the relaxation response
	Problem solving	Help manage day-to-day stress of neurological condition and its impact on current functioning
	Self-monitoring	
MODULE 2: Managing mood	Activity scheduling	Help patients increase activity level, increase pleasant events, help patients identify and modify negative thinking patterns, improve communication
	Cognitive restructuring	
	Interpersonal skills	
MODULE 3: Coping with chronic and progressive stress	Cognitive restructuring	Manage longer term emotional effects of neurological condition (uncertainty, acceptance, disease progression)
	Mindfulness	
MODULE 4: Managing neurocognitive and neurobehavioral symptoms	Problem solving	Manage neurocognitive and neurobehavioral impairment
	Activity scheduling	
	Regulating emotions	
	Cognitive restructuring	
	Interpersonal skills	
	Mindfulness	

for executive dysfunction is to teach patients that when their attention veers off track (and they or someone else points it out), they can notice it and return to the present moment without judging it as "bad" or "good." When therapists bring up the concept of mindfulness and nonjudgment, patients often respond with "I'm terrible at meditation/relaxation/mindfulness," "I don't like meditating," or "I've tried it before and I just can't do it." Thus, finding neutral language to discuss the underlying skill, and staying firm on the need to practice before assessing its utility, is a useful way to help patients to approach learning this strategy. Integrating this skill with a patient's interests (e.g., favorite tastes or smells) also helps build practice into a patient's daily activities.

A summary of the CBT modules for treating patients with neurological conditions is presented in Table 9.1. Table 9.2 presents a selection of self-report measures that can be given to patients as part of the initial assessment process. Giving self-report measures to patients with neurological conditions has its challenges and is sometimes not the right choice for patients. Many patients are frustrated by the cognitive demand (focused attention, memory, decision making, etc.) of having to complete self-reports. Very often completion of self-reports can be a time-consuming process, which is challenging when there are time constraints. It can be difficult for patients to select the "best" option to describe their symptoms and the information collected may not be accurate. Completing self-report forms can also be exhausting for patients, making it more difficult for the patient to participate fully during the

Table 9.2 Sample intake and self-report assessments

Component	Measure	Sample tests
Mental status, brief cognitive screen	Orientation, basic attention, memory, expressive and receptive language, visuoconstruction, cognitive flexibility	Mini-Mental Status Examination (MMSE) [47]
		Montreal Cognitive Assessment [48], Addenbrooke's Cognitive Estimation Test [49]
Psychiatric status	Mood, anxiety	Beck Depression Inventory-II [50], Beck Anxiety Inventory, Brief Symptom Inventory-18 [51], Geriatric Depression Scale [52], Brief Symptom Inventory 18 (BSI-18)
Stress level	Degree to which situations are experienced as unpredictable, uncontrollable, and overloading	Perceived Stress Scale (PSS) [53]
Executive functions	Apathy; behavioral regulation; ability to prioritize, organize, and plan; mental flexibility; memory	Frontal Systems Behavior Scale (self and other report) [54], Behavioral Ratings of Executive Functions (self and other report) [55]
Insight and awareness	Appreciation of deficit, insight into functioning, anosognosia	Awareness Questionnaire, Frontal Systems Behavior Scale (comparison of self to other report) [56], Behavioral Ratings of Executive Functions (comparison of self to other report) [55]

assessment interview. It can be more difficult to build rapport when patients are frustrated within the first 15 min of meeting their therapist. Sending self-reports home to be completed can be an option for some patients. Often the information gained from self-reports is duplicated in a thorough clinical interview and assessment. As mentioned previously, the assessment process is a critical component of CBT treatment with this population and can take several sessions. The assessment is often when patients become aware of the specificity of their symptoms and how their symptoms are connected to feelings of "stress." If a patient becomes overly frustrated, it can be more challenging to conduct a productive assessment and can impact development of the solid rapport that is so essential in the beginning of treatment. Thus, it is recommended that the therapist carefully evaluate the pros/cons of giving self-report measures and assess whether the benefits truly outweigh the costs.

In conclusion, the skills described in these four modules have hopefully provided useful clinical information for therapists to do be able to do a CBT informed psychological treatment with patients with neurological conditions. Just as CBT teaches patients to have a number of different psychological tools in their toolbox, therapists who work with a neurological population also need a toolbox with a variety of skills and different ways of teaching them. CBT with this population requires that the therapist has a directive yet flexible style toward accomplishing therapy goals. This work also lends itself well to therapists who are creative, patient, and think outside the box. It can be challenging work, but the rewards for both patients and therapist far outweigh any difficult moments.

9.4   Case Illustration

Joanne is a 45-year-old divorced woman who was referred for CBT by her psychiatrist, who thought she might benefit from learning concrete strategies to cope with her depressed mood. Joanne sustained a traumatic brain injury (TBI) about 6 months prior to her intake assessment and was having an increasingly difficult time coping with its effects.

Prior to her injury, the patient had worked as a nurse at a nearby community hospital where she had a successful career for 15 years. She worked hard and had excellent relationships with both her colleagues and patients. She was proud to be a nurse and felt this was the job she was always meant to do. Joanne had no psychiatric history and no therapy experience prior to her injury. She described always having had a solid support system, which included her siblings and her ex-husband, who all lived nearby. She saw her family several times a week. Joanne and her husband were married for 10 years before their marriage ended amicably. They did not have children. Joanne's work and her family were the most important things to her. She loved her job and got tremendous satisfaction from helping people feel better, and as she gained seniority, she also enjoyed the administrative and teaching aspects of her work.

Six months ago, when she was visiting her niece at a nearby college, she was physically assaulted and sustained significant injuries including significant TBI, facial fractures, bruises, broken ribs, and injuries to her neck and back. Joanne's medical course included several surgeries, 3 weeks at a rehabilitation facility, followed by in home PT and OT. Neuropsychological testing at 3 months postinjury showed Joanne had significant cognitive deficits in memory, attention, and executive functioning. At the time of our intake, Joanne was receiving outpatient PT. She reported that she noticed her depression worsened after her therapies slowed down and visitors came less frequently. Her mood symptoms were further exacerbated by chronic pain and medication side effects (most notably, fatigue).

Intake assessment included a clinical interview with Joanne and her sister, a thorough review of her medical and neurological history, as well as completion of several self-report questionnaires. Joanne met criteria for Major Depressive Disorder—single episode. Her symptoms included feeling depressed and discouraged most of the day, every day, decreased interest in seeing family and friends, 25-lb weight loss, frequent crying spells, feeling easily frustrated and irritable, decreased sleep (2–4 h/night on average), and feeling discouraged about the future. She also reported near-constant pain and needed to take pain medication several times a day. However, even with medication, she experienced significant pain. Joanne's sister reported that she spends her days at home, watching TV or sleeping. Joanne's family was concerned because her depression was getting worse, not better, and they wanted her to get out of the house and start trying to find a way to live again. They also noticed that Joanne had difficulty remembering things and staying focused for a long period of time. Joanne was often irritable and easily frustrated by these cognitive changes. Joanne was on leave from her job, but kept cancelling meetings with her supervisor about whether and in what capacity she could return to work. The cognitive, emotional, and behavioral deficits exhibited by Joanne were consistent with a TBI and it was clear that her symptoms were affecting her life at home in a number of important ways.

The initial phase of CBT involved teaching Joanne skills to help improve depression and address the immediate stressors created by her TBI. These skills were taught over the course of approximately four CBT sessions. Activity scheduling was the first skill that the patient learned. Specifically, Joanne learned the benefits of having a planned daily routine and a list of tasks to accomplish. She also learned the importance of balancing the "have to do" activities (doctor's appointments, household tasks) with the "want to do" tasks (spending time at her sister's house with her nieces and nephews, cooking together, and attending church with her family). During this phase, she learned to use self-monitoring records, which helped her identify and monitor patterns in her mood, pain, and fatigue levels. Joanne found it helpful to be able to identify windows of time when she felt better than others, even if they were brief, so she could optimize times in which to do certain tasks. She also learned how to identify factors that made her more vulnerable to negative feelings (such as increased pain, poor sleep, feeling sorry for herself, etc.). She began to notice that when she was feeling depressed, her pain also felt worse, and she was more likely to withdraw from her family and friends. This social isolation further worsened her mood and increased her negative self-talk.

The second phase of CBT involved identifying the stresses associated with having a TBI and learning more adaptive coping strategies. This phase of therapy was approximately six sessions which included two family sessions. Joanne had been relying on her siblings and friends to help drive her to her appointments, but it was getting more challenging for them to help out because of their own busy work and family lives. Joanne also experienced deficits in executive functioning which were very frustrating for her. For example, she described a recent situation in which she was trying to rehang a picture that had fallen off the wall in her home. When she set out to accomplish this task, she went to the hardware store to get the wire and hook to hang the picture. When she came home, she realized that the glass in the frame had chipped so she also had to get a new frame before she could hang it up again. She then spent a long time trying to decide if she should replace just the glass (and where she would go to get it) or if she should get a new frame altogether. After another trip to get a new frame, she went to hang the picture on the wall and realized that when the old picture fell, it tore a large chunk of plaster off the wall that would need to be patched and dried before she could hang the picture. This would require a third trip to the store and extra time for the plaster to dry. After all the time and energy Joanne spent trying to accomplish this seemingly straightforward task, she was no closer to completing it. In her frustration, she never hung up the picture. When her sister came over and mentioned the blank space where the picture had hung, Joanne became very frustrated and angry with her sister. Every time Joanne passed by the wall, she was reminded of how difficult things were and felt she will never be the person she was before her injury. As seen in this example, Joanne had difficulty assessing a task/situation, breaking it down into smaller steps, and then sequencing the necessary steps in order to accomplish the task. Joanne's experience demonstrates the impact of executive deficits in a person's daily life.

Helping Joanne manage the direct effects of her TBI involved teaching her how to monitor and regulate her emotions so she could effectively use problem-solving skills. She was taught a brief relaxation exercise that focused on slowing down her breathing (extensive PMR was unable to be done because of her neck and back pain). This allowed her to recognize when she was getting frustrated, take a pause, and then try strategies for problem solving such as assessing the situation, identifying her goals, and then breaking tasks into small steps (e.g., What am I trying to do? What do I need to do first? Second?). Joanne also routinely kept a calendar for appointments and a daily task list which helped structure her days and remember the tasks to be completed. Over time, Joanne got into a routine of using these cognitive strategies and with cognitive restructuring practice, was able to think about the benefits of using strategies, not only the frustration of needing to use them.

The final phase of therapy involved helping Joanne develop and adjust to a new and different life. This part of therapy was approximately six sessions and took place over a 3–4 month span. Unfortunately, the cognitive effects of Joanne's head injury made it impossible for her to provide direct nursing care safely. Her supervisor initially assigned her to administrative tasks only, but it soon became clear that this was not the right fit for her either. Joanne was unable to learn a new computer program for inputting medical information, she had trouble concentrating for more than 15 min without feeling exhausted, and wasn't retaining the information she learned. She also had trouble sitting comfortably at a desk for a few hours without having to stand up or take medicine for pain. After two difficult weeks, it was determined that Joanne would not be able to continue to work at her old job. Understandably, she was devastated by this news and viewed it as a significant setback. She said that it confirmed her beliefs that she would never be who she was before and that she couldn't contribute anything positive to other people's lives. Joanne only saw losses. During this phase of treatment, her therapist used acceptance-based cognitive restructuring techniques. Slowly, over time, she could identify the basics of what she loved about nursing and the qualities that made her a dedicated employee, sister, friend, and aunt. She explained that helping patients through difficult times had been the most meaningful part of her job. She also enjoyed being part of a larger team that cared for a patient. In final few months of therapy, Joanne began volunteering in pediatric oncology at the hospital where she worked. She did this at the suggestion of her supervisor and was an enormous breakthrough. As a volunteer, she would sit and talk with children and their parents about what they were going through. She listened to their stories and felt useful again. She found purpose and meaning in her days again. She felt that in some ways, she was even better at listening and understanding the effects of illness because of what she lived through. During this time, Joanne found a deeper connection to the mindfulness skills she learned.

As CBT neared to an end, Joanne's mood was less depressed, her affect was brighter, and her family reported that she was less irritable. She still had legitimate frustrations and stressors that required extra time and emotional effort to cope with, but she had a better understanding of how to do this. Most notably, she found a way to use cognitive restructuring so that it worked best for her. Instead of writing down negative thoughts, feelings, and behaviors, she would "talk out" the thoughts, feelings, and behaviors/urges to act with one of her sisters, who would then help her find another perspective. In fact, her sisters even started using it themselves and it became a "family strategy."

Joanne's course of CBT was complicated by the variability in her pain, as well as whether she was able to get a ride to therapy (driving was painful because of her back injuries), which contributed to missed sessions. When she would miss a session, a brief phone check-in would be scheduled in order to assess what skills she was using and troubleshoot any difficulties. While this between-session contact took an extra step on the part of the therapist, it helped Joanne to view CBT as a continuous process of skill learning, even if there were breaks in session frequency. Ultimately, Joanne was able to find components of her old life that reflected core aspects of who she was (caring about people, helping people, being connected to family) and was able to take these parts of herself and find new places for them to take root. Joanne completed CBT knowing that she had options for controlling many parts of her life.

9.5 Future Directions

Using CBT skills with patients who have neurological conditions can be an important part of a patient's overall treatment plan. In cases where patients have mild symptoms or mild impairment, only a few sessions might be necessary in order to teach some practical coping strategies. Too often, the referrals that come to psychologists are for patients whose symptoms have become too challenging for their physicians. By the time these individuals meet with a therapist, they have already experienced significant stress and frustration. Thus, patients with neurological conditions could benefit from being referred for CBT earlier in the course of their medical treatment, not only after their providers have identified them as challenging. If there is a social worker who is part of a patient's treatment team, CBT could be an adjunctive component of the work they do. In the future, it would be helpful to train other psychological providers, such as social workers, nursing staff, and mental health counselors, how to do these interventions so a wider range of patients could be seen. This could also allow patients to coordinate CBT visits with neurology visits, thereby improving attendance rates. Furthermore, patients in smaller or more rural communities may have more limited access to individual psychological services and could benefit from such multifaceted care. Typically, when patients are discharged home after rehabilitation or hospitalization, they are at the greatest risk for psychological distress as they adjust to how their symptoms impact daily activities at home. Ideally, outpatient CBT could be initiated immediately after discharge. Because patients are also vulnerable to social isolation once they return home, early

CBT could also include educating family or other supports about skills, so they may practice the techniques at home. While patients and their families may meet with their treatment team for a discussion of the discharge plan, these visits are packed with information to be learned. Thus, having an outpatient CBT visit shortly after discharge could help highlight priorities and reinforce learning of the psychological and cognitive treatment goals. For those patients who have difficulty coming for appointments because of pain or other limitations, the use of video CBT and phone apps can be employed to facilitate or maintain outpatient treatment. Finally, in the future, graduate programs could recruit the next generation of students interested in studying and providing this type of therapy to patients with neurological conditions. As part of earning their degree, students could be the ones to directly provide these services (under appropriate supervision) and be an additional member of the treatment team.

9.6   Conclusion

The skills described in these four modules hopefully provides useful clinical information for therapists to do be able to do a CBT informed psychological treatment with patients with neurological conditions. The case illustration provides clinicians with an example of how to apply CBT interventions with a patient who sustained a Traumatic Brain Injury (TBI). While there are diverse neurological conditions, the cognitive and emotional aspects of coping are often similar across conditions. The four modules consist of specific CBT strategies and how these skills can be applied to common symptoms. CBT strategies can also be adapted to a patient's unique symptoms and situation and is appropriate for patients with mild–moderate cognitive deficits. CBT with this population is most efficacious when the therapist uses a directive yet flexible style. Because neurological conditions can be associated with physical, emotional, and/or cognitive changes, symptoms can be extremely stressful for both patients and their caregivers. Thus, CBT can play an integral role in the treatment of patients with neurological conditions and comorbid psychological distress.

References

1. Williams LS, Jones WJ, Shen J, Robinson RL, Weinberger M, Kroenke K. Prevalence and impact of depression and pain in neurology outpatients. J Neurol Neurosurg Psychiatry. 2003;74:1587–9.
2. Mrabet S, Ben Ali N, Kchaou M, Belal S. Depression in multiple sclerosis. Rev Neurol (Paris). 2014;170(11):700–2.
3. Perez LP, Gonzales RS, Lazaro EB. Treatment of mood disorders in multiple sclerosis. Curr Treat Options Neurol. 2015;17(1):323.

4. Siegert RJ, Abernethy DA. Depression in multiple sclerosis: a review. J Neurol Neurosurg Psychiatry. 2005;76:469–75.
5. Lincoln NB, Flannaghan T. Cognitive behavioral psychotherapy for depression following stroke. Stroke. 2003;34:111–5.
6. Dobkin RD, Menza M, Bienfait KL. CBT for the treatment of depression in Parkinson's disease: a promising non-pharmacological approach. Expert Rev Neurother. 2008;8(1):27–35.
7. Rihmer Z, Gonda A, Dome P. Depression in Parkinson's disease. Ideggogy. 2014;7–8:229–36.
8. Lambert MV, Robertson MM. Depression in epilepsy: etiology, phenomenology, and treatment. Epilepsia. 1999;40:S21–47.
9. Bromfield NM, Quinn TJ, Abdul-Rahm AH, Walters MR, Evans JJ. Depression and anxiety symptoms post-stroke/TIA: prevalence and association in cross sectional data from regional stroke registry. BMC Neurol. 2014;24:198.
10. Rao V, Lyksetsos C. Neuropsychiatric sequelae of traumatic brain injury. Psychosomatics. 2000;41:95–103.
11. Tellez-Zenteno JF, Patten SB, Jetté N, Williams J, Wiebe S. Psychiatric comorbidity in epilepsy: a population-based analysis. Epilepsia. 2007;48(12):2336–44.
12. Au A, Chan F, Li K, Leung P, Li P, Chan J. Cognitive-behavioral group treatment program for adults with epilepsy in Hong Kong. Epilepsy Behav. 2003;4(4):441–6.
13. Hind D, Cotter J, Thake A, Bradburn M, Cooper C, Isaac C, et al. Cognitive behavioural therapy for treatment of depression in people with multiple sclerosis: a systematic review and meta-analysis. BMC Psychiatry. 2014;14:5.
14. Kanner AM. Should neurologist be trained to recognize and treat comorbid depression of neurological disorders? Yes. Epilepsy Behav. 2005;3:303–11.
15. Davies RD, Gabbert SL, Riggs PD. Anxiety disorders in neurologic illness. Curr Treat Options Neurol. 2001;3:333–46.
16. Hermann BP, Seidenberg M, Bell B. Psychiatric comorbidity in chronic epilepsy: identification, consequences, and treatment of major depression. Epilepsia. 2000;41 Suppl 2:S31–41. Review.
17. Kale R. Global campaign against epilepsy: the treatment gap. Epilepsia. 2002;43 Suppl 6:31–3.
18. Reuber M, Andersen B, Elger CE, Helmstaedter C. Depression and anxiety before and after temporal lobe epilepsy surgery. Seizure. 2004;13(2):129–35.
19. Altshuler LL, Devinsky O, Post RM, Theodore W. Depression, anxiety, and temporal lobe epilepsy. Laterality of focus and symptoms. Arch Neurol. 1990;47(3):284–8.
20. Hu X, Song X, Yuan Y, Li E, Liu W, Liu Y. Abnormal functional connectivity of the amygdala is associated with depression in Parkinson's disease. Mov Disord. 2015;30(2):238–44.
21. Nigro S, Passamonti L, Riccelli R, Toschi N, Rocca F, Valentino P, et al. Structural "connectomic" alterations in the limbic system of multiple sclerosis patients with major depression. Mult Scler. 2014;21(8):1003–12.
22. Paulsen JS, Ready RE, Hamilton JM, Mega MS, Cummings JL. Neuropsychiatric aspects of Huntington's disease. J Neurol Neurosurg Psychiatry. 2001;71:310–4.
23. Schmahmann JD, Sherman JC. The cerebellar cognitive affective syndrome. Brain. 1998;121:561–79.
24. Jorge RE, Robinson RG, Moser D, Tateno A, Crespo-Faccoro B, Arndt S. Major depression following traumatic brain injury. Arch Gen Psychiatry. 2004;61:42–50.
25. Levin HS, McCauley SR, Pedroza-Josic C, Boak J, Brown SA, Goodman HS, et al. Predicting depression following mild traumatic brain injury. Arch Gen Psychiatry. 2005;62:523–8.
26. Ramaratnam S, Baker GA, Goldstein LH. Psychological treatments for epilepsy. Cochrane Database Syst Rev. 2005;4.
27. Ortega V, Qazi A, Spector AE, Orrell M. Psychological treatments for depression and anxiety in dementia and mild cognitive impairment. Cochrane Database Syst Rev. 2014;1:CD009125.

28. Cosio D, Jin L, Siddique J, Mohr DC. The effect of a telephone-administered cognitive-behavioral therapy on quality of life among patients with multiple sclerosis. Ann Behav Med. 2011;41(2):227–34.
29. Gandy M, Sharpe L, Perry KN. Cognitive behavior therapy for depression in people with epilepsy: a systematic review. Epilepsia. 2013;54:1725–34.
30. Kneebone II, Jeffries FW. Treating anxiety after stroke using cognitive-behaviour therapy: two cases. Neuropsychol Rehabil. 2013;23(6):798–810.
31. Soo C, Tate R. Psychological treatment for anxiety in people with traumatic brain injury. Cochrane Database Syst Rev. 2007;(3):CD005239.
32. Waldron B, Casserly LM, O'Sullivan C. Cognitive behavioural therapy for depression and anxiety in adults with acquired brain injury: what works for whom? Neuropsychol Rehabil. 2013;23(1):64–101.
33. Gandy M, Sharpe L, Nicholson Perry K, Thayer Z, Miller L, Boseri J, et al. Cognitive behavioral therapy to improve mood in people with epilepsy: a randomized controlled trial. Cogn Behav Ther. 2014;43:153–66.
34. Ownsworth T, Fleming J. The relative importance of metacognitive skills, emotional status, and executive function in psychosocial adjustment following acquired brain injury. J Head Trauma Rehabil. 2005;20:315–32.
35. Mohlman J, Gorenstein EE, Kleber M, de Jesus M, Gorman JM, Papp LA. Standard and enhanced cognitive-behavioral therapy for late-life generalized anxiety disorder: two pilot investigations. Am J Geriat Psychiatry. 2003;11(1):24–32.
36. Safren S, Perlman C, Sprich S, Otto M. Mastering your adult ADHD: therapist guide. New York: Oxford University Press; 2005.
37. Safren S, Sprich S, Perlman C, Otto M. Mastering your adult ADHD: client workbook. New York: Oxford University Press; 2005.
38. Safren S. Cognitive-behavioral approaches to ADHD treatment in adulthood. J Clin Psychiatry. 2006;67 Suppl 8:46–50.
39. Krasny-Pacini A, Chevignard M, Evans J. Goal Management Training for rehabilitation of executive functions: a systematic review of effectiveness in patients with acquired brain injury. Disabil Rehabil. 2014;36(2):105–16.
40. Anson K, Ponsford J. Evaluation of a coping skills group following traumatic brain injury. Brain Inj. 2006;20:167–78.
41. Mateer CA, Sira CS, O'Connell ME. Putting Humpty Dumpty together again: the importance of integrating cognitive and emotional interventions. J Head Trauma Rehabil. 2005;20:62–70.
42. Benson H, Klipper MZ. The relaxation response. London: Collins; 1976.
43. Beck JS. Cognitive therapy: basics and beyond. New York: Guilford; 1995.
44. Kabat-Zinn J. Wherever you go, there you are: mindfulness meditation in everyday life. New York: Hyperion; 1994.
45. Miller WR, Rollnick S. Motivational interviewing. 3rd ed. New York: Guilford; 2013.
46. Linehan MM. DBT skills training manual. 2nd ed. New York: Guilford; 2015.
47. Folstein MF, Folstein SE, Fanjiang G. Mini-mental state examination: clinical guide. Odessa: Psychological Assessment Resources; 2001.
48. Nasreddine ZS, Phillips NA, Bédirian V, et al. The Montreal Cognitive Assessment (MoCA): a brief screening tool for mild cognitive impairment. J Am Geriatr Soc. 2005;53:695–9.
49. Mioshi E, Dawson K, Mitchell J, et al. The Addenbrooke's Cognitive Examination Revised (ACE-R): a brief cognitive test battery for dementia screening. Int J Geriatr Psychiatry. 2006;21(11):1078–85.
50. Beck AT, Steer RA, Brown GK. Beck depression inventory. 2nd ed. San Antonio: The Psychological Corporation; 1996.
51. Beck AT, Steer RA. Beck anxiety inventory. San Antonio: The Psychological Corporation; 1993.

52. Brink TL, Yesavage JA, Lum O, et al. Screening tests for geriatric depression. Clin Gerontol. 1982;1:37–44.
53. Cohen S, Kamarck T, Mermelstein R. A global measure of perceived stress. J Health Soc Behav. 1983;24:385–96.
54. Grace J, Malloy PF. Frontal systems behavior scale. Lutz: Psychological Assessment Resources; 2001.
55. Roth RM, Isquith PK, Gioia GA. Behavior rating inventory of executive function—adult version. Lutz: Psychological Assessment Resources; 2005.
56. Sherer M, Bergloff P, Boake C, High Jr W, Levin E. The Awareness Questionnaire: factor structure and internal consistency. Brain Inj. 1998;12(1):63–8.
57. Derogatis LR. Brief symptom inventory 18. Minneapolis: NCS Pearson; 2004.
58. Mohlman J, Gorman JM. The role of executive functioning in CBT: a pilot study with anxious older adults. Behav Res Ther. 2005 Apr; 43(4): 447–65.
59. Cicerone K, Levin H, Malec J, Stuss D, Whyte J. Cognitive rehabilitation interventions for executive function: moving from bench to bedside in patients with traumatic brain injury. J Cogn Neurosci. 2006 July; 18(7): 1212–22.

Resources

MGH Department of Neurology. http://www.massgeneral.org/neurology/
National Institute of Neurological Disorders and Stroke. http://www.ninds.nih.gov/
American Stroke Association. http://www.strokeassociation.org/STROKEORG/
Brain Injury Association of America. http://www.biausa.org/
Epilepsy Foundation. http://www.epilepsy.com/
ALS Association. http://www.alsa.org/
National MS Society. http://www.alsa.org/
Huntington's Disease Society of America. http://hdsa.org/

Chapter 10
Psychosocial Management of Patients with Heart Disease

Rachel A. Millstein and Jeff C. Huffman

10.1 Introduction

10.1.1 Prevalence of Cardiovascular Disease (CVD)

In the United States, heart disease is the leading cause of death for both men and women [1]. Approximately 600,000 people die of heart disease in the United States annually, representing 1 in every 4 deaths. In addition, about 720,000 Americans suffer a heart attack, also known as a myocardial infarction (MI) [1], a condition that requires hospitalization and acute treatment.

Though patients with CVD can suffer acute events like MI, cardiac disease for many is a chronic condition. Patients with coronary artery disease (CAD) may be limited by chest pain, shortness of breath, or other symptoms, and typically require numerous medications for symptom control and prevention of acute episodes. Patients with a more progressive condition, known as heart failure (HF), often have substantial functional limitations caused by their illness, and rates of mortality for this condition continue to be high. Finally, patients with heart rhythm disorders, such as atrial fibrillation (a condition affecting nearly three million Americans) or ventricular arrhythmias, likewise require medications to prevent complications or acute events, and often have impaired quality of life [2].

R.A. Millstein, Ph.D., M.H.S.
Behavioral Medicine Service, Department of Psychiatry, Massachusetts General Hospital,
Harvard Medical School, Boston, MA, USA
e-mail: ramillstein@mgh.harvard.edu

J.C. Huffman, M.D. (✉)
Department of Psychiatry, Massachusetts General Hospital,
55 Fruit St., Warren 1220/Blake 11, Boston, MA 02114, USA
e-mail: jhuffman@mgh.harvard.edu; jhuffman@partners.org

© Springer Science+Business Media New York 2017
A.-M. Vranceanu et al. (eds.), *The Massachusetts General Hospital Handbook of Behavioral Medicine*, Current Clinical Psychiatry,
DOI 10.1007/978-3-319-29294-6_10

10.1.2 Prevalence of Psychological and Psychiatric Comorbidities

Depression is prevalent in cardiac patients, with 20–40 % meeting criteria for major depressive disorder (MDD) or experiencing an elevation in depressive symptoms [3, 4]. Such depressive symptoms are often chronic and persistent, and are associated with progression of CVD, worse health-related quality of life (QoL), poor physical functioning, recurrent cardiac events, and a 1.5- to 2.5-fold increased risk of mortality [4, 5]. These associations between depression and clinical outcomes are independent of sociodemographic factors as well as severity of cardiac illness and related comorbidities.

Rates of MDD are elevated across various cardiac illnesses. Among patients who have had an MI or related condition known as unstable angina, approximately 15–20 % meet criteria for MDD 1–2 weeks after the event and up to 45 % have some depressive symptoms [6]. Among patients with HF, approximately 20 % have MDD. Likewise, 15–20 % of patients undergoing coronary artery bypass graft (CABG) surgery for serious CAD have depression both prior to surgery and postoperatively. Unfortunately, despite the high prevalence and serious consequences of depression, the vast majority of cardiac patients with MDD go unrecognized and untreated, especially in those with acute cardiac conditions [7].

Anxiety disorders, including generalized anxiety disorder (GAD), panic disorder (PD), and post-traumatic stress disorder (PTSD), also occur at higher rates in cardiac patients than in the general population [8, 9], and have been associated with adverse cardiac outcomes, often independent of depression [10–12]. Furthermore, comorbid depression and anxiety in cardiac patients may magnify the risk of adverse outcomes, compared to having either condition alone [13].

Adverse physiological effects, including elevated levels of circulating inflammatory markers, abnormal activity of platelets, and autonomic nervous system abnormalities, may link depression and anxiety with adverse cardiac outcomes [6, 14]. However, it is likely that important mediators of this relationship are health behaviors. Depression in particular has been associated with impaired participation in vital health behaviors, such as healthy eating, smoking cessation, physical activity, and taking medication as prescribed, among patients with acute or chronic cardiac conditions [6]. Not engaging in these health behaviors is associated with an increased risk of cardiovascular events and mortality. In addition, neuro-vegetative symptoms of depression (i.e., low activation, withdrawal, anhedonia, impaired concentration) may be further associated with poor cardiac outcomes.

10.1.3 The Biopsychosocial Model in CVD

The biopsychosocial model acknowledges the interrelationships among biological, psychological, and social-level factors in disease progression and maintenance, which can be particularly useful in considering CVD. Biologically, genetic risk factors can play a role in the development of both depression and CVD, explaining the high rates of co-occurrence of these conditions. Some genetic factors increase the risk of developing both conditions, and depression and cardiovascular disease may be different manifestations of the same genetic substrates [15]. Furthermore, depression has biological effects that can have adverse consequences on the cardiovascular system (e.g., elevated levels of inflammatory markers). In turn, the inflammation associated with CVD can have far-reaching biological and behavioral consequences including physical symptoms and fatigue. These in turn can lead to behavioral challenges such as poor sleep hygiene and reduced physical activity, increasing risk for depression.

From a psychological standpoint, having cardiovascular disease can precipitate or exacerbate depression. For those experiencing an acute cardiac event, the realization that one has heart disease may come suddenly and without warning. Fears of recurrence are common, as is uncertainty about a "safe" level of activity. Other common concerns linked with heart disease include worries about financial status (especially if one's employment involves physical labor), self-image, and identity issues (especially patients who saw themselves as the breadwinner or emotional bedrock of a family), and the emotional recalibration that comes with having to manage a chronic illness, including making long-term lifestyle changes and taking multiple medications on a regular basis.

Finally, objective and perceived social support is an important factor in people's well-being and recovery after a cardiac event. Social support has been linked to superior cardiovascular outcomes, and such support can be critical in managing the psychological effects of heart disease described above [16]. In addition, social support encourages behavior changes necessary for optimal management of CVD. Support can facilitate greater participation in physical activity and healthy eating. Cardiac rehabilitation programs leverage this concept by employing group-based programs that focus on health behaviors, using social support from peers to encourage ongoing healthy behavior.

10.1.4   Evidence Base for Cognitive-Behavioral Interventions to Manage Comorbid Psychiatric Conditions Among Cardiac Patients

Managing psychiatric illnesses in patients with heart disease has been the focus of much research attention. A meta-analysis evaluating the benefits of psychological treatments in cardiac populations found significant reductions in mortality, particularly among men [17]. This meta-analysis included numerous studies with different modalities of psychotherapy, making it difficult to identify one particular form of therapy that was helpful in improving cardiovascular outcomes. Recent research has examined more structured psychotherapeutic interventions such as cognitive behavioral therapy (CBT) and problem-solving therapy (PST). Both of these types of short-term manualized psychotherapies are effective and frequently used in the non-pharmacological treatment of depression [18–21]. CBT is also well known to be effective for numerous anxiety disorders though it is less studied for these conditions in cardiac patients. While the remainder of this chapter will focus on cognitive, behavioral, and psychosocial interventions for comorbid mental health conditions, we acknowledge that antidepressant medications such as selective serotonin reuptake inhibitors (SSRIs) are well tolerated and effective in patients with heart disease [4, 22] and represent a useful intervention strategy when appropriate.

CBT is the best-studied psychological intervention in cardiac populations. CBT in this population involves identifying and modifying distorted thoughts about one's illness and coping behaviors. CBT was evaluated in the largest randomized controlled trial of treatment for depression in cardiac patients. In a trial of about 2500 MI patients with depression and/or low social support, CBT was associated with significant improvement in depressive symptoms though it was not associated with changes in cardiac outcomes [19]. A second trial of CBT for depression among post-CABG patients found that those in both the CBT and supportive stress management groups experienced significantly higher rates of remission from depressive symptoms at 3 months compared with a usual care group (71 % vs. 57 % vs. 33 %, respectively). However, only patients in the CBT group maintained improvements in depression at 9 months, suggesting that the skills aspects of the intervention lead to long lasting effects [18]. The CBT intervention in this study also resulted in greater improvements in anxiety, hopelessness, perceived stress, and mental health-related QoL compared with usual care. These findings suggest that CBT is an effective treatment for depression in post-MI and post-CABG patients.

CBT for anxiety disorders comorbid with CVD has been less studied compared to depression. However, CBT has been used frequently as a component of a care management program for cardiac patients with GAD and PD [23]. In addition, CBT has been used to target psychological adaptation for patients with serious cardiac arrhythmias (abnormal heartbeat) who required an implanted cardioverter defibrillator. This type of defibrillator is a device that is surgically implanted in the chest to regulate heartbeats. If a patient develops a serious arrhythmia, electrical shock may be required to correct the heartbeat. In this case, the defibrillator "fires," providing a life-saving electrical stimulation. These shocks are sudden and very painful for patients. As such, despite their life-saving nature, having a serious arrhythmia and defibrillator can be very distressing for patients. A randomized controlled trial found that CBT was associated with improved psychological functioning 1 year following defibrillator surgery [24].

PST is the other form of short-term, manualized therapy that has been studied in this population. It is a practical, problem-focused, and easily administered therapy that aims to help patients systematically solve problems in their psychosocial environment that contribute to depression [25, 26]. PST has been used effectively in two collaborative care management studies of depression in heart disease (COPES, CODIACS), resulting in significant improvement in depression [20, 21]. In both collaborative care trials, though medications were offered to patients, the majority elected treatment with PST. In these studies, PTS was well tolerated, and most patients experienced a reduction in depression symptoms. The COPES care management trial for depressed cardiac patients also demonstrated that patients in the care management program (the majority of whom received PST) were less likely to suffer a major cardiac event [20]. These findings suggest that PST is a useful therapy for ongoing and collaborative management of mental health in cardiac patients.

Another avenue of potential benefit of CBT, PST, and other therapeutic interventions may be increased adherence to cardioprotective health behaviors (i.e., diet, physical activity, smoking cessation, medication adherence). As noted, depressed cardiac patients exhibit significantly lower adherence to preventive health behaviors compared to nondepressed patients [27]. Research has shown that among depressed cardiac patients, improvement in depression is associated with superior improvements in medication adherence, diet, physical activity, and stress reduction 6 months after a cardiac event [28]. Another study showed that increased patient activation, a key component in behavioral treatment of anxiety, depression, and disease self-management, was associated with improved health behaviors such as physical activity, dietary awareness, stress reduction, and medication adherence [29].

10.2   Specific CBT Approach, Goals, and Skills

CBT in cardiac populations is often used as part of a collaborative treatment program and does not necessarily proceed in a standard linear fashion. First, we will identify overall cardiac disease management strategies that can impact cognitions; second, we will address common cognitions that lead to anxiety and depression among cardiac patients; and finally, we will address CBT-based treatment options. See Table 10.1 for suggested uses of CBT techniques for different patient issues.

10.2.1   Providing Medical Information and Psychoeducation

Among cardiac patients, medical understanding of their disease and psychoeducation can play important roles in reducing cardiac-related anxiety. Providers can first help patients develop a sense of confidence about the way they perceive their disease. A basic understanding of the illness, mechanisms, and treatment approaches can alleviate and prevent much anxiety. Many self-report measures are available to help patients and providers understand and classify common physical and emotional symptoms (see Table 10.2). Patients should understand which common symptoms are normal and which are abnormal. To that end, symptom monitoring can be useful for patients with more ongoing illnesses (i.e., arrhythmias, chronic HF) to help determine antecedents, timing of symptoms, and significant changes that require medical attention [30]. Such medical information may be beyond the scope of behavioral interventionists, but therapists should encourage patients to obtain such information from their medical providers. Therapists should also speak with the cardiology team to better understand which symptoms are of concern from a medical standpoint, as described further below.

Table 10.1 CBT components and recommendations for specific patient problems

Component	Strategies	Recommended for	Goals
Psychoeducation	Collaborate with MD	For all patients	Provide cardiac-specific educational information
	Understand common versus uncommon symptoms		Provide educational information about the CBT model and skills
			Introduce symptom self-monitoring
Behavioral	Activity scheduling	For patients with depression	Help patients reengage in pleasant activities/decrease avoidance
	Behavioral exposure	For patients with anxiety or agoraphobia	Approach increasingly feared situations with lower anxiety
	Activity pacing/physical activity, nutrition planning, medication adherence planning	For patients able to increase physical activity, improve diet, improve medication adherence	Help patients increase meaningful activity within the confines of cardiac limitations
			Help patients gradually reengage in physical activity (per MD's recommendations)
			Help patients set behavioral nutrition goals (i.e., low sodium, low fat diets)
			Help patients set up a reminder system for taking prescribed medications
Cognitive	Traditional cognitive restructuring	For patients with cardiac anxiety/depression	Help patients identify negative automatic thoughts, decide whether they are distorted or not
			Use thought records to modify distorted thoughts
	Acceptance-based cognitive therapy	For patients with realistic negative thoughts that can't be problem solved	Practice acceptance of current situation while helping patient move in valued directions
	Problem solving	For patients with realistic negative thoughts that can be problem solved	Choose between traditional cognitive restructuring and acceptance-based cognitive restructuring, with or without problem solving. Help patients choose distinct problems to solve one at a time
Physiological	Breath awareness	Beneficial for all cardiac patients	Help patient elicit the relaxation response, decrease reactivity to physical symptoms
	Guided imagery	For patients who are overly reactive to cardiac symptoms or have comorbid anxiety	
	Biofeedback		
	Progressive muscle relaxation		
	Mindfulness		
Cardiac health and family dynamics	Partner education	For patients having difficulty with role shifts related to cardiac-related physical/occupational limitations	Improved communication around patient's limitations
	Communication boundaries		Delegation of household and work-related tasks
			Gradual planning to increase range of activities
Acceptance versus control	Pros and cons	For patients feeling frustrated by the sick role or with difficulty accepting health status/limitations	Help patients understand the futility of fighting against their diagnosis
			Help patients move toward increasing functionality within cardiac-related activity limitations

Table 10.2 Self-report measures for cardiac patients

Measure	Variable	Description
Depression and anxiety		
Patient Health Questionnaire (PHQ-9) [56]	Depression	Nine items assessing major depression symptoms
Beck Depression Inventory (BDI-II) [57]	Depression	Commonly used 21-item measure of depression in general and medical settings
Hospital Anxiety and Depression Scale (HADS) [58]	Anxiety and depression	14 items total, split into two 7-item subscales to assess anxiety and depression, originally designed to assess medically ill patients
Quality of life (QoL)		
Medical Outcomes Study Short Form-12 (SF-12) [59]	Health-related QoL	Mental and physical health status as components of QoL, 12 items
Perceived Stress Scale (PSS) [60]	Stress-related QoL	10-item measures of the degree to which life situations are appraised as stressful
Disease-specific or medically oriented		
Duke Activity Status Index (DASI) [61]	Functioning	12-item measure of patients' functional capacity
Kansas City Cardiomyopathy Questionnaire (KCCQ) [62]	Heart failure-specific QoL	23-item disease-specific health status measure for patients with congestive heart failure
Seattle Angina Questionnaire (SAQ) [63]	Angina-specific QoL	19 items assessing five dimensions of coronary artery disease: physical limitations, anginal stability, anginal frequency, treatment satisfaction, and disease perception
Medical Outcomes Study-Specific Adherence Scale (MOS-SAS) [64]	Adherence to medical recommendations	Eight items measuring self-reported frequency of adherence (i.e., diet, physical activity, medication compliance)
Cardiac Anxiety Questionnaire [65]	Cardiac anxiety	18 items measuring fear of cardiac-related stimuli and sensations in three domains: heart-related fear, avoidance, and attention
Cardiac Depression Scale [66]	Cardiac depression	26-item cardiac-specific measure of depression

10.2.2   Common Distressing Concerns

One of the most common anxiety-provoking cognitions is the fear of having a recurrent cardiac event. This is a normal concern that dissipates over time for most patients. However, when this fear becomes long-standing or pervasive, it can lead to heightened anxiety. Such anxiety can lead to avoidance of important physical, social, and occupational behaviors that could in turn increase cardiac risk and cause functional impairment; this presents an opportunity to intervene using CBT. A second set of common and potentially problematic cognitions involves perceptions about medical illness. During and after a cardiac event, patients' physical functioning is often at least temporarily compromised, and they are placed in the sick role, sometimes unexpectedly. This role may challenge self-perceptions of being strong, independent, and competent, leading to increased depression or anxiety. A third main type of concern involves financial strain. People who experience a cardiac event often have to take time off of work or alter their work routine to accommodate medical appointments, a cardiac rehabilitation program, or reduced work duties. Adjustment to a new work situation and any associated financial changes can bring about or perpetuate feelings of anxiety or depression.

10.2.3   CBT-Based Treatment

The first step in using CBT with cardiac patients is consulting with their medical team to rule-out physical or cardiac symptoms that could be mistaken for mental health symptoms. For instance, panic symptoms often resemble cardiac symptoms, including chest tightness, shortness of breath, or dizziness, and MDD symptoms may overlap with the fatigue and anergia of some cardiac diagnoses [30]. As previously stated, symptom self-monitoring can play an important role in helping patients distinguish between types and nature of symptoms. However, new cardiac patients, particularly those with a somatic focus, may be prone to symptom over-monitoring and hypervigilance to internal stimuli. Patients should be encouraged to find a balance between vigilance and trust in their bodies that can lead to reduced anxiety, especially when it is clear that the existence of symptoms is related to anxiety and not their underlying cardiac condition. A decision tree can be used to make the distinction: a symptom is appropriate for vigilance when it is different or severe, versus chronic and/or established to be noncardiac.

Psychoeducation about the nature of anxiety/depression and CBT is an important next step when working with cardiac patients, some of whom may not have previously experienced mental health concerns. Normalizing the experience of fear or distress is therapeutically useful. As it is central to CBT formulation and treatment, identifying automatic thoughts is a key step toward providing effective therapy [19]. In the case of these three main sources of concern listed above, catastrophic thinking (or fortune telling), is the primary cognitive distortion. Catastrophic thinking involves believing that a poor (or worst) possible outcome is likely to occur in a given situation [31]. A salient example is the automatic thought upon having any cardiac symptom like chest pain, shortness of breath, or palpitations, "This is it, I'm having the big one [heart attack]." This type of thinking can lead to heightened distress, pessimism, and further avoidance of activities. Other cognitive distortions that can play a role for cardiac patients include all-or-nothing thinking, emotional reasoning, and probability overestimation [31]. All-or-nothing thinking might be expressed in thoughts such as, "If I haven't taken all of my medications for a day, I've blown it and may as well not take them anymore." Emotional reasoning automatic thoughts may include, "I always feel so tired, I'm not going to get any better." An example of probability overestimation might be, "If I leave my house I'll have another heart attack." Each of these automatic thoughts can be restructured using CBT strategies. For patients, the first step in restructuring is to recognize antecedents, behaviors, and consequences (A-B-Cs) of distorted forms of thinking. Once patients can identify distorted thoughts, they can begin to evaluate each thought's accuracy, and in turn modify thoughts that are not useful or fully accurate. The use of manuals (i.e., Oxford University Press's *Treatments that Work* series or Greenberger and Padesky's *Mind Over Mood*) can be helpful for guiding patients through CBT protocols, with therapist assistance and tailoring to cardiac-specific concerns (see Resources section below).

CBT offers several strategies to promote more balanced thinking. Table 10.3 provides several questions that patients can ask themselves to identify and correct distortions using objective evidence rather than fear or other emotions. For example, if a medically stable cardiac patient was avoiding normal daily activities for fear of having another heart attack, a therapist might ask, "How many other times have you left your house? How many of those times have you had a heart attack? Do you know what to do if you were experiencing symptoms? Who could help you if you were to experience symptoms?" As in any CBT protocol, patients respond best when they are able to elicit their own solutions through Socratic questioning. Therapists or care providers are encouraged to help patients move toward independence in this type of cognitive restructuring, as CBT-based interventions tend to be time limited. Thought records can be helpful in encouraging patients to practice cognitive restructuring on their own.

As previously described, behaviors are a key component of recovery from a cardiac event, including health behaviors (diet, physical activity, smoking cessation, medication adherence) and reintegration into one's social and family life. If anxiety-related behavioral avoidance or depression-related anergia or amotivation are interfering with recovery, the therapist can include exposure hierarchies, behavioral activation, and/or pleasant event scheduling to increase patients' engagement in their lives. In the case of depression, one of the most important recovery strategies is behavioral activation to bring patients back into contact with reinforcing and satisfying people and activities [32]. In addition to behavioral activation's emotional benefits, it can also be very useful in helping people begin or resume physical activity, which offers independent cardioprotective value. In sum, these cognitive and

Table 10.3 Cognitive strategies to correct distorted thinking and arrive at more balanced thinking

Questions for patients to arrive at balanced thinking
What evidence do I have for this fear or belief?
Am I 100 % sure these awful consequences will occur?
Have I been able to cope with _____ in the past?
What happened in the past in this situation?
Do I have a crystal ball? How can I be sure that I know the answer?
Could there be any other explanations?
How much does it feel like _____ will happen?
What is the true likelihood that _____ will happen?
Is my negative prediction driven by the intense emotions I'm experiencing?

behavioral techniques in cardiac populations involve fluid use of medical- and psychoeducation, identifying and restructuring distorted cognitions, resuming previously meaningful activities, and initiating or resuming healthy behaviors [30].

10.3 Other Behavioral and Therapeutic Interventions

10.3.1 Problem-Solving Therapy

Problem-solving therapy (PST) is a research-supported brief therapy (6–8 sessions) that teaches systematic, practical strategies for patients who are managing a new illness or mental health symptoms [33]. Its advantages include that it is easy to teach and learn and fits in well with integrated care models that may use nurses or social workers to deliver the intervention [20, 21]. A general structure for PST in a medical context is: (1) build rapport and explain the treatment to a patient, (2) help the patient clearly describe the problem or break a large problem into smaller ones, (3) create objective and achievable goals, (4) generate a list of as many solutions as possible, (5) identify pros and cons of each solution, (6) choose an achievable solution to enact, (7) identify steps toward the selected solution, and (8) review the outcome and possibly use a different solution in the same process the next time. A different problem or different aspects of the initial problem should be addressed at each session [34]. Pleasant activity scheduling is another useful aspect of PST. Ongoing depression and anxiety symptom monitoring also provides useful feedback for patients and providers. The principles of PST can be used alone or combined with cognitive restructuring or other CBT modules, as needed.

10.3.2 Relaxation and Mindfulness-Based Treatments

Mindfulness-based stress reduction (MBSR) and relaxation programs can provide anxiety and depression relief as well as cardioprotective effects by reducing stress and related physiological responses, including inflammation [35]. MBSR is an 8-week structured program designed for patients with physical and mental health conditions, or for those who wish to deepen a mindfulness meditation practice [36]. MBSR promotes relaxation and present-moment focus through guided and imaginal exercises and mind–body-based meditations. It has demonstrated efficacy in reducing pain, physical symptoms, and anxiety (http://www.mindfullivingprograms.com/relatedresearch.php). Components of MBSR have been shown to be beneficial in cardiac populations [37]. Many cardiac patients who experience anxiety or depression can benefit from a present-moment focus and the relaxation and mindfulness meditation skills taught in MBSR.

Meditation and relaxation programs, alone or as part of MBSR, have been shown to be effective in reducing stress in the general population [38] and cardiac patients [39]. Such relaxation programs involve holistic and research-based strategies for inducing the parasympathetic nervous system's relaxing effects. Techniques involve guided imagery, mindfulness meditations, deep breathing, and muscle relaxation. A series of steps to induce a relaxation response are as follows: have the patient sit quietly with eyes closed, and intentionally, progressively scan the body and relax all muscles. Patients are then instructed to inhale through the nose and exhale slowly while focusing on one soothing word, such as "peace" or "one." Patients are instructed to continue in this manner for 10–20 min 1–2 times per day and to adopt a nonjudgmental stance [40]. This approach allows cardiac patients the opportunity to learn and self-induce the relaxation response.

10.3.3 Additional Therapeutic Interventions

Interpersonal Therapy (IPT) is a brief strengths-based therapy (IPT-B: 8 weeks) that focuses on improving depressive symptoms, self-esteem, and interpersonal relationships [41]. IPT has been implemented for managing depression in the context of cardiac disease, but was not found to be superior to standard clinical management [42]. IPT involves assisting patients in resolving and rebuilding social connections, self-esteem, and valued behaviors and interactions. It is well accepted and short term, allowing for brief interventions for cardiac patients with mild–moderate depressive symptoms [43].

Though less well studied in this population, Acceptance and Commitment Therapy (ACT) may also provide benefit for cardiac patients in terms of mental health and adherence to health behaviors [44]. The focus on acceptance of one's present life circumstances may be useful for newly diagnosed patients who are struggling to adapt to their illness. Further, ACT's emphasis on pursuing valued action in the context of physical or emotional limitations could provide cardiac patients with a framework and optimism to overcome perceived barriers and live a full and meaningful life. ACT can also be useful when dealing with negative thoughts that are realistic and thus not amenable to cognitive restructuring.

Another promising intervention is positive psychology (PP), which aims to improve the frequency and intensity of positive cognitions and emotions through intentional actions [45]. Increased attention to positive thoughts and feelings through positive psychology exercises can improve patients' feelings of optimism, gratitude, and emotional well-being. Positive psychological states have been shown to impact health behavior adherence like healthy diet, reduced smoking, and improved physical activity, independent of negative emotions [46]. Further, higher optimism and positive affect have been associated with lower rates of cardiac disease and cardiac mortality [47]. PP exercises are easy for patients to complete and well accepted, with little provider training required. Early studies have found that a PP intervention is associated with improved mood and positive affect in cardiac populations, and PP appears to be a novel and efficacious intervention modality [48]. Examples of PP exercises are asking patients to recall three events that were associated with gratitude, happiness, pride, or other positive states in the past week [49] or completing three acts of kindness in the next 2 days [50].

10.3.4   Integrated Care Models

In addition to being used as stand-alone treatments for medical patients with mental health conditions, behavioral interventions are increasingly being used as part of integrated care models for patients with physical health disorders. For example, collaborative care models use a nurse or social work care manager to coordinate care between clinicians (psychiatrists and psychologists) who serve as consultants, and patients' primary medical providers. In this model, the care manager completes diagnostic assessments for patients in medical clinics, and for those identified as having a mood or anxiety disorder, the care manager provides psychoeducation, obtains treatment recommendations from the collaborative care team, and conveys those recommendations (e.g., for psychiatric medications) to the patient and his/her primary medical provider. Increasingly, care managers in this role are trained to encourage behavioral activation or deliver manualized psychotherapeutic interventions, such as PST or CBT, to patients who enroll in these programs. The team psychologistor psychiatrist often serves as a supervising clinician for the care manager.

These models have now been studied extensively in cardiac patients, including hospitalized cardiac patients [23, 51], those with recent heart surgery [51], and those with a recent ACS [21]. These models have been found to have high acceptability and lead to superior outcomes compared to patients receiving medical treatment as usual. In the most contemporary models, care managers also provide motivational interviewing for health behavior change, and one such study of this "blended" care management model led to improvements in blood pressure and blood glucose in patients with diabetes and/or CAD [52].

10.4   Future Directions

Technology can be very useful for delivering mental health care in a cardiac population. In addition to phone-based interventions, internet or web-based CBT has been more recently tested, with good initial results [53]. Internet or web-based CBT is appealing for patients with chronic medical illness because they are less able to present in person for regularly scheduled therapy sessions. Phone and video interventions are nonintrusive, well accepted, and effective. Smartphone-based applications (apps) can also be useful for patients managing anxiety or depression. Several applications have been developed for the general population. The focus of these applications includes helping patients with psychoeducation, symptom monitoring and assessment, tracking treatment progress, CBT skills, and guided imagery or relaxation breathing. Newer applications can also facilitate feedback from providers regarding treatment progress and may be more appealing to younger patients with heart disease [54]. While they may be helpful for patients, few applications are yet evidence based, which represents a new field of research [55].

10.5   Case Illustration

Brenda was a married, retired, 66-year-old woman with a history of MI who had been recently hospitalized for chest pain. She underwent coronary catetherization and had two stents placed to open partially blocked arteries and was cleared for normal activity upon discharge. She had experienced episodes of anxiety in the past but never previously met criteria for an anxiety disorder. Several weeks after she got home from the hospital, she began to notice distressing symptoms: shortness of breath, racing heart, sweating, chest pain, and dizziness. She immediately presented to the ER. Further evaluation revealed clean (unblocked) coronary arteries, and her providers informed her that she had experienced a very typical panic attack. The health professionals explained how her symptoms were different from those of an MI. Brenda was highly distressed by this information, as she had never experienced a panic attack before, and was certain that these symptoms were related to her heart. As a result, she began to have difficulty leaving her house, and she was reluctant to attend to her daily tasks for fear of exerting stress on her heart or having another panic attack. She became reliant on her husband and adult children to manage her responsibilities in and outside of the home. This role shift was upsetting for Brenda, who had been used to providing for her family. At the suggestion of her PCP and urging of her family, she agreed to begin a brief course of CBT with a psychologist for 6–8 sessions.

In session 1, the therapist gave Brenda the HADS self-report anxiety and depression measure designed for medical patients. Her scores were indicative of moderate anxiety and mild depression. First, the therapist introduced psychoeducation about the nature of panic attacks versus the likelihood of another heart attack given Brenda's recent diagnostic evaluations. They then reviewed problem solving in the event that she experiences true cardiac symptoms. The homework for week 1 was symptom self-monitoring, including the A-B-Cs: antecedents, behaviors, and consequences of her panic symptoms. In session 2, the therapist and Brenda collaboratively determined her patterns of panic and anxiety based on the log from last week. The therapist introduced the concept of cognitive distortions and taught deep breathing for inducing relaxation. The homework for week 2 was for Brenda to notice and self-monitor her cognitive distortions and use deep breathing daily to relax. In session 3, Brenda and her therapist reviewed her logs of cognitive distortions related to heart disease and reinforced her coping resources. They attempted to expand the range of possible distortions being used, based on her self-monitoring. As appropriate, the therapist introduced the concepts of an agoraphobia exposure hierarchy. The homework for this session was to continue self-monitoring, use deep breathing daily, and generate and rank agoraphobic situations with accompanying distress ratings. In session 4, the therapist gave Brenda another HADS assessment, and her scores indicated symptom improvements (mild anxiety, mild depression). The therapist introduced the idea of alternative hypotheses based on her commonly used cognitive distortions, and Brenda and her therapist generated alternative hypotheses, especially regarding catastrophizing, overgeneralization, and all-or-nothing thinking. The homework for this week was continued self-monitoring of cognitive distortions, coming up with alternate thoughts for each, and practicing entering situations at a low level of distress on her hierarchy. For instance, Brenda chose going to the grocery store with her husband and then alone, as low-level exposures to begin with. In session 5, Brenda continued to review her strategies for generating alternative cognitions, including reviewing questions to help with that process (see Table 10.1), i.e., "How likely is it that these symptoms are due to panic versus a heart attack?" or "What would you tell a friend in this situation?" They discussed progress on Brenda's agoraphobia hierarchy. Her exposures had gone well the previous week, and Brenda was cautiously optimistic about continuing to approach feared situations. Homework was continued self-monitoring and practicing generating alternative hypotheses, in addition to ongoing exposure hierarchy progression. Her exposure for this week was to go to the bank during a busy time, having to wait in line for at least 10 min and noticing her anxiety rise and fall. In session 6, in addition to continued review of CBT self-monitoring worksheets and exposure planning, the therapist introduced guided imagery and progressive muscle relaxation. Homework was ongoing practice with alternative thoughts, agoraphobia hierarchy, and daily relaxation practice including guided imagery or progressive muscle relaxation. In session 7, the therapist continued to present options for inducing the relaxation response in a 10-min meditation involving either focusing on one's breathing, body scan, or single-pointed attention. In this session, Brenda's HADS anxiety and depression scores had both fallen out of the "case" range, indicating occasional mild symptoms. Based on Brenda's symptom reduction, therapy could have terminated at this point, as she was no longer experiencing panic attacks and was able to attend to her affairs outside of the home. Further, she had a behavioral and cognitive plan for approaching her remaining anxiety-provoking situations. Brenda elected to include a session 8 with a wrap-up, reflection on her progress, and discussion of her comfort level with distinguishing panic from cardiac symptoms. Booster sessions at monthly intervals were scheduled as appropriate.

10.6 Conclusions

In sum, psychiatric conditions and coping challenges are common in patients with heart disease, and these often go unaddressed. Fortunately, a wide variety of therapeutic approaches are effective in this population, and a substantial number of studies have found that mental health treatment in patients with heart disease is well tolerated, effective, and often linked to better health status. Innovations in mental health care, such as collaborative care models and telehealth interventions, may allow for even greater use of behavioral treatments for heart disease patients, and novel approaches focused on mindfulness and resilience may provide additional tools for health psychologists.

References

1. Roger V, Go A, Lloyd-Jones D, Adams R, Berry J, Brown T, et al. Heart disease and stroke statistics—2011 update: a report from the American Heart Association. Circulation. 2011;123(4):e18–209.
2. Thrall G, Lane D, Carroll D, Lip GY. Quality of life in patients with atrial fibrillation: a systematic review. Am J Med. 2006;119(5):448.e1–19.
3. Davidson KW, Kupfer DJ, Bigger JT, Califf RM, Carney RM, Coyne JC, et al. Assessment and treatment of depression in patients with cardiovascular disease: National Heart, Lung, and Blood Institute Working Group Report. Psychosom Med. 2006;68(5):645–50.
4. Celano CM, Huffman JC. Depression and cardiac disease: a review. Cardiol Rev. 2011;19(3):130–42.
5. Meijer A, Conradi HJ, Bos EH, Thombs BD, van Melle JP, de Jonge P. Prognostic association of depression following myocardial infarction with mortality and cardiovascular events: a meta-analysis of 25 years of research. Gen Hosp Psychiatry. 2011;33(3):203–16.
6. Huffman JC, Celano CM, Beach SR, Motiwala SR, Januzzi JL. Depression and cardiac disease: epidemiology, mechanisms, and diagnosis. Cardiovasc Psychiatry Neurol. 2013;2013:695925.
7. Ziegelstein RC, Kim SY, Kao D, Fauerbach JA, Thombs BD, McCann U, et al. Can doctors and nurses recognize depression in patients hospitalized with an acute myocardial infarction in the absence of formal screening? Psychosom Med. 2005;67(3):393–7.
8. Huffman JC, Celano CM, Januzzi JL. The relationship between depression, anxiety, and cardiovascular outcomes in patients with acute coronary syndromes. Neuropsychiatr Dis Treat. 2010;6:123–36.
9. Bankier B, Januzzi JL, Littman AB. The high prevalence of multiple psychiatric disorders in stable outpatients with coronary heart disease. Psychosom Med. 2004;66(5):645–50.
10. Huffman JC, Pollack MH, Stern TA. Panic disorder and chest pain: mechanisms, morbidity, and management. Prim Care Companion J Clin Psychiatry. 2002;4(2):54–62.
11. Roest AM, Zuidersma M, de Jonge P. Myocardial infarction and generalised anxiety disorder: 10-year follow-up. Br J Psychiatry. 2012;200(4):324–9.
12. Tulloch H, Greenman PS, Tasse V. Post-traumatic stress disorder among cardiac patients: prevalence, risk factors, and considerations for assessment and treatment. Behav Sci. 2014;5(1):27–40.
13. Watkins LL, Koch GG, Sherwood A, Blumenthal JA, Davidson JR, O'Connor C, et al. Association of anxiety and depression with all-cause mortality in individuals with coronary heart disease. J Am Heart Assoc. 2013;2(2):e000068.

14. Lett HS, Blumenthal JA, Babyak MA, Sherwood A, Strauman T, Robins C, et al. Depression as a risk factor for coronary artery disease: evidence, mechanisms, and treatment. Psychosom Med. 2004;66(3):305–15.
15. Bondy B, Baghai TC, Zill P, Bottlender R, Jaeger M, Minov C, et al. Combined action of the ACE D- and the G-protein beta3 T-allele in major depression: a possible link to cardiovascular disease? Mol Psychiatry. 2002;7(10):1120–6.
16. Rozanski A, Blumenthal JA, Davidson KW, Saab PG, Kubzansky L. The epidemiology, pathophysiology, and management of psychosocial risk factors in cardiac practice: the emerging field of behavioral cardiology. J Am Coll Cardiol. 2005;45(5):637–51.
17. Linden W, Phillips MJ, Leclerc J. Psychological treatment of cardiac patients: a meta-analysis. Eur Heart J. 2007;28(24):2972–84.
18. Freedland KE, Skala JA, Carney RM, Rubin EH, Lustman PJ, Davila-Roman VG, et al. Treatment of depression after coronary artery bypass surgery: a randomized controlled trial. Arch Gen Psychiatry. 2009;66(4):387–96.
19. Berkman LF, Blumenthal J, Burg M, Carney RM, Catellier D, Cowan MJ, et al. Effects of treating depression and low perceived social support on clinical events after myocardial infarction: the Enhancing Recovery in Coronary Heart Disease Patients (ENRICHD) Randomized Trial. JAMA. 2003;289(23):3106–16.
20. Davidson KW, Rieckmann N, Clemow L, Schwartz JE, Shimbo D, Medina V, et al. Enhanced depression care for patients with acute coronary syndrome and persistent depressive symptoms: coronary psychosocial evaluation studies randomized controlled trial. Arch Intern Med. 2010;170(7):600–8.
21. Davidson KW, Bigger JT, Burg MM, Carney RM, Chaplin WF, Czajkowski S, et al. Centralized, stepped, patient preference-based treatment for patients with post-acute coronary syndrome depression: CODIACS vanguard randomized controlled trial. JAMA Intern Med. 2013;173(11):997–1004.
22. Glassman AH, O'Connor CM, Califf RM, Swedberg K, Schwartz P, Bigger Jr JT, et al. Sertraline treatment of major depression in patients with acute MI or unstable angina. JAMA. 2002;288(6):701–9.
23. Huffman JC, Mastromauro CA, Beach SR, Celano CM, Dubois CM, Healy BC, et al. Collaborative care for depression and anxiety disorders in patients with recent cardiac events: the Management of Sadness and Anxiety in Cardiology (MOSAIC) randomized clinical trial. JAMA Intern Med. 2014;174(6):927–35.
24. Irvine J, Firestone J, Ong L, Cribbie R, Dorian P, Harris L, et al. A randomized controlled trial of cognitive behavior therapy tailored to psychological adaptation to an implantable cardioverter defibrillator. Psychosom Med. 2011;73(3):226–33.
25. Berman MI, Buckey Jr JC, Hull JG, Linardatos E, Song SL, McLellan RK, et al. Feasibility study of an interactive multimedia electronic problem solving treatment program for depression: a preliminary uncontrolled trial. Behav Ther. 2014;45(3):358–75.
26. Choi NG, Hegel MT, Marinucci ML, Sirrianni L, Bruce ML. Association between participant-identified problems and depression severity in problem-solving therapy for low-income homebound older adults. Int J Geriatr Psychiatry. 2012;27(5):491–9.
27. Ziegelstein RC, Fauerbach JA, Stevens SS, Romanelli J, Richter DP, Bush DE. Patients with depression are less likely to follow recommendations to reduce cardiac risk during recovery from a myocardial infarction. Arch Intern Med. 2000;160(12):1818–23.
28. Bauer LK, Caro MA, Beach SR, Mastromauro CA, Lenihan E, Januzzi JL, et al. Effects of depression and anxiety improvement on adherence to medication and health behaviors in recently hospitalized cardiac patients. Am J Cardiol. 2012;109(9):1266–71.
29. Hibbard JH, Mahoney ER, Stock R, Tusler M. Do increases in patient activation result in improved self-management behaviors? Health Serv Res. 2007;42(4):1443–63.
30. Sears SF, Woodrow L, Cutitta K, Ford J, Shea JB, Cahill J. A patient's guide to living confidently with chronic heart failure. Circulation. 2013;127(13):e525–8.
31. Burns DD. The feeling good handbook. New York: Plume; 1999.

32. Burg MM, Abrams D. Depression in chronic medical illness: the case of coronary heart disease. J Clin Psychol. 2001;57(11):1323–37.
33. Unützer J, Katon W, Callahan CM, Williams Jr JW, Hunkeler E, Harpole L, et al. Collaborative care management of late-life depression in the primary care setting: a randomized controlled trial. JAMA. 2002;288(22):2836–45.
34. Arean P, Hegel M, Vannoy S, Fan M-Y, Unuzter J. Effectiveness of problem-solving therapy for older, primary care patients with depression: results from the IMPACT project. Gerontologist. 2008;48(3):311–23.
35. Gallegos AM, Hoerger M, Talbot NL, Krasner MS, Knight JM, Moynihan JA, et al. Toward identifying the effects of the specific components of mindfulness-based stress reduction on biologic and emotional outcomes among older adults. J Altern Complement Med. 2013;19(10):787–92.
36. Kabat-Zinn J. Mindfulness-based interventions in context: past, present, and future. Clin Psychol Sci Pract. 2003;10(2):144–56.
37. Addis M, Davis M. Meditation may reduce heart attack and stroke risk. Lancet. 2000;355.
38. Chang BH, Dusek JA, Benson H. Psychobiological changes from relaxation response elicitation: long-term practitioners vs. novices. Psychosomatics. 2011;52(6):550–9.
39. Chang BH, Hendricks A, Zhao Y, Rothendler JA, LoCastro JS, Slawsky MT. A relaxation response randomized trial on patients with chronic heart failure. J Cardiopulm Rehabil. 2005;25(3):149–57.
40. Herbert Benson M, Klipper MZ. The relaxation response. New York: Harper Collins; 1992.
41. Swartz HA, Frank E, Shear MK, Thase ME, Fleming MA, Scott J. A pilot study of brief interpersonal psychotherapy for depression among women. Psychiatr Serv. 2004;55(4):448–50.
42. Lespérance F, Frasure-Smith N, Koszycki D, Laliberté M-A, van Zyl LT, Baker B, et al. Effects of citalopram and interpersonal psychotherapy on depression in patients with coronary artery disease: the Canadian Cardiac Randomized Evaluation of Antidepressant and Psychotherapy Efficacy (CREATE) trial. JAMA. 2007;297(4):367–79.
43. Lett HS, Davidson J, Blumenthal JA. Nonpharmacologic treatments for depression in patients with coronary heart disease. Psychosom Med. 2005;67 Suppl 1:S58–62.
44. Goodwin CL, Forman EM, Herbert JD, Butryn ML, Ledley GS. A pilot study examining the initial effectiveness of a brief acceptance-based behavior therapy for modifying diet and physical activity among cardiac patients. Behav Modif. 2012;36(2):199–217.
45. Sin NL, Lyubomirsky S. Enhancing well-being and alleviating depressive symptoms with positive psychology interventions: a practice-friendly meta-analysis. J Clin Psychol. 2009;65(5):467–87.
46. Chida Y, Steptoe A. Positive psychological well-being and mortality: a quantitative review of prospective observational studies. Psychosom Med. 2008;70(7):741–56.
47. Scheier MF, Matthews KA, Owens JF, Schulz R, Bridges MW, Magovern GJ, et al. Optimism and rehospitalization after coronary artery bypass graft surgery. Arch Intern Med. 1999;159(8):829–35.
48. Huffman JC, Mastromauro CA, Boehm JK, Seabrook R, Fricchione GL, Denninger JW, et al. Development of a positive psychology intervention for patients with acute cardiovascular disease. Heart Int. 2011;6(2):e14.
49. Seligman ME, Steen TA, Park N, Peterson C. Positive psychology progress: empirical validation of interventions. Am Psychol. 2005;60(5):410–21.
50. Lyubomirsky S, Layous K. How do simple positive activities increase well-being? Curr Direct Psychol Sci. 2013;22(1):57–62.
51. Rollman BL, Belnap BH, LeMenager MS, Mazumdar S, Houck PR, Counihan PJ, et al. Telephone-delivered collaborative care for treating post-CABG depression: a randomized controlled trial. JAMA. 2009;302(19):2095–103.
52. Katon WJ, Lin EH, Von Korff M, Ciechanowski P, Ludman EJ, Young B, et al. Collaborative care for patients with depression and chronic illnesses. N Engl J Med. 2010;363(27):2611–20.
53. Spurgeon JA, Wright JH. Computer-assisted cognitive-behavioral therapy. Curr Psychiatry Rep. 2010;12(6):547–52.

54. Luxton DD, McCann RA, Bush NE, Mishkind MC, Reger GM. mHealth for mental health: integrating smartphone technology in behavioral healthcare. Prof Psychol Res Pract. 2011;42(6):505.
55. Donker T, Petrie K, Proudfoot J, Clarke J, Birch MR, Christensen H. Smartphones for smarter delivery of mental health programs: a systematic review. J Med Internet Res. 2013;15(11):e247.
56. Kroenke K, Spitzer RL, Williams JB. The PHQ-9: validity of a brief depression severity measure. J Gen Intern Med. 2001;16(9):606–13.
57. Beck A, Steer R, Brown G. Manual for beck depression inventory-II (BDI-II). San Antonio: Psychology Corporation; 1996.
58. Zigmond AS, Snaith RP. The hospital anxiety and depression scale. Acta Psychiatr Scand. 1983;67(6):361–70.
59. Ware Jr J, Kosinski M, Keller SD. A 12-Item Short-Form Health Survey: construction of scales and preliminary tests of reliability and validity. Med Care. 1996;34(3):220–33.
60. Cohen S, Kamarck T, Mermelstein R. A global measure of perceived stress. J Health Soc Behav. 1983;24(4):385–96.
61. Hlatky MA, Boineau RE, Higginbotham MB, Lee KL, Mark DB, Califf RM, et al. A brief self-administered questionnaire to determine functional capacity (the Duke Activity Status Index). Am J Cardiol. 1989;64(10):651–4.
62. Green CP, Porter CB, Bresnahan DR, Spertus JA. Development and evaluation of the Kansas City Cardiomyopathy Questionnaire: a new health status measure for heart failure. J Am Coll Cardiol. 2000;35(5):1245–55.
63. Spertus JA, Winder JA, Dewhurst TA, Deyo RA, Prodzinski J, McDonell M, et al. Development and evaluation of the Seattle Angina Questionnaire: a new functional status measure for coronary artery disease. J Am Coll Cardiol. 1995;25(2):333–41.
64. DiMatteo MR, Hays RD, Sherbourne CD. Adherence to cancer regimens: implications for treating the older patient. Oncology (Williston Park). 1992;6(2 Suppl):50–7.
65. Eifert GH, Thompson RN, Zvolensky MJ, Edwards K, Frazer NL, Haddad JW, et al. The cardiac anxiety questionnaire: development and preliminary validity. Behav Res Ther. 2000;38(10):1039–53.
66. Hare DL, Davis CR. Cardiac Depression Scale: validation of a new depression scale for cardiac patients. J Psychosom Res. 1996;40(4):379–86.

Resources

American Heart Association. Coping with feelings. http://www.heart.org/HEARTORG/Conditions/More/CardiacRehab/Coping-with-Feelings_UCM_307092_Article.jsp

American Heart Association. Stress and heart health. http://www.heart.org/HEARTORG/GettingHealthy/StressManagement/HowDoesStressAffectYou/Stress-and-Heart-Health_UCM_437370_Article.jsp

Anxiety and Depression Association of America. Managing stress for heart health. http://www.adaa.org/about-adaa/press-room/press-releases/managing-stress-for-heart-health

Oxford University Press. Treatments that work series. http://global.oup.com/us/companion.websites/umbrella/treatments/

Greenberger D, Padesky CA. Mind over mood. New York: Guilford; 1995.

University of Washington. Problem solving therapy materials. http://impact-uw.org/tools/pst_manual.html

Mindfulness-based stress reduction materials. http://www.mindfullivingprograms.com/index.php

The relaxation response materials. http://www.relaxationresponse.org

Benson H. The relaxation response. New York: Harper Torch; 1975/2000.

Web-based CBT. https://www.beatingthebluesus.com/

Abbreviations

ACS   Acute coronary syndrome
ACT   Acceptance and commitment therapy
CABG   Coronary artery bypass graft
CAD   Coronary artery disease
CBT   Cognitive behavioral therapy
CVD   Cardiovascular disease
GAD   Generalized anxiety disorder
HF   Heart failure
MBSR   Mindfulness-based stress reduction
MDD   Major depressive disorder
MI   Myocardial infarction
PD   Panic disorder
PP   Positive psychology
PST   Problem-solving therapy
PTSD   Post-traumatic stress disorder
QoL   Quality of life
SSRI   Selective serotonin reuptake inhibitor

Chapter 11
HIV

Aaron Blashill, Sannisha Dale, Jonathan Jampel, and Steven Safren

11.1   Introduction

Over 1.2 million individuals in the USA are living with Human Immunodeficiency Virus (HIV) [1] and annually, 50,000 individuals are newly diagnosed [2]. Men who have sex with men (MSM) have the highest risk for HIV infection in the USA and African-American men and women have the highest rate of HIV diagnoses across all racial/ethnic groups [3]. Fortunately, with antiretroviral therapy (ART) and high levels (≥80 %) of adherence, HIV can be a manageable chronic illness, and individuals living with HIV can experience life spans that are similar to the general population [4]. Successful treatment also inhibits the ability of HIV to be spread to sexual partners [5].

A. Blashill (✉)
Department of Psychology, San Diego State University,
6363 Alvarado Court, Suite 103, San Diego, CA 92120, USA
e-mail: ablashill@mail.sdsu.edu

S. Dale
Behavioral Medicine Service, Department of Psychiatry, Massachusetts General Hospital,
Harvard Medical School, Boston, MA, USA
e-mail: skdale@mgh.harvard.edu

J. Jampel
The Fenway Institute, Fenway Health, 1340 Boylston St., Boston, MA 02215, USA
e-mail: jjampel@fenwayhealth.org

S. Safren
Department of Psychology, University of Miami,
5665 Ponce de Leon Blvd., Coral Gables, FL 33124, USA
e-mail: ssafren@miami.edu

© Springer Science+Business Media New York 2017
A.-M. Vranceanu et al. (eds.), *The Massachusetts General Hospital Handbook of Behavioral Medicine*, Current Clinical Psychiatry,
DOI 10.1007/978-3-319-29294-6_11

However, there are common psychiatric/psychological conditions that individuals with HIV experience, and these conditions negatively impact disease management (e.g., medication adherence) and sexual health (managing sexual decisions, sexual satisfaction). There is a growing body of research on the efficacy of cognitive behavioral strategies to improve medication adherence and sexual health and consequently decrease the transmission risk for HIV. In the first half of this chapter, we review the existing literature on common mental health conditions among individuals with HIV, specific population concerns (i.e., sexual health and ART adherence), and research demonstrating the efficacy of cognitive behavioral strategies for these concerns. In the second half of this chapter, we describe a cognitive behavioral therapy (CBT) intervention for HIV medication adherence and depression along with case examples. We conclude by discussing future directions for addressing co-occurring psychological and health conditions for individuals with HIV.

11.1.1 Mental Health Conditions

Individuals living with HIV may struggle with a range of psychiatric issues under the umbrellas of mood and anxiety disorders; however, depression and posttraumatic stress disorder (PTSD) have been especially well documented as key comorbid psychological issues for this population [6–8].

11.1.1.1 Depression

The prevalence of major depressive disorder among persons with HIV is 2–5 times higher than among HIV-negative persons, with the lifetime prevalence among persons living with HIV estimated between 20 and 40 % [9, 10]. In an international sample (including the USA) of people living with HIV, Eller et al. [11] found that 54 % of their sample experienced depressive symptoms in the past week. Individuals with HIV may experience depression as a result of being diagnosed and facing the physical and emotional burdens associated with a long-term illness, and experiencing depression may result in neglect of necessary self-care activities (e.g., medication adherence [12, 13]) for HIV disease management and further exacerbation of symptoms.

11.1.1.2 PTSD

Individuals with HIV are more likely to report histories of sexual abuse (childhood and adult), physical abuse, emotional abuse, intimate partner violence, and other traumatic events in comparison to persons without HIV and are more likely to meet criteria for PTSD as a result of traumatic experiences [14–16]. Indeed, early trauma/stressful life events may place individuals at risk for contracting HIV [16]. Reisner et al. [16] found that each additional early life violent event (i.e., physical abuse, sexual abuse, neglect, verbal violence, or witnessed violence) was associated with elevated odds of HIV infection. In a meta-analysis of HIV-positive women, Machtinger and colleagues [15] reported a 55% rate of intimate partner violence, which is more than double the US national average, and estimated a 30% rate of recent PTSD, which is over 5 times the rate in a national sample. Similarly, Reisner et al. [16] reported that in a sample of men, those living with HIV reported significantly higher rates of trauma histories (physical abuse, 16% vs. 3%; sexual abuse, 12% vs. 2%; neglect, 11% vs. 3%) compared to HIV-negative men. In addition, a higher proportion of HIV-positive men (26%) met criteria for recent PTSD than HIV-negative men (4%) and PTSD is associated with the neglect of self-care behaviors including ART adherence [15].

11.1.2 Specific Population Concerns

11.1.2.1 ART Adherence

Moderate to high levels (at least 80%) of ART adherence is needed to achieve HIV viral suppression [17] although this may vary by regimen and patient factors. ART regimens include once-daily single-tablet, once-daily multi-tablet, and multi-dose multi-tablet [18, 19] and while some studies [18, 20] have shown higher adherence with single-tablet regimens others have not [21, 22]. Viral suppression (i.e., undetectable status) indicates that the HIV virus is under control with minimal or potentially no replication [23, 24]. Lower HIV viral load is associated with higher immune functioning (assessed by CD4 count) and higher immune functioning is linked to lower susceptibility to opportunistic infections and lower morbidity and mortality [25, 26]. Optimal ART adherence is also crucial to public health because HIV viral suppression significantly reduces and possibly eliminates the risk of transmitting HIV [27, 28]. However, ART adherence can be difficult and most individuals struggle with adhering at an optimal level (average ART adherence is approximately 60–70%; [29]). Difficulty with ART adherence has been consistently linked with mental health diagnoses, particularly depression and PTSD [8, 15, 30].

11.1.2.2 Sexual Health and Sexual Risk Behaviors

Improving sexual health practices and behaviors are important factors for HIV-positive persons [31]. Individuals with HIV may contract other sexually transmitted infections (STIs) or additional strains of the HIV virus [32, 33], which may negatively impact their health and the efficacy of their prescribed ART medications [34]. Further, engaging in condomless sexual intercourse may transmit HIV to partners who are HIV negative; and therefore sexual health is not only salient for the individual but also for public health.

Sexual HIV transmission and acquisition risk behaviors have been associated with depression, PTSD, and recent trauma. For example, among HIV-positive men, Wilson, Stadler, Boone, and Bolger [35] reported that the probability of unprotected anal intercourse (UAI) and serodiscordant UAI were higher in weeks when an individual's level of depression was higher than their average level. Similarly, O'Cleirigh, Traeger, Mayer, Magidson, and Safren [36] found that, among HIV-positive men who have sex with men, PTSD was associated with greater odds of UAI with a partner of HIV negative or HIV-unknown status among young gay and bisexual men. In a sample of HIV-positive biological and transgender women, researchers found that women with recent trauma compared to women without recent trauma had more than 3 times the odds of reporting sex and less than 100 % condom use with a partner who was HIV-negative or of unknown status [15]. Similar to how PTSD and depression may impact ART adherence via neglected self-care, they may also negatively influence a patient's ability to take care of their sexual health needs. Further, both depression and PTSD have been linked to diminished self-efficacy and lower self-efficacy is linked to higher engagement in sexual risk behaviors [37, 38].

11.2   Research/Evidence Base for Cognitive/Behavioral Interventions Addressing Sexual Transmission Risk and ART Adherence in HIV

Cognitive behavioral approaches have shown efficacy in improving medication adherence and immune function and lowering sexual transmission risk among individuals with HIV [39–41]. Simoni and colleagues [41] found in a meta-analysis that behavioral interventions were effective in increasing patients' ART adherence or helping patients to attain undetectable viral loads. Another meta-analysis by Crepaz's team [39] on intervention trials to reduce sexual transmission risk behaviors among HIV-positive persons found that interventions that were based on behavioral theory (e.g., CBT), designed to change HIV transmission risk behaviors, and provided skills building were effective in reducing unprotected sex and the risk of becoming infected with STIs. However, while several meta-analyses have concluded that behavioral interventions have shown moderate success in improving ART adherence [41–43] many of the interventions did not explicitly address mental health as part of the intervention per se, or excluded individuals with mental health or substance use problems. Addressing ART adherence, outside the context of mental health issues such as depression, may not work for individuals who experience poor adherence complicated by mental health problems. For instance, Project Enhance [44] provided prevention case management and various modules of intervention on sexual transmission risk to high-risk HIV-positive MSM. The study did not find an overall effect, however it did find that among those with co-occurring depression, the intervention group had significantly greater reductions in condomless sex than those in the control group. However, among participants who were below the cutoff for clinical depression, those in the intervention group did not differ from those in the control group in sexual transmission risk behaviors. Thus, individuals experiencing significant psychological distress may benefit from integrated interventions that simultaneously address sexual risk and mental health.

A limited number of studies specifically addressing both PTSD/trauma and sexual risk among individuals with HIV have shown significant effects on trauma symptoms and sexual risk [45–47]. An 11-session Enhanced Sexual Health Intervention among women with HIV and a history of childhood sexual abuse that incorporated CBT strategies along with cultural- and gender-specific concepts such as collectivism and interconnectedness [47] found a decrease in sexual risk and greater medication adherence among women in the intervention that attended >/= 8 sessions compared to women in the control condition. Similarly, Sikkema and colleagues [45, 46] found that a group coping intervention that included CBT strategies for trauma was effective in lowering sexual risk behaviors and trauma symptoms among women and men living with HIV and a history of childhood sexual abuse. Despite the few number of studies addressing sexual risk and HIV medication adherence in the context of trauma/PTSD, the findings support the usefulness of CBT among HIV-positive individuals.

11.3 Example Intervention: CBT-AD

As mentioned above, traditional behavioral interventions to promote ART adherence typically yield modest effects. One explanation for these findings is that the aforementioned interventions fail to account for the real-life psychosocial stressors that individuals living with HIV face (e.g., depression, a robust predictor of ART non-adherence). These findings, taken in tandem, suggest that an integrated approach is needed. That is, individuals living with HIV who struggle with adherence may benefit from an intervention that simultaneously addressed depression and ART adherence. With this premise in mind, members of our group created an intervention—CBT for HIV medication adherence and depression (CBT-AD [48]) which is based on traditional CBT approaches to the treatment of depression combined with intervention techniques most applicable to persons with chronic illness in general (see [49–51]), and prior clinical experience caring for HIV-infected individuals.

CBT-AD begins with a single-session intervention on HIV medication adherence (LifeSteps [52]), which involves 11 informational, problem-solving, and cognitive behavioral steps (e.g., education about adherence, scheduling, cue control strategies including the use of a watch alarm, adaptive thoughts about adherence, provider communication). In each step, participants and the clinician define the problem, generate alternative solutions, make decisions about the solutions, and develop a plan for implementing them. Participants also receive adherence tools such as assistance with a schedule and a cue-dosing watch that can sound two alarms per day.

The remaining 11 sessions continue to address strategies for and barriers to medication adherence, with a review of adherence at the beginning of each session, and discussion of progress or difficulties with adherence. Session 1 first provides psychoeducation about HIV and depression, and then transitions to motivational interviewing exercises (e.g., pros and cons of changing to improve one's depression and adherence) designed to set the stage for behavioral change interventions to follow. The next several sessions focus on behavioral activation and are designed to increase regularly occurring activities that involve pleasure and mastery. After behavioral activation sessions, adaptive thinking (cognitive restructuring) is usually introduced, with a specific focus on negative automatic thoughts that relate to HIV medication adherence. Problem solving is the next module, with the aims of helping patients engage in a process of identifying a problem, generating possible solutions, evaluating those solutions, selecting the best option, and implementing it. The next module provides progressive muscle relaxation training and diaphragmatic breathing skills, typically across one session. CBT-AD concludes with a session focused on relapse prevention. In this session, patients learn to become their own therapist, reflect on treatment gains, and anticipate future stressors and specific skills that may be applied in those situations. Below is a more comprehensive review, and case examples, of the various CBT-AD modules.

11.3.1   Session 1: LifeSteps

In CBT-AD, LifeSteps is the first session; however, discussion of adherence is integrated throughout all subsequent sessions. Accordingly, the treatment of depression is merged into the treatment of problematic adherence. LifeSteps begins by conducting a motivational exercise in which patients list their thoughts around taking their medications, identifying their barriers to adherence, and highlighting their primary motivations for living a healthy life. These techniques provide important material that will be used throughout treatment to address barriers and increase motivation to change. Next, psychoeducation is provided regarding the importance of adherence and the health risks associated with non-adherence. In the final component of the LifeSteps session, patient and therapist review common barriers to adherence using the "AIM" problem-solving approach (*Articulate* the adherence goal, *Identify* barriers to reaching the goal, and *Make* a plan to overcome the barriers, including a backup plan). The common barriers discussed are: (1) getting to appointments; (2) communicating with treatment team; (3) coping with side effects; (4) obtaining medications and other relevant health-related products; (5) formulating a daily medication schedule; (6) storing medications and medical supplies; (7) cue-control strategies for taking medications; (8) handling slips in adherence; (9) LifeSteps review; and (10) LifeSteps follow-up (occurs during a follow-up phone call or Session 2 of CBT-AD).

11.3.2 Case Example

Jeff is a 46-year-old heterosexual man who lives with his girlfriend, has two children, is on disability, and contracted HIV through injection drug use. On intake, he reported low levels of ART adherence and symptoms of depression. Initially, Jeff had diffi-culty generating thoughts about adherence, a common experience when working with depressed HIV-infected individuals. The clinician used strategies during the motivational exercise to elicit the patient's thoughts, including asking the patient to view his pill bottle and hold several pills in his hands. The thoughts generated through this exercise were negative in nature and were identified as barriers to treatment. Jeff identified many negative thoughts that were barriers to his adherence (e.g., pills are a reminder of being sick, self-blame for acquiring HIV). Jeff further identified several other barriers to adherence that are common to many medical conditions, including forgetting to take doses and having a busy schedule. Next, in order to enhance moti-vation the clinician assisted Jeff in identifying his primary reasons for taking medica-tion. Jeff stated he wanted to watch his children grow up, and that he feels healthier and better about himself when he takes his medication. By the end of the exercise, the patient and therapist have a rich list of barriers to medication adherence and motiva-tions for staying healthy that will be used throughout the various modules of this intervention. Note that the therapist begins to draw connections between the patient's thoughts and his patterns of adherence, which enhances motivation and sets the stage for addressing the 11 LifeSteps later in the session. In this case, the therapist notes that Jeff sometimes stops taking his medications for several days at a time when he feels down or frustrated. Although Jeff meets this statement with some resistance, drawing these connections helps familiarize patients with the types of challenging conversations that may arise later in treatment.

11.3.3 Session 2: Orientation to CBT-AD and Psychoeducation

The primary aim of Session 2 is to provide a theoretical overview of CBT-AD and orient the patient to treatment. As is the case with traditional CBT for depression [53], the core component of this session is to present a three-part model of depression (i.e., the interaction between cognitions/thoughts, behaviors/actions, and physiological reactions), tailored to the unique experiences of the patient. A detailed overview of this procedure can be found elsewhere [54]. Specific to CBT-AD, presentation of a three-part model of depression focuses on eliciting thoughts, behaviors, and physio-logical components that are specific to experiences with HIV infection, as well as ART adherence. By describing these specific aspects of HIV infection and ART adherence when reviewing the three-part model, the patient is able to draw connec-tions between their depressive symptoms and management of their health.

Session 2 ends with a motivational exercise, based on strategies outlined by Miller and Rollnick [55]. The "Pros and Cons of Changing" exercise asks the patient to detail the pros and cons of changing their thoughts and behaviors, as well as the pros and cons of not changing, in order to address the patient's primary motivations for change and the barriers that might be encountered during treatment. Following this exercise, the patient is asked to rate their motivation to change on a scale of 1–10, with higher numbers indicating greater motivation. Based on this score, typically the therapist asks the patient why the score is not lower. This allows the patient to observe their ambivalence about behavior change, but potentially emphasize the primary reasons for making a change, which often pushes the patient toward being more strongly motivated to make changes while acknowledging the barriers they may encounter. Typically, asking about why they did not score a lower number facilitates positive change talk about wanting to change, and asking about why they did not score a higher number facilitates a discussion about barriers.

11.3.4   Case Example

David is a 32-year-old gay man, who is in a romantic relationship with another man, has a long history of depression and substance use and was infected with HIV roughly 2 years ago. His experiences with depression predate his HIV infection, but have subsequently been exacerbated since being diagnosed with HIV. His depressive symptoms are maintained by patterns common to many individuals living with depression, including cognitive distortions and maladaptive behavioral patterns. These patterns further manifest themselves in terms of his thoughts and behaviors associated with his HIV infection. For instance, he notes that when he has negative thoughts and feels hopeless, he does not feel motivated to stay healthy and often skips medication. David is also ambivalent about changing the thoughts and behaviors that are maintaining his depression. Specifically, he reports that he struggles to remove himself from the cycle of drug use that fuels his depression because when he gets in these kinds of "ruts" substance use immediately makes him feel happy. He is able to describe his core motivations for working on depression and improving his health (e.g., spending more time with family and friends), but he is aware of how difficult it will be to engage in change. The clinician continues to elicit examples from the patient that are related to his depression, his health status and ART adherence, and the interrelationships among these conditions.

11.3.5   Sessions 3–12

Sessions 3 through 12 focus on the core skills and techniques that are taught as part of traditional CBT for depression, including (3) activity scheduling (i.e., behavioral activation), (4–5) adaptive thinking (i.e., cognitive restructuring),

(6–7) problem-solving, (8) relaxation, (9–11) flexible sessions, and (12) relapse prevention. Two sessions are devoted to both adaptive thinking and problem solving, leaving three additional sessions in the 12-session protocol to tailor treatment to the needs of the individual patient and spend more time reviewing and practicing the skills that are most relevant to the patient's experiences with depression and ART adherence. While the skills targeted in these sessions are analogous to those found in traditional CBT for depression, CBT-AD emphasizes treatment of depressive symptoms in the context of HIV/AIDS illness and ART adherence. Given this, patient and clinician review depressive symptoms and ART adherence at the beginning of each session, review LifeSteps and adherence problem solving at each session, and the therapist then guides the discussion to include content relevant to the patient's health status and ART adherence, as is relevant to the specific needs of the patient.

11.3.6 Case Example

Patti is a 35-year-old heterosexual woman, is single, and was recently infected with HIV by a male partner. She presented to therapy with moderate levels of ART adherence and many symptoms of depressions, including low mood, anhedonia, loss of energy, guilt, and suicidal ideation. Patti has experienced an improvement in her ART adherence and symptoms of depression during the course of treatment, but she continues to report a number of cognitive distortions related to her HIV status. Patti's presentation highlights a pattern of distorted thinking that is both similar to and distinct from those of patients without HIV infection. Many patients with depression experience loneliness and distress related to lack of a romantic partner, and cognitive distortions may reflect the belief that the patient will never be able to find a significant other. Patti also notes the thought that she will not be able to find a partner because she has HIV. In working to restructure this thought/thoughts like it, it is important that the clinician acknowledge the reality that it may well be more difficult for Patti to find a romantic partner due to the stigma associated with HIV infection. Across all sessions of CBT-AD, it is important for the clinician to have an appreciation for the various ways in which HIV infection may alter the day-to-day life of the patient and therefore changes the approach to intervention. Applied to cognitive restructuring, certain negative thought patterns may be more difficult to challenge for an individual with HIV (e.g., "I am going to die young"; "I will never have children"; "My family will reject me") because although these thoughts are still distorted, certain aspects of these thoughts may be somewhat of a reality for their lives. For example, a more realistic and adaptive thought for "I am going to die young" may be: "I may have more medical struggles due to my HIV infection, but taking my medication will help me stay healthy as long as possible."

11.3.7   Evidence Base for CBT-AD

In 2009, our group [56] published the results of an initial randomized control trial (RCT) that compared CBT for adherence and depression (CBT-AD) vs. an enhanced treatment as usual (ETAU) condition. As described above, both groups received a brief, CBT/problem-solving intervention "LifeSteps" aimed at increasing ART adherence [52], and the experimental intervention received CBT, which integrated the adherence counseling into a modular treatment for depression. Participants were then assessed at 3-, 6-, and 12-month follow-ups. Results revealed that at 3 months, participants in the CBT-AD condition reported greater ART adherence and lower depression compared to participants in the ETAU condition. These results were generally maintained at 6- and 12-month follow-up. This study was the first RCT that we are aware of to integrate evidence-based psychosocial treatment for depression with an intervention to increase ART adherence.

The CBT-AD intervention was also evaluated via an RCT among an opioid-dependent HIV-infected sample [13]. Results indicated that the CBT-AD group reported lower depression at post-treatment, and these gains were maintained at 6- and 12-month follow-up compared to the ETAU condition. The CBT-AD group also reported greater ART adherence throughout active treatment; however, these gains were not maintained at follow-up. Although viral load did not differ between the two conditions at follow-up assessments, the CBT-AD group had significantly improved CD4 cell counts over time compared to the ETAU condition. Currently, our group has completed a multi-site, three-arm RCT for depression and adherence, comparing the CBT-AD intervention to informational and supportive psychotherapy (ISP) and an ETAU condition. These results are pending publication.

11.3.8   Resources

For a more detailed description of CBT-AD, readers are encouraged to consult our therapist manual and patient workbooks [48]. Further, our group has recently published a clinically orientated paper on CBT-AD [57]. This article is novel, in that it includes several videos embedded within the manuscript. These videos are brief, yet illustrative of the various techniques used throughout CBT-AD.

11.4   Future Directions

With new cases of HIV infection occurring each year [2], and the existence of comorbid psychiatric issues (e.g., depression and PTSD) that negatively impact HIV medication adherence and sexual health [8, 15, 30], clinical resources and the dissemination of effective clinical tools are needed as well as ongoing research to develop new tools. While RCTs have demonstrated that CBT strategies are moderately effective in improving HIV medication adherence and sexual health [41, 44], more intensive interventions such as CBT-AD [13, 56] may be needed to address adherence and other health behaviors such as sexual health in the context of comorbid mental health issues. Further, given the limited number of preexisting studies on CBT interventions to improve sexual health and ART adherence in the context of trauma/PTSD [45–47] more research should be conducted. Additional research may highlight clinical tools that can be utilized by clinicians in improving key areas of concern in the lives of HIV-positive individuals.

Beyond enhancing existing CBT tools and developing new strategies to enhance the lives of HIV-positive persons, there is a necessity to disseminate clinical tools that have shown to be effective in RCTs [58–60]. Information is often disseminated via publications, conference presentations, and brief trainings. However, additional dissemination efforts are also important [60] such as (a) active partnerships between researchers and community-based organizations (CBO) who service HIV-positive persons, (b) in-depth training and supervision for CBO clinicians on delivering the tools, and (c) assessments/evaluations of the effectiveness of the trainings on CBO clinicians' competency as well as improvements in the sexual health and medication adherence of HIV-positive clients.

Technological devices (e.g., phone, computer, internet) may be beneficial both to the dissemination of effective CBT tools (e.g., trainings, supervisions) and increasing HIV-positive persons' access to CBT tools (e.g., sessions via video-conferencing) [61, 62]. Although the evidence to support the efficacy of CBT delivered with technological tools and among HIV-positive populations is in the infancy stage [63, 64], it may play out that these technological devices can aid therapy, but not necessarily be a replacement for therapy in certain more complex populations.

Beyond technological advances, current biomedical prevention efforts are helping to improve the sexual health of HIV-negative individuals and decrease their risk of HIV acquisition. Pre- and post-exposure prophylaxis are the key examples of these efforts [65]. Pre-exposure prophylaxis (PrEP) medications are taken once per day by individuals engaging in high HIV-risk behaviors and post-exposure prophylaxis (PEP) medications are taken immediately after high HIV-risk exposures. Both PrEP and PEP have shown efficacy in reducing HIV acquisition (e.g., up to 92 % for PrEP [66, 67]). Future research could explore psychological factors that may influence adherence to PEP and PrEP and investigate the efficacy of CBT tools in improving PrEP and PEP adherence [68]. An intervention such as CBT-AD may be well suited for adaption to address PrEP and PEP adherence among HIV-negative individuals.

See Tables 11.1 and 11.2 for assessments and recommendations.

Table 11.1 Self-report assessments

Measure	Variable	Description
Center for Epidemiologic Studies Depression Scale—CESD	Depression	20-Item self-report scale measuring depressive symptoms, including depressed mood, feelings of guilt and worthlessness, feelings of helplessness and hopelessness, psychomotor retardation, loss of appetite, and sleep disturbance
Adult AIDS Clinical Trials Group (ACTG) Symptoms Distress Module	HIV-related distressing symptoms	20-Item self-report questionnaire that measures physical and psychological symptoms associated with HIV disease and HIV medication
Assessment of Body Change and Distress Questionnaire-Short Form (ABCD-SF)	Appearance-related disturbance	10-Item self-report questionnaire that measures negative affect about appearance, HIV-related outcomes/stigma, exercise/eating behaviors, and HIV medication-related behaviors Available in long and short form
ACTG adherence barriers questionnaire	Barriers to taking HIV medication	27-Item self-report questionnaire that measures beliefs about HIV medications and reasons (if applicable) for missing doses
ACTG dealing with illness questionnaire	Illness coping	22-Item self-report questionnaire addressing coping strategies for HIV infection
ACTG social support questionnaire	Social support	8-Item self-report questionnaire addressing the use of social support in coping with HIV
ACTG brief adherence self-report questionnaire	HIV medication adherence	Self-report percentage scale of adherence to HIV medications over the past month
ACTG substance use self-report	Substance use	13-Item self-report questionnaire of alcohol, tobacco, and illicit substance use
ACTG attitudes about HIV scale	HIV attitudes/beliefs	10-Item self-report questionnaire of attitudes and beliefs related to HIV

Table 11.2 CBT modules and recommendations for specific patient problems

Module	Strategies	Recommendations	Goals
Psychoeducation HIV medication adherence	LifeSteps	General module for all patients	Provide information about the importance of adherence
	Motivational interviewing		Provide general strategies for staying adherent and problem-solving difficulties related to adherence
	AIM problem-solving approach		
Psychoeducation HIV and depression	Motivational interviewing	General module for all patients	Draw connections between depressive symptoms and poor health maintenance that is specific to HIV
	Pros and cons		Help set the stage for behavioral change that follow in the intervention
Behavioral	Activity scheduling	For patients with low physical activity	Help patients reengage in pleasant activities
		For patients interested in increasing activity in spite of depression	Help patients increase activity regardless of depressive symptoms
		For patients with fear avoidance	Help patients gradually reengage in activities avoided
Cognitive	Traditional cognitive restructuring	For patients with automatic negative thoughts related to HIV medication adherence	Help patients identify negative automatic thoughts, with a specific focus on thoughts related to HIV medication adherence
	Automatic thoughts	For patients with realistic negative thoughts that cannot be problem solved	Help patients decide whether thoughts are distorted or not, learn to choose between traditional cognitive restructuring and acceptance-based cognitive restructuring with or without problem solving
		For patients with realistic negative thoughts that can be problem solved	
Problem solving	Problem solving	For patients with realistic negative thoughts that can be problem solved	Help patients identify specific problems and possible solutions, evaluate those solutions, select and implement the best option
Physiological	Progressive muscle relaxation	General module for all patients	Help patients elicit the relaxation response
	Mindfulness		Help patients learn the skill of mindfulness
	Diaphragmatic breathing skills		
Relapse prevention	Applying skills	General module for all patients	Help patients learn to become their own therapists, reflect on treatment gains, anticipate future stressors, and identify specific skills that may be applied in stressful situations

References

1. CDC. Monitoring selected national HIV prevention and care objectives by using HIV surveillance data—United States and 6 dependent areas—2012. HIV Surveil Suppl Rep. 2014;19(3):1–61.
2. CDC. Estimated HIV incidence in the United States, 2007–2010. HIV Surveil Suppl Rep. 2012;17(4):1–26.
3. CDC. HIV surveillance—epidemiology of HIV infection (through 2011). 2013. http://www.cdc.gov/hiv/topics/surveillance/resources/slides/general/index.htm. Accessed Apr 2015.
4. Cohen MS, McCauley M, Gamble TR. HIV treatment as prevention and HPTN 052. Curr Opin HIV AIDS. 2012;7(2):99–105.
5. Rodger A, Bruun T, Weait M, Vernazza P, Collins S, Estrada V, et al. Partners of people on ART—a new evaluation of the risks (The PARTNER study): design and methods. BMC Public Health. 2012;12:296.
6. Blashill AJ, Gordon JR, Mimiaga MJ, Safren SA. HIV/AIDS and depression. In: Richards CS, O'Hara MW, editors. The Oxford handbook of depression and comorbidity. New York: Oxford University Press; 2014.
7. Blashill AJ, Perry N, Safren SA. Mental health: a focus on stress, coping, and mental illness as it relates to treatment retention, adherence, and other health outcomes. Curr HIV/AIDS Rep. 2011;8(4):215–22.
8. Boarts JM, Sledjeski EM, Bogart LM, Delahanty DL. The differential impact of PTSD and depression on HIV disease markers and adherence to HAART in people living with HIV. AIDS Behav. 2006;10(3):253–61.
9. Bing EG, Burnam MA, Longshore D, Fleishman JA, Sherbourne CD, London AS, et al. Psychiatric disorders and drug use among human immunodeficiency virus-infected adults in the United States. Arch Gen Psychiatry. 2001;58(8):721–8.
10. Ciesla JA, Roberts JE. Meta-analysis of the relationship between HIV infection and risk for depressive disorders. Am J Psychiatry. 2001;158(5):725–30.
11. Eller LS, Bunch EH, Wantland DJ, Portillo CJ, Reynolds NR, Nokes KM, et al. Prevalence, correlates, and self-management of HIV-related depressive symptoms. AIDS Care. 2010;22(9):1159–70.
12. Gonzalez JS, Batchelder AW, Psaros C, Safren SA. Depression and HIV/AIDS treatment non-adherence: a review and meta-analysis. J Acquir Immune Defic Syndr. 2011;58(2):181–7.
13. Safren SA, O'Cleirigh CM, Bullis JR, Otto MW, Stein MD, Pollack MH. Cognitive behavioral therapy for adherence and depression (CBT-AD) in HIV-infected injection drug users: a randomized controlled trial. J Consult Clin Psychol. 2012;80(3):404–15.
14. Cohen MS, Deamant C, Barkan S, Richardson J, Young M, Holman S, et al. Domestic violence and childhood sexual abuse in HIV-infected women and women at risk for HIV. Am J Public Health. 2000;90(4):560–5.
15. Machtinger EL, Wilson TC, Haberer JE, Weiss DS. Psychological trauma and PTSD in HIV-positive women: a meta-analysis. AIDS Behav. 2012;16(8):2091–100.
16. Reisner SL, Falb KL, Mimiaga MJ. Early life traumatic stressors and the mediating role of PTSD in incident HIV infection among US men, comparisons by sexual orientation and race/ethnicity: results from the NESARC, 2004–2005. J Acquir Immune Defic Syndr. 2011;57(4):340–50.
17. Panel on Antiretroviral Agents in HIV-Infected Adults and Adolescents. Guidelines for the use of antiretroviral agents in HIV-1 infected adults and adolescents. Department of Health and Human Services. 2009. http://aidsinfo.nih.gov/content-files/adultadolescentGL.pdf. Accessed April 2015.
18. Bangsberg DR, Ragland K, Monk A, Deeks SG. A single tablet regimen is associated with higher adherence and viral suppression than multiple tablet regimens in HIV+ homeless and marginally housed people. AIDS. 2010;24(18):2835–40.

19. Nachega JB, Parienti J-J, Uthman OA, Gross R, Dowdy DW, Sax PE, et al. Lower pill burden and once-daily antiretroviral treatment regimens for HIV infection: a meta-analysis of randomized controlled trials. Clin Infect Dis. 2014;58(9):1297–307.

20. Cohen CJ, Meyers JL, Davis KL. Association between daily antiretroviral pill burden and treatment adherence, hospitalisation risk, and other healthcare utilisation and costs in a US medicaid population with HIV. BMJ Open. 2013;3(8):e003028.

21. Dejesus E, Young B, Morales-Ramirez JO, Sloan L, Ward DJ, Flaherty JF, et al. Simplification of antiretroviral therapy to a single-tablet regimen consisting of efavirenz, emtricitabine, and tenofovir disoproxil fumarate versus unmodified antiretroviral therapy in virologically suppressed HIV-1-infected patients. J Acquir Immune Defic Syndr. 2009;51(2):163–74.

22. Hodder SL, Mounzer K, Dejesus E, Ebrahimi R, Grimm K, Esker S, et al. Patient-reported outcomes in virologically suppressed, HIV-1-Infected subjects after switching to a simplified, single-tablet regimen of efavirenz, emtricitabine, and tenofovir DF. AIDS Patient Care STDS. 2010;24(2):87–96.

23. Arnsten JH, Demas PA, Farzadegan H, Grant RW, Gourevitch MN, Chang C-J, et al. Antiretroviral therapy adherence and viral suppression in HIV-Infected drug users: comparison of self-report and electronic monitoring. Clin Infect Dis. 2001;33(8):1417–23.

24. Ramratnam B, Mittler JE, Zhang L, Boden D, Hurley A, Fang F, et al. The decay of the latent reservoir of replication-competent HIV-1 is inversely correlated with the extent of residual viral replication during prolonged anti-retroviral therapy. Nat Med. 2000;6(1):82–5.

25. Hunt PW, Deeks SG, Rodriguez B, Valdez H, Shade SB, Abrams DI, et al. Continued CD4 cell count increases in HIV-infected adults experiencing 4 years of viral suppression on antiretroviral therapy. AIDS. 2003;17(13):1907–15.

26. Paterson DL, Swindells S, Mohr J, Brester M, Vergis EN, Squier C, et al. Adherence to protease inhibitor therapy and outcomes in patients with HIV infection. Ann Intern Med. 2000;133(1):21–30.

27. Cohen MS, Chen YQ, McCauley M, Gamble T, Hosseinipour MC, Kumarasamy N, et al. Prevention of HIV-1 infection with early antiretroviral therapy. N Engl J Med. 2011;365(6):493–505.

28. Loutfy MR, Wu W, Letchumanan M, Bondy L, Antoniou T, Margolese S, et al. Systematic review of HIV transmission between heterosexual serodiscordant couples where the HIV-positive partner is fully suppressed on antiretroviral therapy. PLoS One. 2013;8(2):e55747.

29. Golin CE, Liu H, Hays RD, Miller LG, Beck CK, Ickovics J, et al. A prospective study of predictors of adherence to combination antiretroviral medication. J Gen Intern Med. 2002;17(10):756–65.

30. Vranceanu AM, Safren SA, Lu M, Coady WM, Skolnik PR, Rogers WH, et al. The relationship of post-traumatic stress disorder and depression to antiretroviral medication adherence in persons with HIV. AIDS Patient Care STDS. 2008;22(4):313–21.

31. Wolitski RJ, Fenton KA. Sexual health, HIV, and sexually transmitted infections among gay, bisexual, and other men who have sex with men in the United States. AIDS Behav. 2011;15 Suppl 1:S9–17.

32. Hague JC, Muvva R, Miazad RM. STD coinfection and reinfection following HIV diagnosis: evidence of continued sexual risk behavior. Sex Transm Dis. 2011;38(4):347–8.

33. Whiteside YO, Merchant AT, Hussey J, Adams SA, Duffus WA. Occurrence of new sexually transmitted diseases in males after HIV diagnosis. AIDS Behav. 2013;17(3):1176–84.

34. Pingen M, Nouwen JL, Dinant S, Albert J, Mild M, Brodin J, et al. Therapy failure resulting from superinfection by a drug-resistant HIV variant. Antivir Ther. 2012;17(8):1621–5.

35. Wilson PA, Stadler G, Boone MR, Bolger N. Fluctuations in depression and well-being are associated with sexual risk episodes among HIV-positive men. Health Psychol. 2014;33(7):681–5.

36. O'Cleirigh CM, Traeger L, Mayer KH, Magidson JF, Safren SA. Anxiety specific pathways to HIV sexual transmission risk behavior among young gay and bisexual men. J Gay Lesbian Ment Health. 2013;17(3):314–26.

37. Alvy LM, McKirnan DJ, Mansergh G, Koblin B, Colfax GN, Flores SA, et al. Depression is associated with sexual risk among men who have sex with men, but is mediated by cognitive escape and self-efficacy. AIDS Behav. 2011;15(6):1171–9.
38. Brown LK, Lourie KJ, Zlotnick C, Cohn J. Impact of sexual abuse on the HIV-risk-related behavior of adolescents in intensive psychiatric treatment. Am J Psychiatry. 2000;157(9):1413–5.
39. Crepaz N, Lyles CM, Wolitski RJ, Passin WF, Rama SM, Herbst JH, et al. Do prevention interventions reduce HIV risk behaviours among people living with HIV? A meta-analytic review of controlled trials. AIDS. 2006;20(2):143–57.
40. Johnson WD, Diaz RM, Flanders WD, Goodman M, Hill AN, Holtgrave D, et al. Behavioral interventions to reduce risk for sexual transmission of HIV among men who have sex with men. Cochrane Database Syst Rev. 2008;3, CD001230.
41. Simoni JM, Pearson CR, Pantalone DW, Marks G, Crepaz N. Efficacy of interventions in improving highly active antiretroviral therapy adherence and HIV-1 RNA viral load. A meta-analytic review of randomized controlled trials. J Acquir Immune Defic Syndr. 2006;43 Suppl 1:S23–35.
42. Amico KR, Harman JJ, Johnson BT. Efficacy of antiretroviral therapy adherence interventions: a research synthesis of trials, 1996 to 2004. J Acquir Immune Defic Syndr. 2006;41(3):285–97.
43. Simoni JM, Amico KR, Pearson CR, Malow R. Strategies for promoting adherence to antiretroviral therapy: a review of the literature. Curr Infect Dis Rep. 2008;10(6):515–21.
44. Safren SA, O'Cleirigh CM, Skeer M, Elsesser SA, Mayer KH. Project enhance: a randomized controlled trial of an individualized HIV prevention intervention for HIV-infected men who have sex with men conducted in a primary care setting. Health Psychol. 2013;32(2):171–9.
45. Sikkema KJ, Hansen NB, Kochman A, Tarakeshwar N, Neufeld S, Meade CS, et al. Outcomes from a group intervention for coping with HIV/AIDS and childhood sexual abuse: reductions in traumatic stress. AIDS Behav. 2007;11(1):49–60.
46. Sikkema KJ, Wilson PA, Hansen NB, Kochman A, Neufeld S, Ghebremichael MS, et al. Effects of a coping intervention on transmission risk behavior among people living with HIV/AIDS and a history of childhood sexual abuse. J Acquir Immune Defic Syndr. 2008;47(4):506–13.
47. Wyatt GE, Longshore D, Chin D, Carmona JV, Loeb TB, Myers HF, et al. The efficacy of an integrated risk reduction intervention for HIV-positive women with child sexual abuse histories. AIDS Behav. 2004;8(4):453–62.
48. Safren SA, Gonzalez J, Soroudi N. Coping with chronic illness: a cognitive-behavioral approach for adherence and depression—therapist guide. New York: Oxford University Press; 2007.
49. Nezu AM, Nezu C, Friedman S, Faddis S, Houts P. Helping cancer patients cope: a problem-solving approach. Washington, DC: American Psychological Association; 1998.
50. Nezu AM, Nezu C, Friedman S, Houts P, Faddis S. Project genesis: application of problem-solving therapy to individuals with cancer. Behav Ther. 1997;20:55–158.
51. Thomason BT, Bachanas PJ, Campos PE. Cognitive behavioral interventions with persons affected by HIV/AIDS. Cogn Behav Pract. 1996;3(2):417–42.
52. Safren SA, Otto MW, Worth JL. Life-steps: applying cognitive behavioral therapy to HIV medication adherence. Cogn Behav Pract. 1999;6(4):332–41.
53. Beck AT. Cognitive models of depression. J Cogn Psychother. 1987;1(1):5–37.
54. Safren SA, Gonzalez J, Soroudi N. CBT for depression and adherence in individuals with chronic illness: therapist guide. New York: Oxford University Press; 2008.
55. Miller WR, Rollnick S. Motivational interviewing: preparing people to change addictive behaviour. New York: Guilford Press; 1991.
56. Safren SA, O'Cleirigh CM, Tan JY, Raminani SR, Reilly LC, Otto MW, et al. A randomized controlled trial of cognitive behavioral therapy for adherence and depression (CBT-AD) in HIV-infected individuals. Health Psychol. 2009;28(1):1–10.
57. Newcomb ME, Bedoya CA, Blashill AJ, Lerner JA, O'Cleirigh CM, Pinkston MM, et al. Description and demonstration of cognitive behavioral therapy to enhance antiretroviral therapy adherence and treat depression in HIV-Infected adults. Cogn Behav Pract. 2015;22(4):430–8.

58. Magidson JF, Seitz-Brown CJ, Safren SA, Daughters SB. Implementing behavioral activation and life-steps for depression and HIV medication adherence in a community health center. Cogn Behav Pract. 2014;21(4):386–403.

59. McHugh RK, Barlow DH. The dissemination and implementation of evidence-based psychological treatments. A review of current efforts. Am Psychol. 2010;65(2):73–84.

60. Wingood GM, DiClemente RJ. The ADAPT-ITT model: a novel method of adapting evidence-based HIV Interventions. J Acquir Immune Defic Syndr. 2008;47 Suppl 1:S40–6.

61. Saberi P, Yuan P, John M, Sheon N, Johnson MO. A pilot study to engage and counsel HIV-positive African American youth via telehealth technology. AIDS Patient Care STDS. 2013;27(9):529–32.

62. Wood JA, Miller TW, Hargrove DS. Clinical supervision in rural settings: a telehealth model. Prof Psychol Res Pract. 2005;36(2):173–9.

63. Khatri N, Marziali E, Tchernikov I, Shepherd N. Comparing telehealth-based and clinic-based group cognitive behavioral therapy for adults with depression and anxiety: a pilot study. Clin Interv Aging. 2014;9:765–70.

64. Tufts KA, Johnson KF, Shepherd JG, Lee J-Y, Bait Ajzoon MS, Mahan LB, et al. Novel interventions for HIV self-management in African American women: a systematic review of mHealth interventions. J Assoc Nurses AIDS Care. 2015;26(2):139–50.

65. Krakower DS, Jain S, Mayer KH. Antiretrovirals for primary HIV prevention: the current status of pre- and post-exposure prophylaxis. Curr HIV/AIDS Rep. 2015;12(1):127–38.

66. Grant RM, Lama JR, Anderson PL, McMahan V, Liu AY, Vargas L, et al. Preexposure chemoprophylaxis for HIV prevention in men who have sex with men. N Engl J Med. 2010;363(27):2587–99.

67. Roland ME, Neilands TB, Krone MR, Katz MH, Franses K, Grant RM, et al. Seroconversion following nonoccupational postexposure prophylaxis against HIV. Clin Infect Dis. 2005;41(10):1507–13.

68. Amico KR, Stirratt MJ. Adherence to preexposure prophylaxis: current, emerging, and anticipated bases of evidence. Clin Infect Dis. 2014;59 Suppl 1:S55–60.

Abbreviations

ART	Antiretroviral therapy
CBO	Community-based organizations
CBT	Cognitive behavioral therapy
CBT-AD	Cognitive behavioral therapy for HIV medication adherence and depression
ETAU	Enhanced treatment as usual
MSM	Men who have sex with men
PEP	Post-exposure prophylaxis
PREP	Pre-exposure prophylaxis
PTSD	Posttraumatic stress disorder
RCT	Randomized control trial
UAI	Unprotected anal intercourse

Part III
Emerging Areas

Part III
Emerging Areas

Chapter 12
Women's Health: Behavioral Medicine Interventions for Women During Childbearing and Menopause

Christina Psaros, Jocelyn Remmert, Nicole Amoyal, and Rebecca Hicks

12.1 Introduction

After decades of health-related research that focused predominantly on males, the field of women's health is now well established. Reproductive events can bring women into contact with the medical system and serve as opportunities to enhance health and well-being. While women's health encompasses a broad array of topics, the present chapter will focus on behavioral medicine approaches to working with women during childbearing and menopause. Specifically, this chapter will review the prevalence of the most common psychiatric disorders as they occur during childbearing-related events and the menopausal transition, discuss the evidence base for cognitive behavioral therapy (CBT)-based interventions as well as specific population concerns, and conclude with a case study of how CBT might be used in women with a history of depression who hope to conceive.

C. Psaros, Ph.D. (✉) • J. Remmert • N. Amoyal
Behavioral Medicine Service, Department of Psychiatry, Massachusetts General Hospital,
Harvard Medical School, Boston, MA, USA
e-mail: cpsaros@mgh.harvard.edu

R. Hicks
Behavioral Medicine, Department of Psychiatry, Massachusetts General Hospital,
One Bowdoin Square, 7th Floor, Boston, MA 02114, USA

12.1.1   Prevalence of Depression and Anxiety
During Pregnancy and Postpartum

Depression and anxiety are the most prevalent and well-studied psychiatric conditions during pregnancy and the postpartum. While pregnancy was once considered a time of emotional well-being, data now suggest that women are vulnerable to both new and recurrent episodes of depression and anxiety during both pregnancy and the postpartum [1, 2]. Even when pregnancy is desired, pregnancy and adjusting to becoming a parent can result in significant stress. For example, both pregnancy and parenthood can result in sleep disruption. Parenthood results in role changes, such as how partners relate to one another in the context of parenthood and how women make decisions about returning to the workplace. In addition to these significant life changes, pregnancy and delivery produce dramatic changes in estrogen and progesterone levels as well as suppression along the Hypothalamic-Pituitary-Adrenal axis, all of which have been implicated as contributors to a biological vulnerability to depression and anxiety in the perinatal period [3]. Approximately 10–15 % of women experience depression during pregnancy [4–6]. Further, women who discontinue antidepressant treatment during pregnancy are 5 times as likely to relapse during pregnancy compared to women who maintain antidepressant treatment [2]. Similarly, up to 10–15 % of women will experience depression during the first year postpartum [7].

Anxiety during pregnancy and the postpartum period has been less well-studied relative to depression. A community-based study in Australia found elevated rates of anxiety symptoms during the first trimester of pregnancy among 15 % of the sample [8]. An Italian study investigating the risk of Panic Disorder during pregnancy found that 7.5 % of the sample met diagnostic criteria at any point during pregnancy [9], while 9.5 % of a US-based sample experience diagnostic criteria for Generalized Anxiety Disorder (GAD) at any point during pregnancy [10]. A recent meta-analysis concluded that pregnant and postpartum women are more likely to suffer from Obsessive Compulsive Disorder (OCD) than the general population, with average prevalence rates of 2.7 % during pregnancy and 2.43 % during the postpartum [11].

12.1.2   Prevalence of Depression and Anxiety Associated
with Infertility

Infertility is defined as the inability to conceive after 12 consecutive months of unprotected intercourse [12, 13]. Approximately 6.7 million U.S. couples, or about 11 % of the reproductive-age population, are affected by infertility [12]. Both the diagnosis of and treatment for infertility can be stressful as childbearing is a milestone to which many individuals and couples aspire. A diagnosis of infertility can result in challenges to identity, particularly as cultural, family, and social expectations and pressures dictate when and how an individual or couple should conceive. Medical treatment for female factor infertility varies from relatively noninvasive (e.g., stimulating the ovaries with oral medication) to invasive (e.g., in vitro fertilization). Treatment is time-intensive and usually requires frequent monitoring and contact with the healthcare system including office visits, blood work, and transvaginal ultrasounds. Treatment success varies widely based on factors such as age and diagnosis, but approximately 31.6% of IVF procedures will result in a live birth [14]. Among women seeking infertility treatment, approximately 8.5–17% meet criteria for Major Depression [15] and 25.7% have elevated levels of anxiety [16]. Nearly one quarter (23.2%) of a sample of women seeking infertility treatment met criteria for GAD [17].

12.1.3   Complicated Pregnancy, Pregnancy Loss, and Mental Health

While pregnancy alone can serve as a stressful life event, several medical conditions that co-occur with pregnancy may be interrelated with maternal mental health [18]. A pregnancy can become complicated or high risk in the presence of gestational diabetes, hypertension, preeclampsia, obesity, placenta previa, and cervical incompetency [18]. Kozhimannil, Pereira, and Harlow [19] found an association between diabetes and perinatal depression in low-income mothers, but a larger review found that there is an overall elevated depression rate in low-income women [20], suggesting that gestational diabetes as a risk factor for perinatal and postpartum depression (PPD) needs further exploration. Stress in general is associated with increased risk of gestational hypertension and preeclampsia; specifically, work-associated stress and anxiety or depression are associated with increased risk of preeclampsia [21]. Women with preeclampsia were found to have worse quality of life, especially mental health, both during the pregnancy and later in life [22, 23]. Drug dependence and mental disorders were found to be strongly associated with preterm premature rupture of membranes and spontaneous preterm birth [24]. The relationship between obesity and maternal mental health during pregnancy is understudied, but in one study women who had a higher pre-pregnancy body mass index (BMI) were more likely to experience major depressive disorder (MDD) during pregnancy than women who gained within and above recommended gestational weight gain guidelines [25]. Providers might consider extra vigilance with respect to screening patients with complicated pregnancies for symptoms of depression and anxiety in order to provide treatment as soon as possible.

Rates of miscarriage are approximately 10–20% [26]. Overall, many women and families who experience miscarriage are not satisfied with the usual procedures of care and may experience perceived negative attitudes from healthcare providers, insufficient information on their miscarriage and next steps, and inadequate follow-up care [18]. Miscarriage is associated with increased risk for anxiety and depressive symptoms in the immediate 4 months following the loss. Disorders such as OCD, Acute Stress Disorder (ASD), and Post-Traumatic Stress Disorder (PTSD) specifically show elevated rates in the 4 months postpartum; data beyond this timeframe are less clear as many women become pregnant again within 6 months after the loss [27]. In subsequent pregnancies, women are at increased risk of psychological symptoms such as anxiety and sadness/depression, but overall the subsequent pregnancy does not lead to psychopathology and can actually be healing for parents [28–31]. Because of the increased risk of grief, anxiety, and depressive symptoms immediately following a miscarriage and in the subsequent pregnancy, clinicians should provide not only medical support but also psychological support as needed [18, 30].

12.1.4 Prevalence of Depression and Anxiety Associated with Menopause

Menopause, defined as the absence of menstruation for 12 successive months, signifies the culmination of fertility and is accompanied by a decline in functioning of the ovaries. The average age for women reaching menopause is 47.5 years in the United States [32]. Common symptoms of menopause include vaginal dryness, hot flashes, night sweats, sleep problems, mood changes, weight gain and slowed metabolism, thinning hair and dry skin, and loss of breast fullness [32–34]. Besides physiological changes, midlife is often filled with many life changes and stressors, such as fertility loss, role changes in household, and caretaking of parents that are aging, among others [32, 35]. As a result of physiological and psychosocial changes, depression and anxiety can also occur during menopause.

Although the majority of women transition well into menopause and do not experience depression [32], overall women transitioning to menopause (perimenopause) and postmenopause are 4–5 times more likely to develop major depression and depressive symptoms when compared to premenopausal women [36], independent of a prior history of depression. For women with a prior history of major depression, a 5 times increased risk is observed [35]. Similarly, women with a history of bipolar disorder have an increased risk of heightened symptoms during menopause [32]. The evidence base for dysthymia and menopause is limited; however, in a review of mood disorders and menopause; one study showed a 4.5 % prevalence rate of dysthymia in menopausal women [37].

The link between anxiety and menopause is inconsistent, partly because physiological symptoms such as hot flashes can mimic symptoms of anxiety (e.g., hyperarousal, panic attack), thus making it difficult to tease apart the cause of the symptom [38]. Although authors of a recent systematic review of the literature concluded that a clinically significant link between menopause and clinical anxiety disorders is not evident [39], other studies do show that anxiety [40] and panic disorder [32] are associated with greater experience of physiological symptoms during menopause. In a 10-year follow-up study including annual assessments for mood and menopausal symptoms, symptoms of anxiety were more robustly linked to vasomotor symptoms (e.g., hot flashes, night sweats) compared to other menopausal symptoms [41].

In the same study, participants with low anxiety symptoms at baseline were more likely to experience high anxiety symptoms during peri and postmenopause compared to premenopause [41]. Stage of menopause was not significantly associated with high anxiety for women who began the study with high symptoms of anxiety [41]. In one study examining OCD and menopause, 7.1% of the sample reported OCD with 0.7% reporting new onset OCD after menopause [42].

12.2   Specific Population Concerns

12.2.1   Medication Use During Pregnancy: Weighing the Risks

For many women with chronic or acute psychiatric disorders, psychotropic medications play a critical role in maintaining emotional health, psychological well-being, and cognitive functioning. Treatment decisions regarding psychiatric medications during pregnancy are challenging for women and clinicians alike and require careful treatment planning including a thorough and individualized risk/benefit analysis. These decisions must take into account not only a woman's current psychiatric health, but also her past psychiatric history, including the severity and chronicity of her illness, as well as any known past psychiatric episodes related to reproductive events [43]. Clinical research over the past 20 years has shown that pregnancy is a time of increased risk for relapse of mood and anxiety disorders in women with a history of these illnesses [2, 44]. Particularly vulnerable are those women who discontinue psychotropic medications during or proximate to pregnancy, with relapse rates increased as high as fivefold in women with MDD who discontinue antidepressant medications during pregnancy and with an even higher relapse rate (85%) for pregnant women with bipolar disorder who discontinue mood stabilizers [44].

Despite a growing appreciation of the clinical risk associated with discontinuing psychiatric medications during pregnancy, treatment decisions for pregnant women remain complex due to varying levels of evidence regarding the safety of fetal exposure to psychiatric medications. While fetal exposure to some psychotropic medications, like Selective Serotonin Reuptake Inhibitors (SSRIs) or Tricyclic Antidepressants (TCAs), has been evaluated in large population-based birth registries and prospective clinical trials, some commonly prescribed psychiatric medications are lacking the safety data necessary to properly assess their use in pregnant women, and others have demonstrated clear contraindications for use in pregnancy [45–47]. The extensive literature evaluating the risk of teratogenicity, neonatal toxicity, and long-term neurobehavioral sequelae of the various classes of psychiatric medications in pregnancy is beyond the scope of this chapter, but is critical to consider while creating a comprehensive treatment plan aimed at promoting the psychiatric health and well-being of both a woman and her developing fetus throughout the course of pregnancy and beyond. Clinicians may find a consultation with an expert in Perinatal Psychiatry to be helpful in weighing various treatment strategies, including medications and behavioral interventions, to reduce the risk of relapse associated with psychiatric disorders in pregnancy while making treatment decisions that minimize risk for both mother and child.

12.2.2   Pregnancy and the Postpartum

While often a desired event, childbearing can be a stressful life experience and can exacerbate or precipitate subthreshold or clinical levels of anxiety. Therefore, this next section will focus on several specific concerns that may worsen during pregnancy (e.g., body dissatisfaction and specific phobias) and also specific treatment adaptations that may be necessary during this time of potential medical stress.

12.2.2.1   Body Dissatisfaction

Pregnancy is a unique time for women with respect to body image and weight, as weight gain is expected, and even accepted [48]. Although pregnant women are generally protected from the societal norms about weight [48], research suggests that body dissatisfaction is still prevalent among pregnant women [49]. Body dissatisfaction is generally defined as discontentment associated with specific aspects of one's body [50]. While there are no community prevalence studies of body image dissatisfaction during pregnancy, Fairburn and Welch [51] found that 40 % of pregnant women expressed fear of weight gain in pregnancy, and 72 % expressed fear of not being able to return to their pre-pregnancy body weight. Often pregnant women are not dissatisfied with regard to increased size in expected areas such as the belly, but are dissatisfied with weight gain in other areas such as the face and arms [48].

Body dissatisfaction during pregnancy is linked with adverse health outcomes such as obesity and excessive gestational weight gain and is also associated with depressed mood, stress, and maternal fetal attachment issues [49, 52]. Breastfeeding and body dissatisfaction are also related, in that women in their third trimester with higher body dissatisfaction were less inclined to breastfeed [53]. The relationship between body image during pregnancy and gestational weight gain is also complex. Due to a general acceptance of weight gain during pregnancy, women may overestimate how much weight is healthy to gain, leading to excessive gestational weight gain [48]. For example, in late pregnancy women who have lower feelings of fatness were found to have greater gestational weight gain, which subsequently may lead to increased risk for pregnancy-associated hypertension, gestational diabetes, complications during labor and delivery, postpartum weight retention, unsuccessful breastfeeding, and subsequent maternal obesity [49, 54]. However, pregnant women are generally more receptive to conversations about healthy weight management, and therefore pregnancy can be used as a "teachable moment" to decrease excessive gestational weight gain and improve health outcomes [48, 55]. Many postpartum women have high, even unrealistic, expectations for losing weight accrued during pregnancy, which can result in stress and body dissatisfaction [48, 56]. As the time from the birth of the child passes, body dissatisfaction can increase due to the perception that it is less acceptable to carry "baby weight" [57], as well as societal pressures.

Eating disorders, such as anorexia nervosa and bulimia, may also present specific concerns during pregnancy. Pregnant women with anorexia nervosa or bulimia may be at increased risk for spontaneous abortion, preterm birth, and PPD when compared to the pregnant women without eating disorders [58–62]. Babies born to mothers with anorexia or bulimia are at risk for developmental delays [63–65]. A team approach is most effective treatment for all disorders during pregnancy. Effective treatment for patients with anorexia includes a combination of renourishment and psychotherapy, such as CBT or interpersonal therapy (IPT), although no one treatment has been shown to be superior at this point [66, 67]; effective treatments for bulimia also include CBT and IPT [66].

12.2.2.2   Specific Phobias

Needle phobias can be a barrier to receiving medical care in general, but particularly during pregnancy and possibly infertility treatment when routine blood tests are an integral part of care. Pregnant women with needle phobias were more likely to register for antenatal care later in pregnancy [68], have a significant delay in blood tests [68], and consent less often to blood tests [68]. Despite later entry into antenatal care and fewer blood tests, women with needle phobias did not differ in adverse birth outcomes from women without needle phobias [68]. Key clinical considerations for pregnant women with needle phobias include finding a healthcare provider with whom the patient feels comfortable and who understands needle phobia and learning mind-body therapies (visualization, relaxation) to reduce stress and anxiety [69]. Although there are no trials to date of any intervention for pregnant women with needle phobia, traditional exposure treatment for needle phobia is likely to also be effective in this population.

Emetophobia, or fear of vomiting, includes avoidance of situations that may lead to vomiting. As such, in a population of people who self-identify as having emetophobia, nearly half of the women reported avoiding or delaying pregnancy because of their phobia [70]. Overall, empirical literature is lacking on how emetophobia affects pregnancy, and future research should be directed to elucidate the relationship between this phobia and the mental and physical effects it has on pregnancy. Cognitive-behavioral treatments such as graded exposure to vomit (and scents that may cause nausea), relaxation, and cognitive restructuring, which have been used in case reports and small nonrandomized studies with the general population, are likely to be useful for women who wish to conceive [71, 72].

12.2.3   Menopause

12.2.3.1   Sexual Dysfunction

Sexual dysfunction is common during menopause and occurs in 15–55 % [73, 74] of middle-aged women. Symptoms of sexual dysfunction are most commonly related to lack of estrogen production during menopause, which results in vaginal dryness and can lead to vaginal atrophy, as well as pain and bleeding during intercourse. In addition, loss of libido and difficulty achieving orgasm are common symptoms of sexual dysfunction in women during menopause [75].

While sexual dysfunction is common in postmenopausal women and can significantly impact satisfaction with life, sexual dysfunction is often not identified and as a result is left untreated [76]. Related research in the field of gynecologic oncology has indicated that providers may lack training in addressing and treating sexual dysfunction while patients often feel uncomfortable about discussing symptoms [77, 78]. If left untreated, vulvovaginal atrophy is unlikely to resolve on its own [76]. While hormonal factors can directly relate to sexual dysfunction, sexual dysfunction can also be impacted by psychological factors (e.g., depression, anxiety), psychosocial stressors (e.g., life changes, relationship issues), and general aging [79]. Sexual side effects that are not directly related to hormonal changes in women after menopause can include, but are not limited to, lower self-esteem, relationship dissatisfaction, and decreased libido and arousal [79]. Thus, treatment of sexual dysfunction after menopause should include a comprehensive biopsychosocial approach (e.g., medications, behavioral, and communication strategies).

Treatment of sexual dysfunction during menopause should include an assessment of physiological symptoms (e.g., vaginal dryness, pain during intercourse), as well as difficulty reaching orgasm, lowered libido and arousal, and other psychosocial symptoms related to sexual dysfunction (e.g., satisfaction with partner, body image, confidence). The Female Sexual Function Index is a comprehensive, reliable, and valid measure of sexual dysfunction [80] and can ideally be used in conjunction with a validated assessment of menopausal symptoms (e.g., The Greene Climacteric Scale; [81]) to assess both menopausal symptoms and sexual dysfunction. Taken together, these assessments can provide a thorough understanding of what is contributing to sexual dysfunction during menopause and can further guide treatment. For example, if a woman is experiencing problems with lubrication, but no decrease in arousal or libido, the treatment may simply require effective lubricants (e.g., over-the-counter moisturizers and lubricants or prescription strength; [76]). However, if a woman is experiencing low libido, arousal, and desire, along with trouble with lubrication, a more comprehensive assessment and treatment may be required. In the latter case, further inquiry about symptoms of depression, relationship dissatisfaction, and stressful life events may ensue. In the case that depression symptoms are significant, a referral for treatment of depression may be provided. In two studies, CBT for menopausal depression had beneficial effects on menopausal symptoms (e.g., hot flashes) [33]. However, more research is needed to understand whether CBT for depression can have residual benefits for sexual dysfunction. Other modes of treatment can include exercise, counseling, anti-depressants, and estrogen therapy.

12.2.3.2 Sleep Disturbance

Sleep disturbance is a common symptom among menopausal women [82]. Sleep disturbance during menopause can have many contributing factors. Hormonal changes specific to menopause, vasomotor symptoms, mood disturbance, lifestyle changes, and other medical conditions during midlife can all impact sleep quality [82]. In efforts to combat sleep disturbance, hormone replacement therapies have been tested due to changes in estrogen and progesterone (and their relationship to sleep cycles) during menopause, though the findings are mixed. In a review of randomized controlled trials of hormone therapies to treat sleep disturbance, the majority of studies showed small positive effects on decreasing arousal and alertness [82, 83]. Other treatments for sleep disturbance during menopause have included sleep hygiene and behavioral therapy, antidepressants, and circadian rhythm training [82]. To date, no CBT intervention solely targeting sleep disturbance in menopausal women exists. However, sleep disturbance is a common symptom of depression, anxiety, and menopause and is part of other, more comprehensive assessments and treatments of menopausal symptoms and depression. Evidence-based strategies for sleep disturbance in the general population include sleep hygiene (e.g., set bedtimes and wake times, avoidance of caffeine later in the day, eliminate naps, etc.), stimulus control, and general CBT for sleep skills. One randomized controlled trial of CBT for menopause study found improvements in sleep in both the treatment and self-help treatment group compared to control group [84, 85]. Overall, CBT treatments for depression and menopausal symptoms are in their infancy, and the focus is on demonstrating efficacy first, before isolating specific pathways (e.g., sleep, sexual dysfunction).

12.2.3.3 Psychosocial Treatments for Depression and Anxiety During Infertility, Pregnancy, the Postpartum, and Menopause

Psychosocial treatments for the entire spectrum of women's health issues are best delivered as part of an integrated team approach, incorporating the obstetrician/gynecologist, psychiatrist, psychologist, and other appropriate physical and mental health professionals (i.e., nutritionist, social worker) [86–88]. This model of care is consistent with evidence-based biopsychosocial models of care, and communication should be fostered among all providers who can together encourage patients' progress toward goals.

12.2.3.4 Psychosocial Treatment for Infertility

Much of the research focused on alleviating infertility-related distress is based on mind-body interventions for women or couples with infertility. In general, mind-body interventions seek to reduce stress and other negative psychological symptoms through techniques such as relaxation training, meditation, and psychoeducation to support healthy lifestyle changes. Cognitive-based mind-body interventions for infertility can aid in managing negative emotions (such as shame, feelings of inadequacy, depression) that accompany the infertility experience by teaching techniques such as role-playing to practice both interactions with the partner and others (such as discussing infertility with family members) and yoga to increase the mind-body connection and help with relaxation [89, 90]. In several trials of mind-body interventions for infertility, participants experienced increased social support, decreased depressive symptoms, and decreased stress [90, 91]. Investigators have examined a range of interventions for women and couples with infertility, from supportive counseling to the aforementioned mind-body interventions. Boivin [92] found that interventions focused on education and skills training (i.e., relaxation training), such as mind-body interventions, were significantly more effective in producing positive change across outcomes such as depression and anxiety, when compared to counseling interventions that focused on emotional expression of topics related to infertility [92]. While psychosocial interventions for infertility have been widely studied and applied [92], the majority of studies have many methodological limitations, including lack of randomization, inadequate control groups, and inadequate follow-up periods, thus making any conclusions about their efficacy in increasing fertility difficult to ascertain [93].

12.2.3.5 Psychosocial Treatments for Depression During Pregnancy and the Postpartum

Among the plethora of psychosocial treatments for depression, IPT and CBT have received the most attention and research support in this population. These treatments are effective when they are delivered both individually and in a group format.

IPT is a time-limited and present-focused psychotherapy that emphasizes the interpersonal context of depression, specifically, how an individual's personal relationships and environment affect their individual depression experience. In an IPT-based model, clinical manifestations of PPD include affective, cognitive, neurovegetative, and behavioral, which can all disrupt interpersonal relationships and social functioning at multiple levels [94]. IPT treatment can include techniques such as demystifying and externalizing the current problem as something the patient has rather than defining aspect of who she is (i.e., "I will always be a depressed mother" could change to "I have depression right now, but it is not necessarily permanent"). IPT utilizes the "sick role" (the mother has an illness, the PPD, which is like other illnesses that may not be permanent) to decrease guilt of past failures and burdens of current expectations and to increase motivation to change (i.e., "I am sick currently, but I can work to get better"). IPT can be utilized in both individual and group settings [94]. A review of 11 studies on IPT for PPD found that IPT was more effective than waitlist controls or treatment as usual in improving depression symptoms [94]. Many of the IPT treatments for PPD focus on relationships and partner involvement, in order to aid in the potentially upsetting changes in personal relationships and social functioning that PPD can cause.

CBT for depression during pregnancy and postpartum is not delivered in a uniform fashion; rather, it is individualized to the specific symptoms and goals with which women present. Typical symptoms of PPD include anger/irritability, impaired concentration, and anxiety, particularly around child safety. Insomnia can also be a difficulty for mothers who have PPD, particularly in adjusting to a baby with inconsistent sleep schedules. CBT techniques such as activity scheduling (for example, attending a mother baby exercise class), cognitive restructuring of distortions, particularly as they relate to mothering (i.e., "I'll never breastfeed successfully") and problem solving (i.e., ways to preserve sleep), would be effective components of CBT for PPD.

Regardless of the approach, treatments are complicated by difficulties with child care. Providers need to be flexible and able to incorporate the baby into the treatment. Additionally, treatments delivered via videoconferencing can be particularly useful for this population as it decreases the burden on patients and may increase likelihood of adherence to treatment. Programs in which therapists travel to patients' homes have been used in Australia and the United Kingdom and found to be efficacious in decreasing depression, increasing overall mental health, and improving satisfaction with community health services [95–97]. Although such programs are not currently covered by insurance in the United States, they represent an important area for research.

Group CBT is an effective treatment for PPD, shown to significantly improve symptoms of depression in a wide variety of settings as compared to routine primary care and waitlist groups [98]. Mothers experiencing PPD may feel isolated and need additional peer social support; group-based interventions address these needs in a supportive and therapeutic environment where mothers can learn from and teach each other [98, 99]. Group treatments in general are also more cost-effective and practical, given limited mental health resources and the wide prevalence of PPD. Group CBT for PPD has the added benefit of normalizing difficulties and adjustments to motherhood in general, and other activities to foster social support and normalize mothers' experiences. Delivery of therapy via telemedicine platforms can be particularly helpful in reducing burden of traveling to clinic, as well as reaching women in rural setting where evidenced-based CBT treatments might not be available.

CBT is also used in depressed pregnant women to prevent PPD [100, 101]. A review of 28 trials (involving almost 17,000 women) across countries such as Australia, United Kingdom, Ireland, Canada, United States, and China showed that women who received a psychosocial or psychological intervention of any kind during pregnancy were significantly less likely to develop PPD [100]. Effective interventions included CBT (individual and group) and individualized postpartum home visits by a public health nurse or midwife. Overall, CBT can be an effective treatment to both prevent and treat PPD, particularly for women who wish to opt out of pharmacological treatment during this time. Moreover, preventing symptoms is generally easier and more cost-effective than treating the disorder.

12.2.3.6 Exposure Treatment for Anxiety Disorders During Pregnancy

Exposure-based CBT is the most empirically supported treatment for anxiety disorders in the general adult population. However, pregnant women have often been excluded from exposure efficacy trials due to assumptions that exposure would stress or harm the fetus [102]. While there is a paucity of research on exactly what occurs in the fetus during exposure therapy in pregnant women, the available evidence suggests that exposure-based CBT on pregnant women is likely to be safe, particularly relative to the alternatives of medication and not treating the anxiety disorder [102]. The risks of untreated anxiety-related disorders during pregnancy include preterm birth, small-for-gestational-age infants, and risky maternal health behaviors, such as smoking, alcohol consumption, and substance use [102–105]. Additionally, a past or current anxiety disorder is a risk factor for developing PPD [102, 105]. While exposure-based CBT does increase heart rate and blood pressure in the moment, evidence suggests that this physiological arousal is not long-lasting [102]. Additionally, exposure is an extremely powerful and effective tool in CBT and can decrease anxiety symptoms rapidly, after only a few sessions [102]. Overall, the current body of research indicates that exposure-based CBT during pregnancy is likely to be safe, particularly in comparison with the alternatives of pharmacotherapy and untreated anxiety disorders [102]. Modifications to utilizing exposures with pregnant women in the clinical setting are recommended; for example, instead of spinning standing to induce dizziness and light headedness, the patient could spin in an office chair [102].

12.2.3.7   Treatment for OCD in Pregnancy and Postpartum

OCD during pregnancy occurs in 0.2–3.5 % of women [106, 107]. Often obsessional ideation in pregnancy relates to concerns about the health of the fetus, fears related to harming the fetus, worries related to the physical changes associated with pregnancy, and the physical process of childbirth. Often obsessions related to disease and contamination become prominent fears associated with unintentionally harming the infant. Compulsions can include cleaning and organizing the home, seeking reassurance from healthcare providers and loved ones, as well as the range of myriad compulsive behaviors associated with the illness.

OCD in the postpartum occurs in 2.43 % of women [108]. Similar to OCD during pregnancy, women with a history of OCD are at greater risk for developing OCD during the postpartum [109]. Fairbrother and Abramowitz propose a CBT-based model of postpartum OCD, focused on three parameters: (1) there is an abrupt increase in responsibility for a vulnerable and highly valued infant; (2) this increase of responsibility can lead to the misinterpretation of normally occurring infant-related thoughts which feel threatening, and subsequently leads the parent to feel like these thoughts need additional attention to prevent the feared negative behavior, thus eventually becoming the obsessions; (3) then overt and covert behaviors, the compulsions, develop in response to the obsessions (e.g., checking the baby, avoidance of the child, thought suppression attempts) [110]. OCD in the postpartum period can be either abrupt in onset or can result from pre-existing clinical or subclinical symptoms that intensify postpartum [110, 111]. OCD in postpartum women is primarily comprised of intrusive thoughts around the safety of the baby such as accidentally harming the baby via contamination or being capable of deliberately harming the infant [111–113]. Similar to pregnancy, compulsions can include excessive hand washing and cleaning the home [111, 113].

CBT is a widely studied and proven effective treatment for OCD in the general population and shows feasibility and preliminary effectiveness in pregnant and postpartum women. Pregnant women at risk for OCD who participated in a traditional childbirth education class combined with CBT modules on OCD experienced significantly lower levels of compulsions and obsessions than women who participated in a time-matched control of childbirth education plus general psychoeducation, thus demonstrating CBT's preliminary effectiveness in preventing postpartum OCD [114]. There is limited research on CBT for OCD during the postpartum, but as noted above, exposure treatments are likely to be safe during pregnancy. Several case studies on CBT for OCD in postpartum women report significant improvement and clinical remission in OCD symptoms [111, 115]. These studies include modules similar to CBT for OCD in the general population, such as psychoeducation, exposure and response prevention, and cognitive restructuring; a clinician would use these modules along with relevant examples to a postpartum mother, such as exposure to fear of contamination or fear of hurting the child, in the overall context of CBT for OCD.

12.2.3.8 Interventions for Menopause

Cognitive behavioral interventions for menopause have been investigated and yield support for their usage to mollify the physiological symptoms of menopause [74, 116–118] and symptoms associated with menopause (e.g., mood symptoms, sexual dysfunction, sleep disorders, and life stressors). In a review of psychosocial treatments targeting depression in menopausal women [33], only two studies were identified as targeting depression specifically for peri and post-menopausal women. One study included 16 sessions of individual CBT, and almost one third of perimenopausal and postmenopausal participants experienced remission in depression, and 50 % of post and perimenopausal women reported at least a 50 % reduction in depression assessment ratings [119]. In another study that included 16, twice-weekly group therapy sessions, perimenopausal women experienced significant reductions in depression scores at follow-up [120]. There have been several cognitive-behavioral, behavioral, and mindfulness-based treatments targeting menopausal symptoms that have yielded beneficial effects on depression. In a review of psychosocial treatments for menopause, 12 interventions were identified, and 9 of the 12 studies yielded significant reductions in depression scores following treatment [33]. Overall, the most useful interventions are comprehensive and include cognitive-behavioral and mindfulness-based strategies in addition to psychoeducation, in either an individual or group format.

There is one comprehensive and manualized treatment specifically for menopause that targets depression, anxiety, and physiological menopausal symptoms [121]. The Cognitive Behavioral Workbook for Menopause treatment manual [121] includes step-by-step, self-help sections. The workbook provides psychoeducation about menopausal symptoms, an opportunity to create an individualized treatment plan, coping strategies for physiological symptoms of menopause (e.g., hot flashes, sleeping problems) and mood symptoms (e.g., depression and anxiety), information about alternative treatment options, and suggestions for other healthy lifestyle changes. For example, readers are instructed on how to complete a symptom diary that includes listing symptoms and their related maladaptive thoughts, feelings, and behaviors. Then readers can prioritize by listing their symptoms in order after rating severity and interference with life. These monitoring exercises provide a way to plan treatment according to personalized preferences. Then, subsequent chapters teach strategies about managing various symptoms (e.g., depression, anxiety, sleep problems, sexual dysfunction). Unfortunately, this manualized treatment has yet to be tested for efficacy in a randomized controlled trial; however, the content and strategies are largely informed by evidence-based cognitive-behavioral therapy approaches to treat menopausal symptoms and mood disorders.

12.3 Conclusions and Future Directions

In summary, while many women will experience the range of reproductive events without incident, a sizeable minority of the population will experience new or recurrent episodes of mood and/or anxiety disorders. The use of psychotropic medication can be an important and even life saving component of treatment for women with psychiatric disorders, particularly during times of vulnerability-associated pregnancy and the postpartum period. Weighing the risks and benefits of pharmacotherapy must be considered on an individual basis for each woman, taking into account both the risks associated with fetal exposure to medication, as well as the risks that untreated psychiatric disorders may pose to both mother and child. While psychotherapies such as CBT have some evidence for use during pregnancy, the postpartum, and menopause, greater research is required. Specifically, research utilizing control groups, examining who is best able to deliver treatment, and research with minority women is needed. See Tables 12.1 and 12.2.

12.4 CBT for the Prevention of Depressive Recurrence: Case Illustration

Because many women with a diagnosis of depression will discontinue their antidepressant medication either in preparation for or upon learning of pregnancy independent of their risk for recurrence [2], the scientific community is compelled to identify non-pharmacologic treatments for depression during the perinatal period. A few studies have attempted to utilize CBT to protect against depressive recurrence in the general population [122–127], and a recent pilot study examined the potential efficacy of CBT for the prevention of depressive recurrence among euthymic women who wished to discontinue their antidepressant in order to conceive [90]. What

Table 12.1 Self-report assessments

Measure	Variable	Description
Fertility Problem Inventory (FPI)	Stress specific to infertility	5 Domain scale (social concerns, sexual concerns, relationship concerns, need for parenthood, and rejection of a childfree lifestyle) assessing stress on a six point Likert scale [128]
Perinatal Grief Intensity Scale	Grief intensity	14 Item questionnaire identifying intensity of grief in pregnancy subsequent to a miscarriage, stillbirth, or neonatal death [129]
Perinatal Anxiety Screening Scale (PASS)	Anxiety symptoms	31 Item scale screening for anxiety during pregnancy [130]
Pregnancy-Related Anxiety Questionnaire-Revised (PRAQ-R)	Pregnancy-related anxiety	10 Item scale that examines the extent to which participants feel anxious, concerned, afraid, and panicky about their pregnancy [131]
Perinatal Obsessive Compulsive Scale (POCS)	OCD symptoms	Screen for perinatal (16 item) and postpartum (33 item) obsessive compulsive thoughts and behaviors, specific to the baby [132]
Edinburgh Postnatal Depression Scale (EPDS)	Depression	10-Item scale assessing depressive symptoms. This scale has been validated in pregnancy through postpartum [133–135]
Greene Climacteric Scale	Menopause symptoms	21 Item scale that assesses three main domains; psychological, physical, and vasomotor symptoms on a four point Likert scale [136]
Menopause Decision Quality Worksheet v2.0	Treatment decisions about how to manage menopausal symptoms	21 Item scale that assesses value of importance for management of menopausal symptoms, knowledge about menopausal symptoms and treatment, and results from talking with healthcare providers [137]

follows is a case illustration of how CBT strategies may be used in order to help women with a history of depression remain well during attempts to conceive.

Andrea is a 35 year old, recently married woman of Mediterranean heritage who was seen in consultation with a reproductive psychiatrist for the purposes of planning pregnancy. She has a history of Major Depressive Disorder and has been well for the past 2 years on 40 mg of fluoxetine. She has had approximately five lifetime episodes of major depression, the first of which occurred during her first year in college. Other episodes have occurred in the context of increased stress or loss, such as the death of her father after a prolonged illness. While Andrea has been under the care of a psychiatrist and has received some supportive psychotherapy, she has never received CBT. She describes a positive relationship with her husband and a

Table 12.2 CBT modules and recommendations for specific patient problems

Problem	Intervention recommendation (interventions with the most evidence)	Key components	Goals
Infertility	Mind-body interventions	Relaxation training, meditation, psychoeducation to support healthy lifestyle changes, role-playing, exercises to promote resiliency	Reduce stress and other negative emotions around infertility, increase comfort in social interactions regarding infertility, minimize impact of infertility on partnership
Perinatal depression	CBT, IPT (group and/or individual)	CBT: activity scheduling, cognitive restructuring, problem solving IPT: "sick role," separate self from illness, improve interpersonal relationships	Reduce depressive symptoms and increase functioning
Perinatal anxiety	CBT	Therapeutic exposure, cognitive restructuring, relaxation training	Reduce anxiety symptoms, minimize avoidance
Eating disorders	CBT, motivational interviewing	Behaviorally change eating habits (either to eat more or stop binge and purge cycle), motivational interviewing to increase self-efficacy around behavioral change	To change eating behaviors to behaviors consistent with a healthy pregnancy and modify cognitions that body is undesirable during pregnancy and the postpartum
Specific phobias	CBT	Visualization, relaxation, exposure treatment, cognitive restructuring	To reduce stress and anxiety around specific phobias to decrease avoidant behavior
OCD	CBT	Exposure and response prevention, psychoeducation, cognitive restructuring	Reduce obsessive thoughts and compulsive behaviors
Mood and physiological symptoms of menopause	CBT, psychoeducation (group/or individual)	Mindfulness, relaxation strategies, cognitive restructuring, healthy lifestyle changes	To cope with and reduce distress associated with the physiological and mood symptoms associated with menopause

close relationship overall with her family of origin. She completed an advanced degree and works in a competitive business position. She would like to start trying to become pregnant as soon as she has fully tapered her antidepressant.

After a comprehensive psychosocial assessment, a medication taper schedule was determined by her consulting psychiatrist. Treatment began with psychoeducation on CBT for depression. Using an approach grounded in motivational interviewing, a pros and cons matrix of medication continuation versus discontinuation (in the context of receiving CBT) during attempts to conceive was completed. Andrea's most prominent concern with respect to medication continuation was fear of harm to the fetus and ability to breastfeed (despite relatively encouraging reproductive safety data). She also expressed a strong preference to avoid the use of psychotropic mediations during pregnancy, if at all possible. Potential cons of medication discontinuation included the fear and possibility of relapse, uncertainly around the effectiveness of CBT, and the effort involved in adhering to CBT skills.

The CBT model for depression was then reviewed using examples from Andrea's most recent depressive episode. The therapist and Andrea also discussed her understanding of her depressive disorder and its current remission (including etiology and triggers, maintaining factors, and factors that contributed to remission), as well as her expectations for therapy. Andrea was able to articulate that some of her triggers for depressive symptoms involved taking on too much and losing time for self care, feeling criticized or not good enough, and feeling out of control. Lastly, the ways in which planning a pregnancy may exacerbate these triggers or lead to vulnerabilities for depressive symptoms were discussed. Andrea acknowledged that not being fully in control around the timing of pregnancy would likely be difficult for her. She also acknowledged that she was more of a "planner" than her husband, and she worried about the potential for conflict around attempts to conceive given their difference in styles. The therapist and Andrea then generated a series of treatment goals.

The first skill covered in treatment was relaxation training, specifically, diaphragmatic breathing, guided imagery, and progressive muscle relaxation. Andrea was given a compact disc of recorded relaxation exercises to practice at home. Finding time to practice the exercises was a barrier to utilization; Andrea ultimately scheduled 15 min of relaxation practice into her work day 3–5 times per week.

Activity scheduling was introduced next. While Andrea's report of her current well-being and self-report questionnaires suggested that she was currently euthymic with only a few, mild symptoms of depression, monitoring of her daily activities revealed that she was engaging in minimal activities that had the potential to yield feelings of pleasure and/or mastery. Andrea was not enthusiastic about her current job; she did not find the work meaningful, it was demanding, and she worked long hours. She had started to use ovulation prediction kits in order to aid conception and felt that sexual activity with her husband now felt "scheduled" and lacked intimacy. Andrea noted that her organization had a mentoring program for junior employees with protected time for mentors and mentees. She signed up for the program as a way to add more meaning to her current job and allowed herself to acknowledge that while there were real reasons to stay with her current company at this time (e.g., competitive salary while her husband was starting his own business), she would think about a career move when things at home felt more stable. She noted that she used to enjoy cooking dinner and taking hikes with her husband, but that these activities occurred only rarely as a result of increased demands on her time. By committing to working 1–2 h in the evening after dinner on some occasions, she was able to leave work earlier and work less on weekends to fit these activities back into her schedule.

Cognitive restructuring was conducted in two phases. The first phase involved learning to identify automatic thoughts and cognitive distortions and generating rational responses via a thought record. The second phase involved identifying core beliefs and learning how to challenge them. At the time cognitive restructuring was introduced, Andrea had been trying to conceive over four menstrual cycles and was not yet pregnant. Some of the cognitive errors contained in her automatic thoughts involved black and white thinking ("I will never be a mother"), catastrophizing ("I probably have a fertility problem"), and using should statements and personalizing ("My stress levels at work are making it hard to get pregnant; I should practice relaxation more"). Through cognitive restructuring, Andrea was able to articulate that she would somehow become a mother. In fact, she knew that her husband was open to adoption if they were unable to conceive from conversations they had before their marriage. She was also able to reason that she could not reasonably conclude that she had a fertility problem at this juncture; if she still had not conceived after 6 months of trying, she would contact her primary care physician for a referral to a specialist for evaluation. Lastly, she noted conception was influenced by many processes, some of which she could not control and putting extra pressure on herself to "relax more" was counterproductive.

The CBT protocol used in this study was 12 sessions; thus, extensive core belief work could not be conducted. However, Andrea was able to identify two core beliefs and learned strategies for challenging them. Specifically, Andrea identified a core belief of "I have no control". She felt this was accurate at about 65 % and behaviorally made her attempt to overcompensate, leading to increased stress. She was taught how to design behavioral experiments to test her core beliefs (e.g., identifying what was reasonable to control in a given situation, letting go of the rest, and evaluating the outcome) and encouraged to continue this work over time.

Formal problem-solving skills and assertiveness skills were also introduced. At the time these skills were introduced, Andrea's most salient problem was how to divide care responsibilities of her aging, widowed mother with her siblings. After she chose a solution to implement, cognitive restructuring and assertiveness skills were used to increase the likelihood of a successful outcome. For Andrea, potential barriers to plan implementation included assumptions about what type of daughter and sibling she "should" be, feeling intimidated by her brother, and not having a clear understanding of what care she would like to provide or how to communicate about these concerns effectively.

Andrea successfully tapered her antidepressant and completed the 12-week protocol without a recurrence of depression. She continued monthly booster sessions for the next 8 months as she tried to conceive. Ultimately, she did require fertility treatment, but was able to achieve pregnancy. Booster sessions were spent reviewing CBT skills and applying them to new stressors that emerged as part of the infertility process.

References

1. Altshuler LL, Hendrick V, Cohen LS. Course of mood and anxiety disorders during pregnancy and the postpartum period. J Clin Psychiatry. 1998;59 Suppl 2:29–33.
2. Cohen LS, Altshuler LL, Harlow BL, Nonacs R, Newport DJ, Viguera AC, et al. Relapse of major depression during pregnancy in women who maintain or discontinue antidepressant treatment. JAMA. 2006;295(5):499–507. doi:10.1001/jama.295.5.499.
3. Steiner M, Dunn E, Born L. Hormones and mood: from menarche to menopause and beyond. J Affect Disord. 2003;74(1):67–83.
4. Evans J, Heron J, Francomb H, Oke S, Golding J. Cohort study of depressed mood during pregnancy and after childbirth. BMJ. 2001;323(7307):257–60.
5. O'Hara MW, Zekoski EM, Philipps LH, Wright EJ. Controlled prospective study of postpartum mood disorders: comparison of childbearing and nonchildbearing women. J Abnorm Psychol. 1990;99(1):3–15.
6. Spinelli M, Broudy C. Depression in the context of pregnancy. In: Mann J, McGrath P, Roose S, editors. Clinical handbook for the management of mood disorders. New York: Cambridge University Press; 2013. p. 206–19.
7. O'Hara M, Swain A. Rates and risk of postpartum depression-a meta-analysis. Int Rev Psychiatry. 1996;8:37–54.
8. Rubertsson C, Hellström J, Cross M, Sydsjö G. Anxiety in early pregnancy: prevalence and contributing factors. Arch Womens Ment Health. 2014;17(3):221–8. doi:10.1007/s00737-013-0409-0.
9. Marchesi C, Ampollini P, Paraggio C, Giaracuni G, Ossola P, De Panfilis C, et al. Risk factors for panic disorder in pregnancy: a cohort study. J Affect Disord. 2014;156:134–8. doi:10.1016/j.jad.2013.12.006.
10. Buist A, Gotman N, Yonkers KA. Generalized anxiety disorder: course and risk factors in pregnancy. J Affect Disord. 2011;131(1–3):277–83. doi:10.1016/j.jad.2011.01.003.
11. Russell EJ, Fawcett JM, Mazmanian D. Risk of obsessive-compulsive disorder in pregnant and postpartum women: a meta-analysis. J Clin Psychiatry. 2013;74(4):377–85. doi:10.4088/JCP.12r07917.
12. CDC. Infertility FAQs—reproductive health. 2012. http://www.cdc.gov/reproductivehealth/Infertility/#1files/6/Infertility.html
13. Watkins KJ, Baldo TD. The infertility experience: biopsychosocial effects and suggestions for counselors. J Couns Dev. 2004;82(4):394–402. doi:10.1002/j.1556-6678.2004.tb00326.x.
14. Reproductivefacts.org. Frequently asked questions about infertility. Birmingham: American Society Reproductive Medicine; 2015.
15. Williams KE, Marsh WK, Rasgon NL. Mood disorders and fertility in women: a critical review of the literature and implications for future research. Hum Reprod Update. 2007;13(6):607–16. doi:10.1093/humupd/dmm019.
16. Anderson KM, Sharpe M, Rattray A, Irvine DS. Distress and concerns in couples referred to a specialist infertility clinic. J Psychosom Res. 2003;54(4):353–5.
17. Chen T-H, Chang S-P, Tsai C-F, Juang K-D. Prevalence of depressive and anxiety disorders in an assisted reproductive technique clinic. Hum Reprod. 2004;19(10):2313–8. doi:10.1093/humrep/deh414.
18. Geller PA. Pregnancy as a stressful life event. CNS Spectr. 2004;9(03):188–97. doi:10.1017/S1092852900008981.
19. Kozhimannil K, Pereira MA, Harlow BL. Association between diabetes and perinatal depression among low-income mothers. JAMA. 2009;301(8):842–7. doi:10.1001/jama.2009.201.
20. Barakat S, Martinez D, Thomas M, Handley M. What do we know about gestational diabetes mellitus and risk for postpartum depression among ethnically diverse low-income women in the USA? Arch Womens Ment Health. 2014;17(6):587–92. doi:10.1007/s00737-014-0460-5.

21. Zhang S, Ding Z, Liu H, Chen Z, Wu J, Zhang Y, Yu Y. Association between mental stress and gestational hypertension/preeclampsia: a meta-analysis. Obstet Gynecol Surv. 2013;68(12):825–34. doi:10.1097/OGX.0000000000000001.

22. Hoedjes M, Berks D, Vogel I, Franx A, Duvekot JJ, Steegers EAP, Raat H. Poor health-related quality of life after severe preeclampsia. Birth. 2011;38(3):246–55. doi:10.1111/j.1523-536X.2011.00477.x.

23. Stern C, Trapp E-M, Mautner E, Deutsch M, Lang U, Cervar-Zivkovic M. The impact of severe preeclampsia on maternal quality of life. Qual Life Res. 2014;23(3):1019–26. doi:10.1007/s11136-013-0525-3.

24. Auger N, Le TUN, Park AL, Luo Z-C. Association between maternal comorbidity and preterm birth by severity and clinical subtype: retrospective cohort study. BMC Pregnancy Childbirth. 2011;11:67. doi:10.1186/1471-2393-11-67.

25. Bodnar LM, Wisner KL, Moses-Kolko E, Sit DKY, Hanusa BH. Prepregnancy body mass index, gestational weight gain and the likelihood of major depression during pregnancy. J Clin Psychiatry. 2009;70(9):1290–6. doi:10.4088/JCP.08m04651.

26. Miscarriage: signs, symptoms, treatment and prevention. (n.d.). http://americanpregnancy.org/pregnancy-complications/miscarriage/. Accessed 9 Sep 2015.

27. Geller PA, Kerns D, Klier CM. Anxiety following miscarriage and the subsequent pregnancy: a review of the literature and future directions. J Psychosom Res. 2004;56(1):35–45. doi:10.1016/S0022-3999(03)00042-4.

28. Chojenta C, Harris S, Reilly N, Forder P, Austin M-P, Loxton D. History of pregnancy loss increases the risk of mental health problems in subsequent pregnancies but not in the postpartum. PLoS One. 2014;9(4):e95038. doi:10.1371/journal.pone.0095038.

29. Giannandrea SAM, Cerulli C, Anson E, Chaudron LH. Increased risk for postpartum psychiatric disorders among women with past pregnancy loss. J Womens Health (Larchmt). 2013;22(9):760–8. doi:10.1089/jwh.2012.4011.

30. Klier CM, Geller PA, Ritsher JB. Affective disorders in the aftermath of miscarriage: a comprehensive review. Arch Womens Ment Health. 2002;5(4):129–49. doi:10.1007/s00737-002-0146-2.

31. McCarthy F, Moss-Morris R, Khashan A, North R, Baker P, Dekker G, et al. Previous pregnancy loss has an adverse impact on distress and behaviour in subsequent pregnancy. BJOG. 2015;122(13):1757–64. doi:10.1111/1471-0528.13233.

32. Gramann S, Lundquist R, Langenfeld S, Memon M, Talavera F. Menopause and mood disorders. 2012.

33. Green SM, Key BL, McCabe RE. Cognitive-behavioral, behavioral, and mindfulness-based therapies for menopausal depression: a review. Maturitas. 2015;80(1):37–47. doi:10.1016/j.maturitas.2014.10.004.

34. Terauchi M. Which is worse: old or obese? Menopause. 2013;20(8):802–3. doi:10.1097/GME.0b013e3182966dd5.

35. Freeman EW. Associations of depression with the transition to menopause. Menopause. 2010;17(4):823–7. doi:10.1097/gme.0b013e3181db9f8b.

36. Bromberger JT, Kravitz HM. Mood and menopause: findings from the Study of Women's Health Across the Nation (SWAN) over 10 years. Obstet Gynecol Clin North Am. 2011;38(3):609–25. doi:10.1016/j.ogc.2011.05.011.

37. Llaneza P, García-Portilla MP, Llaneza-Suárez D, Armott B, Pérez-López FR. Depressive disorders and the menopause transition. Maturitas. 2012;71(2):120–30. doi:10.1016/j.maturitas.2011.11.017.

38. Soares CN. Anxiety and the menopausal transition: managing your expectations. Menopause. 2013;20(5):481–2. doi:10.1097/GME.0b013e31828f9ba0.

39. Bryant C, Judd FK, Hickey M. Anxiety during the menopausal transition: a systematic review. J Affect Disord. 2012;139(2):141–8. doi:10.1016/j.jad.2011.06.055.

40. Terauchi M, Hiramitsu S, Akiyoshi M, Owa Y, Kato K, Obayashi S, et al. Associations among depression, anxiety and somatic symptoms in peri- and postmenopausal women. J Obstet Gynaecol Res. 2013;39(5):1007–13. doi:10.1111/j.1447-0756.2012.02064.x.

41. Bromberger JT, Kravitz HM, Chang Y, Randolph JF, Avis NE, Gold EB, Matthews KA. Does risk for anxiety increase during the menopausal transition? Study of women's health across the nation. Menopause. 2013;20(5):488–95. doi:10.1097/GME.0b013e3182730599.

42. Uguz F, Sahingoz M, Gezginc K, Karatayli R. Obsessive-compulsive disorder in postmenopausal women: prevalence, clinical features, and comorbidity. Aust N Z J Psychiatry. 2010;44(2):183–7. doi:10.3109/00048670903393639.

43. Payne JL, Meltzer-Brody S. Antidepressant use during pregnancy: current controversies and treatment strategies. Clin Obstet Gynecol. 2009;52(3):469–82. doi:10.1097/GRF.0b013e3181b52e20.

44. Viguera AC, Whitfield T, Baldessarini RJ, Newport DJ, Stowe Z, Reminick A, et al. Risk of recurrence in women with bipolar disorder during pregnancy: prospective study of mood stabilizer discontinuation. Am J Psychiatry. 2007;164(12):1817–24. doi:10.1176/appi.ajp.2007.06101639.

45. Greene MF. Teratogenicity of SSRIs—serious concern or much ado about little? N Engl J Med. 2007;356(26):2732–3. doi:10.1056/NEJMe078079.

46. Hallberg P, Sjöblom V. The use of selective serotonin reuptake inhibitors during pregnancy and breast-feeding: a review and clinical aspects. J Clin Psychopharmacol. 2005;25(1):59–73.

47. Ross LE, Grigoriadis S, Mamisashvili L, et al. Selected pregnancy and delivery outcomes after exposure to antidepressant medication: a systematic review and meta-analysis. JAMA Psychiatry. 2013;70(4):436–43. doi:10.1001/jamapsychiatry.2013.684.

48. Hodgkinson EL, Smith DM, Wittkowski A. Women's experiences of their pregnancy and postpartum body image: a systematic review and meta-synthesis. BMC Pregnancy Childbirth. 2014;14:330. doi:10.1186/1471-2393-14-330.

49. Fuller-Tyszkiewicz M, Skouteris H, Watson BE, Hill B. Body dissatisfaction during pregnancy: a systematic review of cross-sectional and prospective correlates. J Health Psychol. 2013;18(11):1411–21. doi:10.1177/1359105312462437.

50. Thompson JK, Coovert MD, Stormer SM. Body image, social comparison, and eating disturbance: a covariance structure modeling investigation. Int J Eat Disord. 1999;26(1):43–51.

51. Fairburn CG, Welch SL. The impact of pregnancy on eating habits and attitudes to shape and weight. Int J Eat Disord. 1990;9(2):153–60. doi:10.1002/1098-108X(199003)9:2<153::AID-EAT2260090204>3.0.CO;2-8.

52. Skouteris H, Carr R, Wertheim EH, Paxton SJ, Duncombe D. A prospective study of factors that lead to body dissatisfaction during pregnancy. Body Image. 2005;2(4):347–61. doi:10.1016/j.bodyim.2005.09.002.

53. Foster SF, Slade P, Wilson K. Body image, maternal fetal attachment, and breast feeding. J Psychosom Res. 1996;41(2):181–4.

54. Hill B, Skouteris H, McCabe M, Fuller-Tyszkiewicz M. Body image and gestational weight gain: a prospective study. J Midwifery Womens Health. 2013;58(2):189–94. doi:10.1111/j.1542-2011.2012.00227.x.

55. Phelan S. Pregnancy: a "teachable moment" for weight control and obesity prevention. Am J Obstet Gynecol. 2010;202(2):135.e1–8. doi:10.1016/j.ajog.2009.06.008.

56. Clark A, Skouteris H, Wertheim EH, Paxton SJ, Milgrom J. My baby body: a qualitative insight into women's body-related experiences and mood during pregnancy and the postpartum. J Reprod Infant Psychol. 2009;27(4):330–45. doi:10.1080/02646830903190904.

57. Gjerdingen D, Fontaine P, Crow S, McGovern P, Center B, Miner M. Predictors of mothers' postpartum body dissatisfaction. Women Health. 2009;49(6):491–504. doi:10.1080/03630240903423998.

58. Cardwell MS. Eating disorders during pregnancy. Obstet Gynecol Surv. 2013;68(4):312–23. doi:10.1097/OGX.0b013e31828736b9.

59. Franko DL, Blais MA, Becker AE, Delinsky SS, Greenwood DN, Flores AT, et al. Pregnancy complications and neonatal outcomes in women with eating disorders. Am J Psychiatry. 2001;158(9):1461–6.

60. Franko DL, Spurrell EB. Detection and management of eating disorders during pregnancy. Obstet Gynecol. 2000;95(6 Pt 1):942–6.

61. James DC. Eating disorders, fertility, and pregnancy: relationships and complications. J Perinat Neonatal Nurs. 2001;15(2):36–48.
62. Mazzeo SE, Slof-Op't Landt MCT, Jones I, Mitchell K, Kendler KS, Neale MC, et al. Associations among postpartum depression, eating disorders, and perfectionism in a population-based sample of adult women. Int J Eat Disord. 2006;39(3):202–11. doi:10.1002/eat.20243.
63. Koubaa S, Kouba S, Hällström T, Lindholm C, Hirschberg AL. Pregnancy and neonatal outcomes in women with eating disorders. Obstet Gynecol. 2005;105(2):255–60. doi:10.1097/01.AOG.0000148265.90984.c3.
64. Park RJ, Senior R, Stein A. The offspring of mothers with eating disorders. Eur Child Adolesc Psychiatry. 2003;12 Suppl 1:I110–9. doi:10.1007/s00787-003-1114-8.
65. Patel P, Wheatcroft R, Park RJ, Stein A. The children of mothers with eating disorders. Clin Child Fam Psychol Rev. 2002;5(1):1–19.
66. Kass AE, Kolko RP, Wilfley DE. Psychological treatments for eating disorders. Curr Opin Psychiatry. 2013;26(6):549–55. doi:10.1097/YCO.0b013e328365a30e.
67. Watson HJ, Bulik CM. Update on the treatment of anorexia nervosa: review of clinical trials, practice guidelines and emerging interventions. Psychol Med. 2013;43(12):2477–500. doi:10.1017/S0033291712002620.
68. McAllister N, Elshtewi M, Badr L, Russell IF, Lindow SW. Pregnancy outcomes in women with severe needle phobia. Eur J Obstet Gynecol Reprod Biol. 2012;162(2):149–52. doi:10.1016/j.ejogrb.2012.02.019.
69. Searing K, Baukus M, Stark MA, Morin KH, Rudell B. Needle phobia during pregnancy. J Obstet Gynecol Neonat Nurs. 2006;35(5):592–8. doi:10.1111/j.1552-6909.2006.00076.x.
70. Lipsitz JD, Fyer AJ, Paterniti A, Klein DF. Emetophobia: preliminary results of an internet survey. Depress Anxiety. 2001;14(2):149–52.
71. Boschen MJ. Reconceptualizing emetophobia: a cognitive-behavioral formulation and research agenda. J Anxiety Disord. 2007;21(3):407–19. doi:10.1016/j.janxdis.2006.06.007.
72. Faye AD, Gawande S, Tadke R, Kirpekar VC, Bhave SH. Emetophobia: a fear of vomiting. Indian J Psychiatry. 2013;55(4):390–2. doi:10.4103/0019-5545.120556.
73. Shifren JL, Monz BU, Russo PA, Segreti A, Johannes CB. Sexual problems and distress in United States women: prevalence and correlates. Obstet Gynecol. 2008;112(5):970–8. doi:10.1097/AOG.0b013e3181898cdb.
74. Green SM, Haber E, McCabe RE, Soares CN. Cognitive-behavioral group treatment for menopausal symptoms: a pilot study. Arch Womens Ment Health. 2013;16(4):325–32. doi:10.1007/s00737-013-0339-x.
75. Simon JA. Identifying and treating sexual dysfunction in postmenopausal women: the role of estrogen. J Womens Health (Larchmt). 2011;20(10):1453–65. doi:10.1089/jwh.2010.2151.
76. Krapf JM, Belkin Z, Dreher F, Goldstein AT. Current and emerging treatment options for vulvovaginal atrophy. In: Farage MA, Miller KW, Woods NF, Maibach HI, editors. Skin, mucosa and menopause. Heidelberg: Springer; 2015. p. 229–35.
77. Bober SL, Varela VS. Sexuality in adult cancer survivors: challenges and intervention. J Clin Oncol. 2012;30(30):3712–9. doi:10.1200/JCO.2012.41.7915.
78. Parish SJ, Rubio-Aurioles E. Education in sexual medicine: proceedings from the international consultation in sexual medicine, 2009. J Sex Med. 2010;7(10):3305–14. doi:10.1111/j.1743-6109.2010.02026.x.
79. Graziottin A, Leiblum SR. Biological and psychosocial pathophysiology of female sexual dysfunction during the menopausal transition. J Sex Med. 2005;2 Suppl 3:133–45. doi:10.1111/j.1743-6109.2005.00129.x.
80. Rosen R, Brown C, Heiman J, Leiblum S, Meston C, Shabsigh R, et al. The Female Sexual Function Index (FSFI): a multidimensional self-report instrument for the assessment of female sexual function. J Sex Marital Ther. 2000;26(2):191–208. doi:10.1080/009262300278597.
81. Greene JG. A factor analytic study of climacteric symptoms. J Psychosom Res. 1976;20:425–30.

82. Ameratunga D, Goldin J, Hickey M. Sleep disturbance in menopause. Intern Med J. 2012;42(7):742–7. doi:10.1111/j.1445-5994.2012.02723.x.

83. Joffe H, Massler A, Sharkey KM. Evaluation and management of sleep disturbance during the menopause transition. Semin Reprod Med. 2010;28(5):404–21. doi:10.1055/s-0030-1262900.

84. Hunter MS, Liao KL. Determinants of treatment choice for menopausal hot flushes: hormonal versus psychological versus no treatment. J Psychosom Obstet Gynaecol. 1995;16(2):101–8.

85. Vélez Toral M, Godoy-Izquierdo D, Padial García A, Lara Moreno R, Mendoza Ladrón de Guevara N, Salamanca Ballesteros A, et al. Psychosocial interventions in perimenopausal and postmenopausal women: a systematic review of randomised and non-randomised trials and non-controlled studies. Maturitas. 2014;77(2):93–110. doi:10.1016/j.maturitas.2013.10.020.

86. Becker AE. Outpatient management of eating disorders in adults. Curr Womens Health Rep. 2003;3(3):221–9.

87. Horowitz JA, Goodman JH. Identifying and treating postpartum depression. J Obstet Gynecol Neonatal Nurs. 2005;34(2):264–73. doi:10.1177/0884217505274583.

88. Lagrew Jr DC, Jenkins TR. The future of obstetrics/gynecology in 2020: a clearer vision—finding true north and the forces of change. Am J Obstet Gynecol. 2014;211(6):617–22.e1. doi:10.1016/j.ajog.2014.08.021.

89. Lemmens GMD, Vervaeke M, Enzlin P, Bakelants E, Vanderschueren D, D'Hooghe T, Demyttenaere K. Coping with infertility: a body-mind group intervention programme for infertile couples. Hum Reprod. 2004;19(8):1917–23. doi:10.1093/humrep/deh323.

90. Psaros C, Freeman M, Safren SA, Barsky M, Cohen LS. Discontinuation of antidepressants during attempts to conceive: a pilot trial of cognitive behavioral therapy for the prevention of recurrent depression. J Clin Psychopharmacol. 2014;34(4):455–60. doi:10.1097/JCP.0000000000000158.

91. Frederiksen Y, Farver-Vestergaard I, Skovgård NG, Ingerslev HJ, Zachariae R. Efficacy of psychosocial interventions for psychological and pregnancy outcomes in infertile women and men: a systematic review and meta-analysis. BMJ Open. 2015;5(1), e006592. doi:10.1136/bmjopen-2014-006592.

92. Boivin J. A review of psychosocial interventions in infertility. Soc Sci Med. 2003;57(12):2325–41.

93. Wischmann T. Implications of psychosocial support in infertility—a critical appraisal. J Psychosom Obstet Gynaecol. 2008;29(2):83–90. doi:10.1080/01674820701817870.

94. Miniati M, Callari A, Calugi S, Rucci P, Savino M, Mauri M, Dell'Osso L. Interpersonal psychotherapy for postpartum depression: a systematic review. Arch Womens Ment Health. 2014;17(4):257–68. doi:10.1007/s00737-014-0442-7.

95. Armstrong KL, Fraser JA, Dadds MR, Morris J. A randomized, controlled trial of nurse home visiting to vulnerable families with newborns. J Paediatr Child Health. 1999;35(3):237–44.

96. Fraser JA, Armstrong KL, Morris JP, Dadds MR. Home visiting intervention for vulnerable families with newborns: follow-up results of a randomized controlled trial. Child Abuse Negl. 2000;24(11):1399–429.

97. MacArthur C, Winter HR, Bick DE, Knowles H, Lilford R, Henderson C, et al. Effects of redesigned community postnatal care on womens' health 4 months after birth: a cluster randomised controlled trial. Lancet. 2002;359(9304):378–85.

98. Goodman JH, Santangelo G. Group treatment for postpartum depression: a systematic review. Arch Womens Ment Health. 2011;14(4):277–93. doi:10.1007/s00737-011-0225-3.

99. Clark R, Tluczek A, Wenzel A. Psychotherapy for postpartum depression: a preliminary report. Am J Orthopsychiatry. 2003;73(4):441–54. doi:10.1037/0002-9432.73.4.441.

100. Dennis C-L, Dowswell T. Psychosocial and psychological interventions for preventing postpartum depression. Cochrane Database Syst Rev. 2013;2, CD001134. doi:10.1002/14651858.CD001134.pub3.

101. Sockol LE. A systematic review of the efficacy of cognitive behavioral therapy for treating and preventing perinatal depression. J Affect Disord. 2015;177:7–21. doi:10.1016/j.jad.2015.01.052.

102. Arch JJ, Dimidjian S, Chessick C. Are exposure-based cognitive behavioral therapies safe during pregnancy? Arch Womens Ment Health. 2012;15(6):445–57. doi:10.1007/s00737-012-0308-9.

103. Bánhidy F, Acs N, Puhó E, Czeizel AE. Association between maternal panic disorders and pregnancy complications and delivery outcomes. Eur J Obstet Gynecol Reprod Biol. 2006;124(1):47–52. doi:10.1016/j.ejogrb.2005.04.013.

104. Chen Y-H, Lin H-C, Lee H-C. Pregnancy outcomes among women with panic disorder—do panic attacks during pregnancy matter? J Affect Disord. 2010;120(1–3):258–62. doi:10.1016/j.jad.2009.04.025.

105. Morland L, Goebert D, Onoye J, Frattarelli L, Derauf C, Herbst M, et al. Posttraumatic stress disorder and pregnancy health: preliminary update and implications. Psychosomatics. 2007;48(4):304–8. doi:10.1176/appi.psy.48.4.304.

106. Stein MB, Roy-Burne PP, Hermann R. Obsessive-compulsive disorder in pregnant and postpartum women. UpToDate. 2014. http://www.uptodate.com/contents/obsessive-compulsive-disorder-in-pregnant-and-postpartum-women#H15.

107. Vythilingum B. Anxiety disorders in pregnancy. Curr Psychiatry Rep. 2008;10(4):331–5.

108. Maternal OCD. What is obsessive compulsive disorder? (n.d.). http://www.maternalocd.org/aboutocd.php.

109. Abramowitz JS, Schwartz SA, Moore KM. Obsessional thoughts in postpartum females and their partners: content, severity, and relationship with depression. J Clin Psychol Med Settings. 2003;10(3):157–64. doi:10.1023/A:1025454627242.

110. Fairbrother N, Abramowitz JS. New parenthood as a risk factor for the development of obsessional problems. Behav Res Ther. 2007;45(9):2155–63. doi:10.1016/j.brat.2006.09.019.

111. Challacombe FL, Salkovskis PM. Intensive cognitive-behavioural treatment for women with postnatal obsessive-compulsive disorder: a consecutive case series. Behav Res Ther. 2011;49(6–7):422–6. doi:10.1016/j.brat.2011.03.006.

112. Abramowitz JS, Schwartz SA, Moore KM, Luenzmann KR. Obsessive-compulsive symptoms in pregnancy and the puerperium: a review of the literature. J Anxiety Disord. 2003;17(4):461–78.

113. Speisman BB, Storch EA, Abramowitz JS. Postpartum obsessive-compulsive disorder. J Obstet Gynecol Neonat Nurs. 2011;40(6):680–90. doi:10.1111/j.1552-6909.2011.01294.x.

114. Timpano KR, Abramowitz JS, Mahaffey BL, Mitchell MA, Schmidt NB. Efficacy of a prevention program for postpartum obsessive-compulsive symptoms. J Psychiatr Res. 2011;45(11):1511–7. doi:10.1016/j.jpsychires.2011.06.015.

115. Christian LM, Storch EA. Cognitive behavioral treatment of postpartum onset obsessive compulsive disorder with aggressive obsessions. Clin Case Stud. 2009;8(1):72–83. doi:10.1177/1534650108326974.

116. Allen LA, Dobkin RD, Boohar EM, Woolfolk RL. Cognitive behavior therapy for menopausal hot flashes: two case reports. Maturitas. 2006;54(1):95–9. doi:10.1016/j.maturitas.2005.12.006.

117. Ayers B, Smith M, Hellier J, Mann E, Hunter MS. Effectiveness of group and self-help cognitive behavior therapy in reducing problematic menopausal hot flushes and night sweats (MENOS 2): a randomized controlled trial. Menopause. 2012;19(7):749–59. doi:10.1097/gme.0b013e31823fe835.

118. Keefer L, Blanchard EB. A behavioral group treatment program for menopausal hot flashes: results of a pilot study. Appl Psychophysiol Biofeedback. 2005;30(1):21–30.

119. Brandon AR, Minhajuddin A, Thase ME, Jarrett RB. Impact of reproductive status and age on response of depressed women to cognitive therapy. J Womens Health (Larchmt). 2013;22(1):58–66. doi:10.1089/jwh.2011.3427.

120. Khoshbooii R, Hassan S, Hamzah M, Baba M. Effectiveness of a group cognitive behavioral therapy on depression among Iranian women around menopause. Aust J Basic Appl Sci. 2011;5(11):991–5.
121. Green S, McCabe R, Soares C. The cognitive behavioral workbook for menopause: a step-by-step program for overcoming hot flashes, mood swings, insomnia, anxiety, depression, and other symptoms. Oakland: New Harbinger; 2012.
122. Fava GA, Rafanelli C, Grandi S, Canestrari R, Morphy MA. Six-year outcome for cognitive behavioral treatment of residual symptoms in major depression. Am J Psychiatry. 1998;155(10):1443–5. doi:10.1176/ajp.155.10.1443.
123. Fava GA, Rafanelli C, Grandi S, Conti S, Belluardo P. Prevention of recurrent depression with cognitive behavioral therapy: preliminary findings. Arch Gen Psychiatry. 1998;55(9):816–20.
124. Fava GA, Ruini C, Rafanelli C, Grandi S. Cognitive behavior approach to loss of clinical effect during long-term antidepressant treatment: a pilot study. Am J Psychiatry. 2002;159(12):2094–5.
125. Jarrett RB, Kraft D, Doyle J, Foster BM, Eaves GG, Silver PC. Preventing recurrent depression using cognitive therapy with and without a continuation phase: a randomized clinical trial. Arch Gen Psychiatry. 2001;58(4):381–8.
126. Ma SH, Teasdale JD. Mindfulness-based cognitive therapy for depression: replication and exploration of differential relapse prevention effects. J Consult Clin Psychol. 2004;72(1):31–40. doi:10.1037/0022-006X.72.1.31.
127. Paykel ES, Scott J, Teasdale JD, Johnson AL, Garland A, Moore R, et al. Prevention of relapse in residual depression by cognitive therapy: a controlled trial. Arch Gen Psychiatry. 1999;56(9):829–35.
128. Newton CR, Sherrard W, Glavac I. The fertility problem inventory: measuring perceived infertility-related stress. Fertil Steril. 1999;72(1):54–62.
129. Hutti MH, Armstrong DS, Myers J. Evaluation of the perinatal grief intensity scale in the subsequent pregnancy after perinatal loss. J Obstet Gynecol Neonat Nurs. 2013;42(6):697–706. doi:10.1111/1552-6909.12249.
130. Somerville S, Dedman K, Hagan R, Oxnam E, Wettinger M, Byrne S, et al. The perinatal anxiety screening scale: development and preliminary validation. Arch Womens Ment Health. 2014;17(5):443–54. doi:10.1007/s00737-014-0425-8.
131. Huizink AC, Delforterie MJ, Scheinin NM, Tolvanen M, Karlsson L, Karlsson H. Adaption of pregnancy anxiety questionnaire-revised for all pregnant women regardless of parity: PRAQ-R2. Arch Womens Ment Health 2015. doi:10.1007/s00737-015-0531-2.
132. Lord C, Rieder A, Hall GBC, Soares CN, Steiner M. Piloting the perinatal obsessive-compulsive scale (POCS): development and validation. J Anxiety Disord. 2011;25(8):1079–84. doi:10.1016/j.janxdis.2011.07.005.
133. Cox JL, Holden JM, Sagovsky R. Detection of postnatal depression. Development of the 10-item Edinburgh postnatal depression scale. Br J Psychiatry. 1987;150:782–6.
134. Kernot J, Olds T, Lewis LK, Maher C. Test-retest reliability of the English version of the Edinburgh postnatal depression scale. Arch Womens Ment Health. 2015;18(2):255–7. doi:10.1007/s00737-014-0461-4.
135. Kozinszky Z, Dudas RB. Validation studies of the Edinburgh postnatal depression scale for the antenatal period. J Affect Disord. 2015;176:95–105. doi:10.1016/j.jad.2015.01.044.
136. Greene JG. Constructing a standard climacteric scale. Maturitas. 1998;29(1):25–31.
137. Massachusetts General Hospital. Menopause decision quality worksheet v2.0. 2014. http://www.massgeneral.org/decisionsciences/assets/pdfs/Menopause_DQI_SV.pdf.
138. Psaros C, Kagan L, Shifren JL, Willett J, Jacquart J, Alert MD, et al. Mind-body group treatment for women coping with infertility: a pilot study. J Psychosom Obstet Gynaecol. 2015;36(2):75–83. doi:10.3109/0167482X.2014.989983.

Resources

Domar A. Conquering infertility. New York: Penguin Group; 2002.
Endocrine Society. Hormone Health Network. 2015. http://www.hormone.org/.
Massachusetts General Hospital. MGH Center for Women's Mental Health. 2013. http://womensmentalhealth.org/.
The National Infertility Association. 2015. http://www.resolve.org/.
The North American Menopause Society. 2015. http://www.menopause.org/.

Abbreviations

ASD	Acute Stress Disorder
CBT	Cognitive Behavioral Therapy
GAD	Generalized Anxiety Disorder
IPT	Interpersonal Psychotherapy
MDD	Major Depressive Disorder
OCD	Obsessive Compulsive Disorder
PPD	Postpartum Depression
PTSD	Post-Traumatic Stress Disorder
SSRIs	Selective Serotonin Reuptake Inhibitors
TCAs	Tricyclic Antidepressants

Chapter 13
Early Palliative Care for Patients with Advanced Cancer

Joseph A. Greer, Vicki A. Jackson, Juliet C. Jacobsen, William F. Pirl, and Jennifer S. Temel

13.1 Early Palliative Care for Patients with Advanced Cancer

Cancer is among the leading cause of morbidity and mortality in the USA, with nearly 590,000 Americans expected to die from the disease in 2015 [1]. Patients diagnosed with advanced cancers and their families are confronted with myriad challenges due to high symptom burden, loss of functioning, role transitions, poor prognosis, and difficult treatment decisions, especially toward the end of life. Although cancer care for patients with advanced malignancies has improved in recent decades due to the development of targeted therapeutics, interventions aimed at effective symptom management and quality of life in this population have lagged far behind [2, 3]. In the last decade, however, a novel model of care has emerged with a growing evidence base that supports the delivery of palliative care services early in the course of oncology treatment for advanced cancer [4]. Studies show that patients with advanced cancer who receive palliative care services simultaneously with their oncology care are more likely to report improved quality of life, mood, prognostic awareness, and end-of-life (EOL) care compared to those who do not receive such services [5]. Given these positive results, national professional organizations such as the American Society of Clinical Oncology have recommended consideration of referral to palliative care early in the course of disease for patients diagnosed with metastatic cancer and for those with a high symptom burden [6].

J.A. Greer, Ph.D. (✉)
Center for Psychiatric Oncology & Behavioral Sciences, Massachusetts General Hospital Cancer Center, Yawkey Suite 10B, 55 Fruit Street, Boston, MA 02114, USA
e-mail: jgreer2@mgh.harvard.edu

V.A. Jackson • J.C. Jacobsen • W.F. Pirl • J.S. Temel
Massachusetts General Hospital Cancer Center, Harvard Medical School,
55 Fruit Street, Boston, MA 02114, USA

© Springer Science+Business Media New York 2017
A.-M. Vranceanu et al. (eds.), *The Massachusetts General Hospital Handbook of Behavioral Medicine*, Current Clinical Psychiatry,
DOI 10.1007/978-3-319-29294-6_13

13.1.1 What Is Early Palliative Care?

Palliative care is a specialty-trained medical discipline that focuses on enhancing quality of life, symptom management, coping, treatment decision-making as well as psychosocial and spiritual support for patients with serious illnesses and their caregivers [7]. Often consisting of physicians, nurses, social workers, and chaplains, the multidisciplinary palliative care team aims to help patients with medical illness live as well as possible for as long as possible [8]. Historically, patients and families have received such services late in the course of disease within the inpatient setting as consultations for acute, uncontrolled symptoms or for planning end-of-life care. In contrast, the simultaneous delivery of palliative and standard oncology care in the outpatient setting includes features of clinical practice that are distinct from inpatient palliative care. The focus of care is on enhancing quality of life and adapting to serious illness throughout the disease trajectory for patients and their families, regardless of whether the patient has curable or terminal disease [9]. In this chapter, we describe palliative care services that are fully integrated within the outpatient oncology clinic, allowing for seamless comanagement of patient symptoms, psychosocial concerns, and treatment decisions.

13.1.2 What Is the Purpose of Early Palliative Care?

Given their multidisciplinary, team-based approach and primary aim to improve quality of life, palliative care clinicians are well suited to work collaboratively with oncologists to address the unmet needs of patients with advanced cancer. The demands on oncologists are quite high, as they must attend to the determination of diagnosis, continuous assessment of disease changes, evaluation of clinical trial eligibility, administration of cancer therapies, and monitoring of side effects and toxicities. Thus, a collaborative team approach is maximally beneficial. Specifically, the role of palliative care clinicians in the outpatient oncology setting is to provide assistance with symptoms, coping, psychosocial and spiritual support, as well as illness understanding and treatment decisions for patients, their families, and other healthcare providers [10].

Patients with a diagnosis of advanced cancer often present with variable symptoms such as pain, loss of appetite, weight loss, fatigue, breathlessness, and at times neurologic problems, though these vary by cancer type [11, 12]. In addition, side effects of cancer therapy often exacerbate these symptoms and may also cause nausea, vomiting, body disfigurement, neuropathy, and sleep disturbance, among others [13, 14]. Compounding these physical symptoms is the psychosocial, spiritual, and existential distress related to the diagnosis of advanced cancer, which in many cases is an incurable illness [15–17]. Patients must often make significant shifts in their life roles by taking time off from work and reducing home responsibilities while undergoing cancer treatment. Understandably, within this context, approximately one quarter to one third of patients with advanced cancers experience elevated anxiety and depression symptoms [18]. This burden is shared by family members who are also at increased risk of psychiatric morbidity, in part due to the stress of caregiving [19–22].

To help oncologists manage this medical complexity, palliative care clinicians identify and treat symptoms proactively as they emerge and worsen. In addition, palliative care clinicians bolster adaptive coping with illness, encouraging patients to remain engaged in meaningful life activities to the extent possible [23]. By alleviating symptom burden in real time and promoting effective coping strategies, the palliative care team not only helps improve quality of life for patients and families, but also may enhance patient capacity to adhere to difficult and often toxic cancer therapies.

In addition to managing debilitating symptoms, palliative care clinicians serve as key members of the cancer care team to help patients understand their illness and prognosis more accurately [24]. Such understanding is necessary in order for patients to make treatment decisions that are informed and aligned with their wishes. Although most patients with metastatic cancer and their family members report that they want timely and realistic prognostic information [25–27], the majority fails to understand the terminal nature of the disease and that the goal of cancer therapy is palliative rather than curative [28–30]. As a result, patients with poor prognostic awareness tend to overestimate their chances of survival. With inaccurate prognostic awareness, they are significantly more likely to pursue futile, aggressive cancer therapy at the end of life, with limited discussion of preferences for advance directives and hospice care [31, 32].

Conversations about prognosis and end-of-life care are undeniably challenging for patients and their families, as well as for oncologists [33, 34]. Palliative care clinicians play a key role in facilitating prognostic awareness over time by interpreting and conveying accurate illness information shared between patients and the oncology team. In the outpatient setting, palliative care clinicians also have the opportunity to establish long-standing therapeutic relationships with patients and families. Therefore, when the clinical need arises, palliative care clinicians are able to support the oncology team by drawing on this established trust with patients and families to have conversations about difficult topics such as advance care planning, termination of chemotherapy, and referral to hospice [35]. Studies show that patients who recall having such discussions with their doctors not only receive less aggressive care at the end of life, but also have earlier referral to hospice services and better quality of death [36, 37].

13.1.3   What Is the Evidence Base for Early Palliative Care?

Several prior scholarly reviews of palliative care interventions have shown mixed findings with respect to outcomes, which range from patient quality of life and symptom burden to satisfaction with care and resource utilization [38–40].

These reviews highlight the difficulty of conducting palliative care research and making firm conclusions about the evidence base given methodological weaknesses of studies to date as well as the diversity of patients, interventions, care settings, and treatment targets. However, in the last decade, researchers of early palliative care models have greatly improved the scientific rigor of intervention studies, generally observing a number of positive outcomes for patients with advanced cancer and their families [41]. Specifically, three separate groups of researchers have been testing the efficacy of early palliative care including the work of Dr. Bakitas [42–44], Dr. Zimmermann [45], and our group led by Dr. Temel [46, 47]. All three groups have taken a systematic approach to intervention development and testing, starting with feasibility pilot studies and then conducting larger randomized controlled trials of early palliative care models [48].

Bakitas and colleagues have conducted a series of trials called Project ENABLE (Educate, Nurture, Advise, Before Life Ends) primarily in New Hampshire and Vermont. The early palliative care intervention in Project ENABLE entails a multicomponent, psychoeducational counseling intervention delivered by advanced practice nurses over the telephone. Prior pilot investigation demonstrated that the approach was feasible and acceptable to patients [42]. A subsequent randomized controlled trial of the intervention versus standard care in a largely rural sample of patients ($N=322$) with mixed, newly diagnosed advanced cancers showed improvement in quality of life, with marginal findings for symptom intensity-and patient survival [43]. A more recent follow-up randomized trial ($N=207$) of the same model comparing early palliative care (soon after diagnosis of advanced cancer) versus delayed palliative care (after 3 months) showed no significant effects on patient quality of life, mood, symptom impact, or resource utilization. However, the investigators did observe significantly lower depression scores in family caregivers and higher rates of 1-year survival in the early versus delayed palliative care group [44, 49].

Zimmermann and colleagues recently published the largest trial to date of early palliative care for patients diagnosed with mixed, poor-prognosis advanced cancers ($N=461$) in Toronto, Canada [45]. For this intervention study, participants were randomly assigned either to receive standard care or to meet in person with the palliative care team at least monthly for approximately 4 months. Findings from this trial showed that, compared to those who received standard care, patients in the intervention group reported greater satisfaction with care and had a trend toward improved quality of life at the primary end point (3 months), which became significant at 4 months along with reduced symptom burden [45].

Finally, Dr. Temel and colleagues at Massachusetts General Hospital Cancer Center in Boston, MA have conducted a series of trials examining the feasibility and efficacy of a fully embedded, comanagement model of early palliative care for patients with metastatic non-small cell lung cancer (NSCLC) [46, 47]. Specifically, to test this approach, 151 patients with metastatic NSCLC were randomly assigned to receive at least monthly consultations with a palliative care specialist in addition to standard oncology care from the time of diagnosis until death versus standard oncology care alone. Compared to the control group, patients who received early, integrated palliative care experienced improved quality of life, lower rates of depression, more accurate prognostic awareness, and higher quality care at the end of life [28, 47, 50]. In addition, post hoc analyses showed a survival advantage for those who received early palliative care versus standard care alone. Given these promising findings, we are currently completing a larger randomized trial of this same model of early palliative care in 350 patients with metastatic lung and gastro-intestinal cancers.

Taken together, the clinical trials from three independent research groups demonstrate that early palliative care positively impacts a number of key outcomes including patient-reported quality of life and mood as well as end-of-life care and perhaps even survival, though the latter requires prospective study and confirmation.

13.1.4   What Are the Intervention Components of Early Palliative Care?

The integration of palliative and oncology care in the outpatient setting includes features of clinical practice that expand upon, and at times differ from, the traditional model of inpatient palliative care [51]. In this section, we describe six domains of early palliative care:

- Developing and maintaining the *therapeutic relationship* with patients and caregivers
- Assessing and treating *patient symptoms*
- Promoting and reinforcing adaptive *coping with advanced cancer* in patients and caregivers
- Assessing and enhancing *prognostic awareness and illness understanding* in patients and caregivers
- Assisting with *treatment decision-making*
- Planning for *end-of-life care*

Although palliative care clinicians may focus on the above content domains across multiple clinical visits or address several of these domains within a single consultation, we will present the information according to the targets of palliative care that occur most prominently during the following time frames: (1) initially at the time of cancer diagnosis; (2) throughout the entire course of disease; (3) at clinical turning points (e.g., changing to a new regimen of chemotherapy or after being discharged from the hospital); and (4) upon the conclusion of cancer treatment and/ or transition to hospice services [52]. See Table 13.1.

Table 13.1 Summary of components of early palliative care (PC)

Content domain	Point of care	Interventions
Therapeutic relationship	Emphasis during initial visits	• Conduct joint visit with patient, family, oncologist, and PC clinician, if possible
		• Demystify role of PC and emphasize quality of life goal
		• Assess history including values, life goals, and experiences of patient and family
		• Outline parameters of communication and provide reassurance for patient and family
Patient symptoms	Throughout all visits	• Educate patient and family about symptom trajectories and methods of treatment
		• Collaborate closely with oncologist to work within preferred practice patterns for symptom management
		• Order medications and procedures as clinically indicated
		• Refer to specialty care as clinically indicated
Coping with advanced cancer	Throughout all visits	• Assess and encourage diverse coping strategies, such as:
		– Behavioral approaches
		– Cognitive approaches
		– Acceptance and living with illness
		– Spiritual approaches
		– Social support
		– Life review
		• Assess and bolster caregiver coping
Prognostic awareness & illness understanding	Emphasis during clinical turning points	• Consult with oncologist to develop clear and consistent understanding of prognosis before discussions with patient and family
		• Assess patient understanding of disease and future
		• Consider use of hypothetical questions about "imagining poorer health state"
		• Clarify and provide the type of information patient and family actually want to know
		• Witness and validate emotions of patients and families
		• Emphasize realistic hopes and quality of life goals

Treatment decision-making	Emphasis during clinical turning points	• Assess decision-making style of patient and family
		• Elicit treatment goals and values of patient and family
		• Collaborate closely with oncology team to assist patients with informed decision-making
		• Clarify questions about efficacy, risks and benefits, side effects, quality versus quantity of life concerns, and potential burdens related to cancer therapy
		• Support informed decision-making that is consistent with patient's goals and values while facilitating communication with family and oncology team
End-of-life (EOL) care	Emphasis at end of cancer therapy	• Discuss EOL care wishes incrementally over time, if possible
		• Clarify questions and preferences for advance care planning such as:
		– Selection of healthcare proxy
		– Determination and documentation of resuscitation preferences
		– Location of death and funeral planning
		• Discuss and facilitate transition to hospice services as clinically indicated
		• Provide ongoing resources, support, counseling, and referral for bereaved family members

13.2　Initial Outpatient Palliative Care Visits in the Oncology Setting

13.2.1　Key Domain: Therapeutic Relationship

Certainly, developing and maintaining the therapeutic relationship is essential across all palliative care visits throughout the course of disease. Nonetheless, the prominent focus of initial clinic visits soon after the diagnosis of advanced cancer in the outpatient setting is on building rapport and establishing trust between the palliative care clinician and patient [52].

Given that many patients and families have limited understanding or misconceptions of palliative care, thoughtful introduction of the service is vital for establishing trust and rapport. Specifically, in the context of a new diagnosis of advanced cancer for patients, a referral to outpatient palliative care works best if the oncologist either personally introduces the palliative care clinician during a joint visit or at least discusses the value of the palliative care team and collaborative nature of treatment. The palliative care clinician often begins the first encounter by describing the service and exploring the patient's and caregiver's understanding of palliative care, ideally clarifying any misconceptions about the treatment. To help reduce potential resistance, the palliative care clinician may then emphasize the role of palliative care to help the patient and caregivers achieve the best possible quality of life through expert symptom management, support, and assistance with treatment decision-making. Finally, the palliative care clinician explains the nature of the service as a multidisciplinary team that is available to the patient and caregiver throughout the disease process. This conversation may also need to differentiate the role of palliative care from hospice.

Another key feature of building rapport includes the palliative care clinician learning about the values, life goals, and experiences of patients and their caregivers both prior to and after the cancer diagnosis. The palliative care clinician accomplishes this by first asking about the patient's life experiences outside the context of cancer and then how life has changed since the diagnosis. For example, eliciting information about the patient's work, family, hobbies/interests, social network, spiritual or religious involvement, etc. helps affirm for the patient that he or she has a broader, richer life outside of cancer treatment that is acknowledged and valued by the palliative care clinician. This history taking may occur over multiple visits, during which the palliative care clinician can assess the patient's and caregiver's current wishes, priorities, emotions, and lifestyle changes that have resulted from the diagnosis and treatment of cancer. In these discussions, the palliative care clinician emphasizes that the goal of care is to help the patient to live as well as possible for as long as possible while also supporting caregivers.

Because conversations about the impact of advanced cancer are often difficult, palliative care clinicians foster a trusting alliance with patients and caregivers by outlining the parameters of communication and providing reassurance. For example, palliative care clinicians facilitate trust by clarifying and validating what the patient wishes and does not wish to discuss; encouraging the patient to disclose symptoms and other concerns; and reassuring the patient and caregiver that discussions about end-of-life care or other medical decisions will be raised when necessary. Clinicians also partner with patients and their families by normalizing fears and other feelings associated with the disease while providing support in coping with future uncertainty.

13.3   Outpatient Palliative Care Visits Throughout the Entire Course of Disease

13.3.1   Key Domain: Patient Symptoms

Symptom management is a prominent focus of all palliative care visits from the initial encounter and throughout the course of disease [52]. Assessing and treating symptoms to enhance quality of life is one of the fundamental ways that palliative care clinicians establish trust and credibility with patients and caregivers. In this way, palliative care clinicians demonstrate the collaborative nature of integrated palliative and oncology care. Moreover, through effective symptom management, the palliative care clinicians help patients realize that they can live more fully, even while having advanced cancer.

Patients and families often have concerns about how cancer symptoms change over time and treatment side effects. Palliative care clinicians in the outpatient setting help to forecast and clarify the likely symptoms patients will experience, while offering reassurance about the methods for treating such symptoms as they occur [53]. At every clinic visit, the palliative care clinician conducts a review of systems to elicit existing and new symptom concerns, especially as related to disease and treatment side effects. The common symptoms patients with advanced cancer report in the outpatient setting include pain, dyspnea/cough, fatigue, gastrointestinal symptoms, neurologic symptoms, edema, mood/emotional symptoms, sleep-related symptoms, issues of sexuality, and other symptoms related to pre-existing or comorbid conditions. Drawing upon their expert training and skill in medical management of complex symptom clusters, palliative care clinicians may prescribe opioids, non-opioid analgesics, antiemetic agents, and psychotropic medications, among others.

When working closely with the oncologist, the palliative care clinician will need to maintain ongoing, effective communication with the treatment team to define this mutual collaboration and work within the preferred practice patterns of the oncology team. Specifically, some oncology clinicians may want to take a more or less active role in managing symptoms, and the palliative care clinician will need to adjust his or her role accordingly. Thus, palliative care clinicians provide an extra layer of support for both the oncology team and patient. Although palliative care clinicians possess expertise to assess and treat severe and poorly controlled symptoms, they also emphasize the team approach to comprehensive cancer care by referring to specialty care, mental health (e.g., psychiatry, psychology, social work), integrative medicine (e.g., acupuncture, massage, art therapy), and spiritual support (e.g., chaplaincy) as needed.

13.3.2 Key Domain: Coping with Advanced Cancer

As with symptom management, palliative care clinicians in the outpatient setting continuously assess how patients and caregivers are coping with advanced cancer across clinic visits throughout the course of disease [52]. The provision of early palliative care affords the opportunity and time for counseling patients and caregivers to enhance adjustment and coping with the many existential and lifestyle changes that occur as a result of cancer and its treatment. In particular, the aim is to help patients maintain hope and engagement with life activities to the extent that is possible, despite expected decrements in functioning over time [53].

Palliative care clinicians value and recognize that patients and caregivers bring their own expertise in coping to the current circumstance based on how they have managed difficulties and crises in the past. Thus, the palliative care clinician often begins the discussion of coping by asking patients and caregivers what strategies (e.g., calling upon social support, seeking counseling, increasing self-care activities) they have used to adjust to other life transitions or losses. During this conversation, the palliative care clinician strives to highlight and reinforce all adaptive forms of coping, while also assessing for potentially harmful behaviors (e.g., substance use, social withdrawal). While it is natural in times of crisis to doubt one's capacity to cope, the palliative care clinician communicates to patients and caregivers that they have the strength and abilities to meet their imminent challenges by highlighting successful prior coping efforts. Moreover, by emphasizing the partnership with the treatment team, the palliative care clinician reinforces that patients and caregivers are not alone as they navigate the many treatments, scans, symptoms, and uncertainties related to advanced cancer.

After assessing and validating patients' prior coping efforts, palliative care clinicians may also introduce various strategies to broaden coping resources and improve adjustment and meaning in life depending on the specific needs and interests of patients and their families [23]. For example, the following topics may be explored:

- Behavioral approaches: Specifically, palliative care clinicians may employ evidence-based techniques for stress reduction (e.g., breathing, meditation, and relaxation exercises); behavioral activation (remaining engaged with important activities and sustaining normal life as much as possible even with the disease); sleep hygiene; exercise; and activity pacing as needed due to pain, fatigue, or other symptoms.
- Cognitive approaches: Palliative care clinicians also support the use of diverse cognitive interventions to bolster coping, often brainstorming with patients about ways to generate moments of optimism, gratitude, joy, and being in the "flow." Alternatively, for instances when patients become overwhelmed, simple distraction and practical problem-solving skills may be helpful tools. A noteworthy advantage of cognitive interventions is that patients can often engage with these strategies regardless of health status and level of physical disability.
- Accepting and living with illness: Palliative care clinicians help patients and caregivers understand that accepting and living with illness has cognitive,

emotional, and behavioral elements. For example, although patients may more or less intellectually understand their prognosis and course of disease, they often experience difficulty in emotionally processing this information. By offering a safe venue for patients and caregivers to ask questions about the disease, clarify uncertainties, and experience the related affect, palliative care clinicians facilitate cognitive and emotional acceptance of illness. Also, palliative care clinicians help patients and caregivers live with the illness by defining the parameters of what is in their control, acknowledging the limitations due to disease, and maintaining hope for achieving valued quality of life goals.

- Spiritual approaches: Palliative care clinicians assess the role that spirituality plays in a patient's life in a respectful and nonjudgmental manner and with a broad perspective to incorporate multiple meanings of spirituality (such as religious affiliation and participation in community of faith, personal spiritual beliefs and practices, cultural traditions, etc.). Involvement of chaplaincy as part of the palliative care team is common.
- Social support: Palliative care clinicians help patients and caregivers define the different forms of social support they need, such as informational, instrumental, or emotional support. For example, they work with patients to determine which individuals are able to assist with functional tasks such as making meals, transportation to appointments, and going shopping, as well as those who are available to listen and offer emotional support for discussing the experience of life-limiting cancer. Also, the palliative care clinician works with patients and families to identify and problem-solve any gaps in soliciting needed support.
- Life review: Although not all patients will have the interest or capacity to reflect on their life experiences in a meaningful way, some will appreciate the process of life review as a form of existential coping. Specifically, as patients approach the end of life, some seek to take time to reflect on their life story and experiences, consider their legacy, and explore how they want to spend their remaining time. Such life review work might also include specific activities such as writing letters to loved ones, completing unfinished tasks, reconciling relationships with family and friends, and completing a creative or artistic project (e.g., scrapbook, personal history record) as a representation of who the patient is and expression of love for others.

Finally, research shows that patient distress is highly related to caregiver distress and vice versa [19, 20]. In the outpatient setting, palliative care clinicians have the rare opportunity to fortify caregiver coping by conducting ongoing assessments of burden, enhancing communication between patients and loved ones, and providing recommendations for additional support or referral. The palliative care clinician calls upon other members of the supportive care team as needed for patients and caregivers who may be experiencing complicated or severe distress. Referrals to social work, psychology, psychiatry, and pastoral care may be useful depending on the specific presenting circumstances and concerns.

13.4 Outpatient Palliative Care Visits During Clinical Turning Points

13.4.1 Key Domain: Prognostic Awareness and Illness Understanding

During clinical turning points in the patient's illness trajectory, such as starting a new chemotherapy regimen or after a hospitalization, palliative care clinicians often have discussions about illness understanding and treatment decision-making [52]. A notable benefit of the longer relationship that palliative care clinicians develop in the outpatient setting is that the assessment and discussion of prognosis and illness understanding are not a single event, but rather occur over multiple visits.

Before engaging in detailed communication with patients and families about the likely course of disease, palliative care clinicians must first consult with the primary oncologist to ensure they have an accurate assessment of a patient's prognosis. When possible, joint clinic visits between oncology and palliative care will reinforce the team approach to care and ensure clear and effective communication with patients and caregivers, especially about prognosis.

Palliative care clinicians recognize that patient and caregiver illness understanding often vacillates between more and less realistic expectations, which can be confusing for the medical team. Over time, palliative care clinicians can work with patients to decrease this vacillation and improve prognostic awareness [35]. Specifically, palliative care clinicians first assess prognostic awareness by asking patients and caregivers in an open-ended manner about their understanding of the disease and their future. Patients' responses provide some clarity not only about their level of awareness but also their ability to tolerate discussions regarding prognosis [54, 55]. For those who struggle to have these conversations, it may be helpful to align with patients by hoping for best possible outcome while also framing questions with the hypothetical of "preparing for or imagining a poorer health state" [56]. Additionally, palliative care clinicians attempt to clarify the type of information patients and caregivers want to know, such as expected length of life, possible changes in disease and function, or what the dying process is like. The goal of these discussions is to offer patients an opportunity to talk about aspects of the prognosis at a time when the patient is clinically stable and not pressured by medical decision making.

As patients and caregivers begin to understand and integrate information about prognosis, they will often experience heightened affect such as disbelief, sadness, and anger. Rather than blocking or providing false reassurance, the palliative care clinician's role is to witness and validate these emotions with silence, an empathic touch, restatement of realistic hopes, and "I wish" statements (e.g., "It sounds like that was hard to hear. I wish I had better news") [57, 58]. The palliative care clinician can then use this moment as a starting point to discuss those aspects of care and the disease that can be controlled, emphasizing realistic hopes and quality of life goals (e.g., helping patient to feel well enough to spend valuable time with grandchildren).

13.4.2   Key Domain: Treatment Decision-Making

As noted earlier, although treatment decision-making can occur at any point along the illness trajectory for patients with advanced cancer, such discussions tend to occur more frequently during times of clinical transitions (e.g., when cancer is progressing, after a hospitalization, or when starting or stopping chemotherapy) [52]. The palliative care clinician first aims to elicit information from patients and caregivers regarding their decision-making style, quality versus quantity of life concerns, as well as goals and values for care. The purpose of this assessment is to determine the extent to which patient's preferences and values align with current or potential treatments.

Palliative care clinicians, in close collaboration with the oncology team, provide additional support for patients and caregivers to understand the efficacy, risks and benefits, side effects, and potential burdens associated with different forms of cancer treatment. To do this, palliative care clinicians elicit and emphasize patients' values and goals in making informed treatment decisions. Using their medical expertise, palliative care clinicians then help interpret how patients' goals and values align with the medical options. At multiple points during the course of cancer care, patients must discern whether to start, continue, or stop treatments in collaboration with their cancer care team, as well as decide the extent to which family caregivers are consulted about these decisions [59]. In this context, palliative care clinicians help clarify misunderstandings about treatment, support patient decision-making and freedom to change course, as well as facilitate communication with caregivers and members of the oncology team [53].

13.5   Final Outpatient Palliative Care Visits and Transition to Hospice Services

13.5.1   Key Domain: End-of-Life Care

Palliative care clinicians generally raise the discussion of EOL care incrementally over time and most prominently later in the course of illness, after having established a strong, trusting therapeutic relationship with patients and caregivers. Typically, the final palliative care visits in the outpatient setting focus not only on symptom management, illness understanding, and decisions about stopping cancer therapy but also on the last days of life [52]. Given the longer clinical relationship in the outpatient setting, palliative care clinicians have the opportunity to reduce patients' anxiety in discussing EOL care issues by having such conversations slowly over time. The primary topics for EOL care planning include discussions regarding selection of healthcare proxy, determination of resuscitation preferences, will/estate planning, hospice care, location of death, and funeral planning.

Most patients with advanced cancer will experience progressive decline in their functional status over time. Thus, they often require additional assistance from family and loved ones for personal care and communication of their values and wishes as they approach the end of life. This caregiving role can be both personally meaningful and stressful for family members and loved ones. The palliative care clinician works closely with patients and caregivers to determine the available resources for EOL care and whether it is appropriate for patients to receive their terminal care in the home or other hospice or inpatient settings. Palliative care clinicians can also serve as advocates for family caregivers in making plans for the will/estate and funeral. Palliative care clinicians recognize that their specialized care considers the family unit as the focus of treatment. As such, they continue to provide resources, support, counseling, and referral for bereavement in family caregivers after the patient has died.

13.6   Case Example: "Ruth"

To illustrate the components of early palliative care, we describe the case of Ruth, a 70-year-old woman diagnosed with metastatic lung cancer. Until her cancer diagnosis, Ruth was in generally good health, about to retire from her 40-year career in nursing. She was living alone, as her husband had died 5 years earlier. She otherwise maintained close relationships with her two adult daughters and sister who lived locally in the Boston area. Ruth had begun to have unremitting symptoms of cough and difficulty breathing which prompted her to consult with her primary care doctor. Initial chest X-ray and follow-up CT scan showed a lung mass, at which point the primary care clinician referred the patient to Dr. Temel, a thoracic oncologist, at the Massachusetts General Hospital Cancer Center. Soon after, the patient learned that she had metastatic lung cancer. Within a month of her diagnosis, she enrolled in our clinical trial of early palliative care and was randomly assigned to the intervention group.

Dr. Temel took the opportunity to introduce Ruth to Dr. Jackson from the palliative care team during one of their regularly scheduled oncology visits. They explained the purpose of palliative care and that the patient and Dr. Jackson would be meeting at least monthly throughout the course of treatment. Although Ruth was an experienced nurse, she was somewhat confused about the role palliative care within this context, as she primarily associated the term with hospice care. Dr. Jackson therefore explained the benefits of outpatient palliative care for improving symptoms, managing treatment side effects, and supporting adaptive coping with cancer from the time of diagnosis. For example, during this conversation, the patient and Dr. Jackson identified Ruth's recurrent cough and dyspnea as salient symptoms that were currently interfering with her quality of life. Drs. Temel and Jackson agreed to work together to manage these symptoms as effectively as possible to help Ruth continue to engage in the life activities that were important to her.

During the initial palliative care visits, Dr. Jackson continued to assess for symptoms such as cough and dyspnea, but also spent time getting to know Ruth personally, including her life interests, activities, and priorities. For example, now that Ruth was retiring, she had planned to spend more time with her daughters and grandchildren as well as enjoy her lifelong hobbies of choral singing and swimming on an adult master's team. Ruth also had a strong network of social support in close friends from work and her many activities, with whom she wanted to spend time in the city going to restaurants, museums, and shows. Unfortunately, since her cancer diagnosis, Ruth found herself becoming more isolated, at times avoiding physically demanding activities that made her breathlessness worse. Dr. Jackson encouraged the patient to continue to exercise when possible to prevent deconditioning while also educating her that the symptoms would likely improve some with cancer treatment. She also reassured Ruth that they could use opioid medication in the meantime, which has shown benefit for relieving breathlessness.

Over the course of cancer care, Ruth experienced a number of new symptoms, largely as a result of treatment. Specifically, she began to have chemotherapy-related neuropathy and increased fatigue. Moreover, although she had no significant history of mental health problems prior to her cancer diagnosis, she also noted heightened anxiety symptoms, especially in anticipation of cancer scans every few months. The anxiety only worsened her fatigue and breathlessness, again leading to avoidance of meaningful life activities and social engagements. She tended to interpret new symptoms through the lens of disease progression, which in turn exacerbated her worry about prognosis and limited life expectancy.

Dr. Jackson took a multidisciplinary approach to address the new symptom and anxiety concerns with Ruth. Specifically, in addition to prescribing medications to help with these symptoms, she referred Ruth to Dr. Greer, a clinical psychologist, for cognitive-behavioral therapy to treat the anxiety. Together, they emphasized the importance of using adaptive coping strategies with Ruth. First, the team helped to reframe Ruth's automatic interpretations of new symptoms and medical scan anxiety by considering alternative explanations, helping her to understand that side effects of treatment do not necessarily represent disease progression. They also worked with Ruth to help her scale and pace her physically demanding activities to be more consistent with her changing functional status. For example, rather than avoiding swimming altogether, Ruth was able to resume this activity by moving to a slower lane in the pool and taking breaks as needed. Such functional changes were understandably accompanied by feelings of loss, sadness, and grief, which Ruth also needed to process emotionally with both Drs. Jackson and Greer in their visits.

Ruth's prognostic awareness and illness understanding were generally accurate in that she understood that her cancer was not curable and that the goal of her treatment was to prevent the disease from growing for as long as possible. Nonetheless, early on in care, she was explicit with her oncologist, Dr. Temel, and her palliative care specialist, Dr. Jackson, about her preference not to know any statistics or time frames with respect to life expectancy. On occasion, Ruth had questions about the process and trajectory of getting sicker with metastatic cancer, such as how the team would manage her worsening breathless and any pain symptoms over time.

During these conversations, Drs. Jackson and Temel would offer support and reassure Ruth of their partnership in staying abreast of symptoms as they emerge, effectively treating them with pharmacological and behavioral approaches. Also, recognizing Ruth's expressed boundaries about discussing the end of life, Dr. Jackson told the patient and her family that she would let them know when they need to start having conversations about advance directives and the possibility of transitioning to hospice care. The benefit of their long-standing clinical relationship in the outpatient setting was that Ruth, her family, Dr. Jackson, and the oncology team could have these difficult conversations incrementally over time rather than during an acute medical crisis or hospitalization.

For approximately 2 years, Dr. Temel worked closely with Ruth to monitor changes in her disease status, assess for clinical trial eligibility, administer new chemotherapies as clinically indicated, as well as address any treatment toxicities. During this time, Ruth maintained a fairly high level quality of life, despite fluctuations in symptoms and side effects of treatment. She continued to swim and sing with her choral group, as well as enjoy her family and lifelong friendships. However, after undergoing four successive chemotherapy regimens, Ruth's cancer stopped responding to treatment, and she began to decline. Drs. Temel and Jackson decided it was time to have a family meeting and discuss the possibility of Ruth starting hospice services. During the family meeting, Ruth and her daughters were initially resistant to the idea of stopping chemotherapy and wanted to consider other treatment options. Drs. Temel and Jackson validated and empathized with the family's reaction, also expressing their wish to do more to stop the cancer if they could. However, they went on to explain how another regimen of chemotherapy may actually do more harm than good. They met with the family for over an hour, answering all questions and allowing time for everyone to express their thoughts, feelings, and fears about making this decision. Ruth expressed clearly her wish to die at home rather than at the hospital. After coming to agreement, Dr. Jackson then arranged the referral to have a nurse come to Ruth's home in the next day to discuss enrollment in home hospice services with the family.

Drs. Jackson, Temel, and Greer continued to follow up regularly with Ruth and her daughters after starting hospice services, at times in clinic, often over the telephone, and even in the home. As Ruth stopped the chemotherapy, the side effects subsided, and she started to feel a bit better for a while. She became increasingly reflective during these final months of life. Ruth spoke often of the meaningful relationships that mattered most to her, and she decided to write letters to loved ones expressing her appreciation. In addition, she made a recording of her choral singing and shared copies of the CD with her family and treatment team as part of her legacy. About 4 months into hospice care, Dr. Jackson was able to make a final visit to Ruth's home before she died. During this visit, they had the opportunity to express appreciation for the time they shared with one another over the past 2 and a half years. After Ruth's death, Dr. Jackson continued to offer support to Ruth's family, helping them coordinate funeral planning and offering referral for grief counseling services. Although the loss was poignant, the family was pleased that Ruth was able to die at home as she wished.

13.7   Conclusions

Early palliative care represents a novel model of delivering comprehensive cancer care that has a strong evidence base for improving multiple outcomes for patients with advanced cancer and their families. Patients with advanced cancer who receive this service from the time of diagnosis report improved quality of life, mood, prognostic awareness, and quality of care at the end of life compared to those who receive standard oncology care alone. Palliative care clinicians help patients and their families achieve these beneficial outcomes through multidisciplinary collaboration and comanagement of patient needs with the oncology team. Finally, by developing strong therapeutic relationships, managing symptoms and side effects, cultivating accurate illness understanding, assisting with treatment decisions, and facilitating timely planning of care at the end of life, palliative care clinicians ensure an extra layer of support for patients and families throughout the illness course.

References

1. Society AC. Cancer facts & figures 2015. Atlanta: American Cancer Society; 2015.
2. National Cancer Institute, NIH, DHHS. Cancer trends progress report. Bethesda, MD. 2015. http://progressreport.cancer.gov.
3. Abernethy AP, Aziz NM, Basch E, et al. A strategy to advance the evidence base in palliative medicine: formation of a palliative care research cooperative group. J Palliat Med. 2010;13:1407–13.
4. Parikh RB, Kirch RA, Smith TJ, et al. Early specialty palliative care—translating data in oncology into practice. N Engl J Med. 2013;369:2347–51.
5. Greer JA, Jackson VA, Meier DE, et al. Early integration of palliative care services with standard oncology care for patients with advanced cancer. CA Cancer J Clin. 2013;63:349–63.
6. Smith TJ, Temin S, Alesi ER, et al. American Society of Clinical Oncology provisional clinical opinion: the integration of palliative care into standard oncology care. J Clin Oncol. 2012;30:880–7.
7. National Consensus Project for Quality Palliative Care. Clinical practice guidelines for quality palliative care. 3rd ed. 2013. https://www.hpna.org/multimedia/NCP_Clinical_Practice_Guidelines_3rd_Edition.pdf.
8. World Health Organization. WHO definition of palliative care. http://www.who.int/cancer/palliative/definition/en/.
9. Meier DE, Brawley OW. Palliative care and the quality of life. J Clin Oncol. 2011;29:2750–2.
10. Epstein AS, Morrison RS. Palliative oncology: identity, progress, and the path ahead. Ann Oncol. 2012;23 Suppl 3:43–8.
11. Gilbertson-White S, Aouizerat BE, Jahan T, et al. A review of the literature on multiple symptoms, their predictors, and associated outcomes in patients with advanced cancer. Palliat Support Care. 2011;9:81–102.
12. Cheung WY, Le LW, Zimmermann C. Symptom clusters in patients with advanced cancers. Support Care Cancer. 2009;17:1223–30.
13. Dong ST, Butow PN, Costa DS, et al. Symptom clusters in patients with advanced cancer: a systematic review of observational studies. J Pain Symptom Manage. 2014;48:411–50.

14. Yennurajalingam S, Kwon JH, Urbauer DL, et al. Consistency of symptom clusters among advanced cancer patients seen at an outpatient supportive care clinic in a tertiary cancer center. Palliat Support Care. 2013;11:473–80.

15. Delgado-Guay MO, Hui D, Parsons HA, et al. Spirituality, religiosity, and spiritual pain in advanced cancer patients. J Pain Symptom Manage. 2011;41:986–94.

16. Hui D, de la Cruz M, Thorney S, et al. The frequency and correlates of spiritual distress among patients with advanced cancer admitted to an acute palliative care unit. Am J Hosp Palliat Care. 2011;28:264–70.

17. Lichtenthal WG, Nilsson M, Zhang B, et al. Do rates of mental disorders and existential distress among advanced stage cancer patients increase as death approaches? Psychooncology. 2009;18:50–61.

18. Mitchell AJ, Chan M, Bhatti H, et al. Prevalence of depression, anxiety, and adjustment disorder in oncological, haematological, and palliative-care settings: a meta-analysis of 94 interview-based studies. Lancet Oncol. 2011;12:160–74.

19. Bambauer KZ, Zhang B, Maciejewski PK, et al. Mutuality and specificity of mental disorders in advanced cancer patients and caregivers. Soc Psychiatry Psychiatr Epidemiol. 2006;41:819–24.

20. Hendriksen E, Williams E, Sporn N, et al. Worried together: a qualitative study of shared anxiety in patients with metastatic non-small cell lung cancer and their family caregivers. Support Care Cancer. 2015;23:1035–41.

21. Rhee YS, Yun YH, Park S, et al. Depression in family caregivers of cancer patients: the feeling of burden as a predictor of depression. J Clin Oncol. 2008;26:5890–5.

22. Braun M, Mikulincer M, Rydall A, et al. Hidden morbidity in cancer: spouse caregivers. J Clin Oncol. 2007;25:4829–34.

23. Jacobsen J, Kvale E, Rabow M, et al. Helping patients with serious illness live well through the promotion of adaptive coping: a report from the improving outpatient palliative care (IPAL-OP) initiative. J Palliat Med. 2014;17:463–8.

24. Jacobsen J, Thomas J, Jackson VA. Misunderstandings about prognosis: an approach for palliative care consultants when the patient does not seem to understand what was said. J Palliat Med. 2013;16:91–5.

25. Parker SM, Clayton JM, Hancock K, et al. A systematic review of prognostic/end-of-life communication with adults in the advanced stages of a life-limiting illness: patient/caregiver preferences for the content, style, and timing of information. J Pain Symptom Manage. 2007;34:81–93.

26. Hagerty RG, Butow PN, Ellis PM, et al. Communicating with realism and hope: incurable cancer patients' views on the disclosure of prognosis. J Clin Oncol. 2005;23:1278–88.

27. Steinhauser KE, Christakis NA, Clipp EC, et al. Factors considered important at the end of life by patients, family, physicians, and other care providers. JAMA. 2000;284:2476–82.

28. Temel JS, Greer JA, Admane S, et al. Longitudinal perceptions of prognosis and goals of therapy in patients with metastatic non-small-cell lung cancer: results of a randomized study of early palliative care. J Clin Oncol. 2011;29:2319–26.

29. Weeks JC, Catalano PJ, Cronin A, et al. Patients' expectations about effects of chemotherapy for advanced cancer. N Engl J Med. 2012;367:1616–25.

30. El-Jawahri A, Traeger L, Park ER, et al. Associations among prognostic understanding, quality of life, and mood in patients with advanced cancer. Cancer. 2014;120:278–85.

31. Weeks JC, Cook EF, O'Day SJ, et al. Relationship between cancer patients' predictions of prognosis and their treatment preferences. JAMA. 1998;279:1709–14.

32. Mack JW, Weeks JC, Wright AA, et al. End-of-life discussions, goal attainment, and distress at the end of life: predictors and outcomes of receipt of care consistent with preferences. J Clin Oncol. 2010;28:1203–8.

33. Mack JW, Smith TJ. Reasons why physicians do not have discussions about poor prognosis, why it matters, and what can be improved. J Clin Oncol. 2012;30:2715–7.

34. Jacobsen J, Jackson VA. A communication approach for oncologists: understanding patient coping and communicating about bad news, palliative care, and hospice. J Natl Compr Canc Netw. 2009;7:475–80.
35. Jackson VA, Jacobsen J, Greer JA, et al. The cultivation of prognostic awareness through the provision of early palliative care in the ambulatory setting: a communication guide. J Palliat Med. 2013;16:894–900.
36. Wright AA, Zhang B, Ray A, et al. Associations between end-of-life discussions, patient mental health, medical care near death, and caregiver bereavement adjustment. JAMA. 2008;300:1665–73.
37. Mack JW, Cronin A, Keating NL, et al. Associations between end-of-life discussion characteristics and care received near death: a prospective cohort study. J Clin Oncol. 2012;30:4387–95.
38. Zimmermann C, Riechelmann R, Krzyzanowska M, et al. Effectiveness of specialized palliative care: a systematic review. JAMA. 2008;299:1698–709.
39. Higginson IJ, Evans CJ. What is the evidence that palliative care teams improve outcomes for cancer patients and their families? Cancer J. 2010;16:423–35.
40. El-Jawahri A, Greer JA, Temel JS. Does palliative care improve outcomes for patients with incurable illness? A review of the evidence. J Support Oncol. 2011;9:87–94.
41. Rabow M, Kvale E, Barbour L, et al. Moving upstream: a review of the evidence of the impact of outpatient palliative care. J Palliat Med. 2013;16:1540–9.
42. Bakitas M, Stevens M, Ahles T, et al. Project ENABLE: a palliative care demonstration project for advanced cancer patients in three settings. J Palliat Med. 2004;7:363–72.
43. Bakitas M, Lyons KD, Hegel MT, et al. Effects of a palliative care intervention on clinical outcomes in patients with advanced cancer: the project ENABLE II randomized controlled trial. JAMA. 2009;302:741–9.
44. Bakitas MA, Tosteson TD, Li Z, et al. Early versus delayed initiation of concurrent palliative oncology care: patient outcomes in the ENABLE III randomized controlled trial. J Clin Oncol. 2015;33:1438–45.
45. Zimmermann C, Swami N, Krzyzanowska M, et al. Early palliative care for patients with advanced cancer: a cluster-randomised controlled trial. Lancet. 2014;383:1721–30.
46. Temel JS, Jackson VA, Billings JA, et al. Phase II study: integrated palliative care in newly diagnosed advanced non-small-cell lung cancer patients. J Clin Oncol. 2007;25:2377–82.
47. Temel JS, Greer JA, Muzikansky A, et al. Early palliative care for patients with metastatic non-small-cell lung cancer. N Engl J Med. 2010;363:733–42.
48. Bauman JR, Temel JS. The integration of early palliative care with oncology care: the time has come for a new tradition. J Natl Compr Canc Netw. 2014;12:1763–71. quiz 1771.
49. Dionne-Odom JN, Azuero A, Lyons KD, et al. Benefits of early versus delayed palliative care to informal family caregivers of patients with advanced cancer: outcomes from the ENABLE III randomized controlled trial. J Clin Oncol. 2015;33:1446–52.
50. Greer JA, Pirl WF, Jackson VA, et al. Effect of early palliative care on chemotherapy use and end-of-life care in patients with metastatic non-small-cell lung cancer. J Clin Oncol. 2012;30:394–400.
51. Jacobsen J, Jackson V, Dahlin C, et al. Components of early outpatient palliative care consultation in patients with metastatic nonsmall cell lung cancer. J Palliat Med. 2011;14:459–64.
52. Yoong J, Park ER, Greer JA, et al. Early palliative care in advanced lung cancer: a qualitative study. JAMA Intern Med. 2013;173:283–90.
53. Back AL, Park ER, Greer JA, et al. Clinician roles in early integrated palliative care for patients with advanced cancer: a qualitative study. J Palliat Med. 2014;17:1244–8.
54. Back AL, Arnold RM. Discussing prognosis: "how much do you want to know?" talking to patients who do not want information or who are ambivalent. J Clin Oncol. 2006;24: 4214–7.

55. Back AL, Arnold RM. Discussing prognosis: "how much do you want to know?" talking to patients who are prepared for explicit information. J Clin Oncol. 2006;24:4209–13.
56. Back AL, Arnold RM, Quill TE. Hope for the best, and prepare for the worst. Ann Intern Med. 2003;138:439–43.
57. Campbell TC, Carey EC, Jackson VA, et al. Discussing prognosis: balancing hope and realism. Cancer J. 2010;16:461–6.
58. Clayton JM, Butow PN, Arnold RM, et al. Fostering coping and nurturing hope when discussing the future with terminally ill cancer patients and their caregivers. Cancer. 2005;103:1965–75.
59. Pirl WF, Greer JA, Irwin K, et al. Processes of discontinuing chemotherapy for metastatic non-small-cell lung cancer at the end of life. J Oncol Pract. 2015;11(3):e405–12.

Chapter 14
Task Shifting and Delivery of Behavioral Medicine Interventions in Resource-Poor Global Settings: HIV/AIDS Treatment in sub-Saharan Africa

Jessica F. Magidson, Hetta Gouse, Christina Psaros, Jocelyn E. Remmert, Conall O'Cleirigh, and Steven A. Safren

14.1 Introduction

Task shifting is defined by the World Health Organization (WHO) as the "process of delegation whereby tasks are moved, where appropriate, to less specialized health workers" [1]. This allows, for example, for qualified nurses to prescribe and dispense medications when doctors are not available, and for community workers (who are in greater supply compared to nurses and physicians in resource-limited settings) to deliver a wide range of clinical services that would normally have been delivered by nurses or other professionals. More recently, task shifting models have been re-conceptualized to be instead a "task sharing" approach, as a way to avoid overburdening and over-relying on lower level cadres of workers. Task *sharing* (vs. shifting) involves delineating specific roles and responsibilities for each provider within a clinical team, as well as considering other ways of task sharing with family members and patients themselves [2]. As tasks are shifted and shared across the team, it is also essential to consider the changing roles of the physicians

J.F. Magidson, Ph.D. (✉) • C. Psaros, Ph.D. • J.E. Remmert • C. O'Cleirigh
Behavioral Medicine Service, Department of Psychiatry, Massachusetts General Hospital, Harvard Medical School, Boston, MA, USA
e-mail: jmagidson@mgh.harvard.edu; cpsaros@mgh.harvard.edu; jremmert@mgh.harvard.edu; cocleirigh@mgh.harvard.edu

H. Gouse, Ph.D.
Department of Psychiatry and Mental Health, University of Cape Town, Anzio Road, Cape Town, Western Cape 7925, South Africa
e-mail: Hetta.gouse@uct.ac.za

S.A. Safren, Ph.D.
Department of Psychology, University of Miami, 5665 Ponce de Leon Blvd., Coral Gables, FL 33124, USA
e-mail: ssafren@miami.edu

© Springer Science+Business Media New York 2017
A.-M. Vranceanu et al. (eds.), *The Massachusetts General Hospital Handbook of Behavioral Medicine*, Current Clinical Psychiatry, DOI 10.1007/978-3-319-29294-6_14

and higher level nurses, particularly focusing their attention on complex, treatment resistant patients and also ensuring ongoing supervision and management of the lower level providers [2].

Within the global context of HIV/AIDS and behavioral medicine interventions, task shifting[1] is important because of the lack of specialized professionals relative to the epidemiology of the epidemic. To expand access to biomedical treatment, task shifting has been employed to deliver HIV care and HIV medication because of the shortage of trained physicians. For behavioral medicine, task shifting can be used to deliver psychosocial interventions to improve adherence to HIV medication, as well as to deliver evidence-based mental health interventions [2].

In this chapter, we aim to demonstrate how the use of task shifting for delivering biomedical HIV care in sub-Saharan Africa can inform efforts to use task shifting models to deliver behavioral medicine interventions for individuals living with HIV/AIDS in this setting. In doing so, we first describe the widespread HIV/AIDS epidemic in sub-Saharan Africa and the shortage of trained health care providers to meet the needs of the epidemic. We describe task shifting efforts for expanding access to HIV medication in sub-Saharan Africa, and then illustrate how this approach to task shifting can be used to inform a similar approach for evidence-based behavioral medicine interventions among individuals living with HIV/AIDS in sub-Saharan Africa. We move from a broad overview of task shifting in HIV care in sub-Saharan Africa to specific examples of task shifting efforts to deliver evidence-based cognitive behavioral therapy (CBT) among individuals living with HIV/AIDS in sub-Saharan Africa. These efforts to task shift CBT address HIV medication adherence and commonly co-occurring psychological symptoms that interfere with successful HIV/AIDS outcomes, including depression and substance use. Although at the time of writing there have been few examples of task shifting of CBT to address psychosocial and behavioral medicine issues among individuals living with HIV/AIDS in sub-Saharan Africa, there have been a few promising early examples, including in the treatment of depression in Zimbabwe [3], the treatment of alcohol use in Kenya [4, 5], and integrated interventions for depression and HIV medication adherence in South Africa [6]. From these in-depth examples of task shifting CBT for alcohol use, depression, and integrated adherence interventions, we discuss considerations when adapting and implementing CBT using a task shifting model in this population. Finally, we discuss future directions and novel methodologies, for instance using multimedia-based interventions to promote standardization of task shifting delivery of CBT interventions and/or facilitate the use of these techniques by live interventionists. We also discuss the need to move from efficacy and effectiveness designs to more implementation science focused methods to promote sustainable integration of CBT for behavioral medicine in HIV care in sub-Saharan Africa.

This chapter focuses on HIV/AIDS and task shifting in HIV/AIDS care given its global prevalence, the need for behavioral medicine interventions for HIV medication adherence, self-care, and secondary prevention, and a rich prior history of using task shifting for expanding access to HIV medication in sub-Saharan Africa. Yet, HIV is just one example of a global disease burden that has benefitted from

---

[1] Throughout the chapter we use the term "task shifting" to refer to both task shifting and task sharing.

biomedical and behavioral task shifting efforts. This model and clinical examples provided in the remainder of this chapter are relevant for other diseases that require significant self-care that have increasing prevalence in sub-Saharan Africa, such as cancer and diabetes [7, 8].

14.1.1   HIV/AIDS Epidemic in sub-Saharan Africa

Nearly 71 % (24.7 million) of the total number of people living with HIV/AIDS in the world live in sub-Saharan Africa [9]. In sub-Saharan Africa, nearly 1 in every 25 adults is living with HIV [9]. In this region, ten countries (Ethiopia, Kenya, Malawi, Mozambique, Nigeria, South Africa, Uganda, Tanzania, Zambia, and Zimbabwe) account for 81 % of all individuals living with HIV/AIDS. Collectively, South Africa (SA) (25 %) and Nigeria (13 %) account for half of the HIV-infected population. Between 2005 and 2013, there has been a significant decline (39 %) in AIDS-related deaths in the region as a result of the rapid increase in number of people on HIV treatment [9].

14.1.2   Shortage of Trained Health Care Workers in sub-Saharan Africa

Sub-Saharan Africa has the lowest density of physicians, nurses, and midwives in the world, at 1.33 health workers per 1000 population (3 % of the global health workforce), with large variations between and within countries [10, 11]. Only 8 out of the 49 countries in sub-Saharan Africa have a health force density above the recommendations put forth by the World Health Organization [12]. The density of health workers tends to increase with improved economic status, although this is not always the case (see Ahmat et al. [10] for greater discussion of the relationship between higher economic status and health workforce). Further, in more specialized training areas, such as psychology and behavioral health, there are shortages in all countries in sub-Saharan Africa [13].

14.1.3   Gap Between HIV Treatment Needs and Staff Resources in sub-Saharan Africa

The HIV/AIDS epidemic in sub-Saharan Africa has compounded the need for health providers and has placed additional strain on the health sector that is already facing professional health worker shortages; for example, an estimated minimum of one to two doctors, up to seven nurses, and approximately three pharmacy staff are required per 1000 people for effective provision of HIV treatment [14]. As illustrated above, the reality falls far short of the requirements. These low numbers are further exacerbated by health workers themselves being vulnerable to disease, death, burnout and fatigue [15, 16], and the *brain drain*, or loss of doctors, nurses, and other health professionals by emigration to other, usually better resourced countries ([17, 18]). In addition, many African countries lack institutions and the capacity to train sufficient numbers of doctors [19].

14.1.4   Need for Task Shifting to Address Provider Shortage

WHO noted in 2006 that it was crucial for drastic action to be taken to address the human resource crises in the face of the HIV/AIDS epidemic in sub-Saharan Africa and launched a "Treat, Train, Retrain" plan to upscale and expand the health workforce [1]. WHO aims to get HIV medication to all persons living with HIV/AIDS worldwide. Although in sub-Saharan Africa HIV treatment is now available to approximately 37 % of people, there are significant differences between countries [9]. Universal access to HIV treatment and care services will require health systems capable of delivering quality interventions on a vastly expanded scale, relying heavily on task shifting models [20].

14.1.5   Task Shifting in HIV Care in sub-Saharan Africa

As stated above, in HIV care in sub-Saharan Africa, nurses and/or community health workers can successfully perform tasks such as provision and management of HIV medication, and counseling and screening to facilitate enrollment of HIV-infected patients eligible for treatment [21–23]. For instance, nurses have been successfully used to identify HIV treatment eligible patients, while physicians continued to initiate HIV treatment and prioritize time with HIV treatment eligible patients and those with more complex treatment needs [24]. Community health workers have also proved to contribute to service delivery and human resource capacity in sub-Saharan Africa. By serving as an entry point into HIV care, support, and treatment services, community health workers reduced waiting times, streamlined patient flow, and reduced workload of health workers, thus enhancing reach, uptake, and overall quality of HIV services [23].

14.1.6   Task Shifting HIV Medication Adherence Counseling

After initiating HIV medication, treatment requires lifelong adherence [25], which proves challenging for many; a prior meta-analysis indicated that approximately 23 % of patients in sub-Saharan Africa did not achieve optimal HIV medication adherence [26]. Implications of HIV medication nonadherence are heightened in sub-Saharan Africa where available HIV medication regimens are limited, and developing drug resistance may further eliminate availability of treatment regimens [27]. Task shifting HIV medication adherence counseling to lay health workers aims to increase access to adherence counseling, support, and psychoeducation [21–23]. Lay counselor-delivered HIV medication adherence counseling in HIV care aims to provide treatment preparation and ongoing adherence support to people enrolled in HIV clinic services [28, 29]. Lay counselors frequently remain outside the formal health system and are generally instructed, employed, and managed through nongovernmental intermediaries [29]. Educational requirements for lay health workers differ from country to country, and requirements may also change over time. Lay counselors, like other community health workers, do not have any formal professional or paraprofessional qualifications [30] for the field that they work in and they are generally trained by nongovernmental intermediaries.

14.1.7 Outcomes of Task Shifting

Prior research has suggested the effectiveness of task shifting in the delivery of HIV treatment in Africa, specifically substantial cost savings [21] and physician time savings [21–23, 31]. In settings where tasks have shifted to nurses, there is less loss to follow-up in the nurse-managed groups (vs. physician-managed) with no difference in mortality and equal survival rates at 12 months [32]. Many patients appear to prefer nurse-managed care because of friendlier service, better patient examination and education, and the closer proximity of services to their homes. This result was however not found universally, and some patients feared stigmatization and inadequate care [33] and preferred care from primary health clinics and district management units because of better relationships with providers, friendlier and more supportive care, and better patient education [34, 35].

The presence of community health workers also appears to improve retention in care and the quality of life of people living with HIV/AIDS [23, 36]. However, community health worker programs have not always been successful, and, in particular, larger programs tend to present with sustainability and quality of care challenges [23, 37–39]. In a South African study assessing the impact of a community-based adherence support program on HIV outcomes in government HIV treatment sites, patients with community health worker adherence support more consistently collected their medication and attained a treatment pickup rate of 95 % vs. 67 % of those who did not have community health workers adherence support [40]. Retention in care and adherence are two of the most important issues for long-term success of HIV treatment programs, and both appear to benefit from task shifting and community health worker involvement [23]. As has been suggested by prior researchers, we must leverage the lessons learned from task shifting in HIV care in sub-Saharan Africa for other noncommunicable diseases [41]. More specifically, in this chapter, we will discuss how these lessons can inform efforts to implement other evidence-based behavioral medicine interventions for individuals living with HIV/AIDS in sub-Saharan Africa.

14.2   Applications of Task Shifting for Behavioral Medicine Interventions in HIV Care in sub-Saharan Africa

In addition to the behavioral health needs related to managing HIV/AIDS, such as HIV medication adherence and retention in care, comorbid psychiatric conditions are also common among HIV-infected individuals in sub-Saharan Africa. Two of the most common psychiatric disorders among individuals living with HIV/AIDS in sub-Saharan Africa are depression and substance abuse [42]. Elevated depressive symptom rates are approximately 31 %, and a pooled estimate of major depression is 18 % according to a meta-analysis in sub-Saharan Africa [42]. Alcohol is the most common drug used in sub-Saharan Africa [43], and rates of alcohol use disorders range from 7 to 31 % [42]. When untreated, depression and substance use are significantly associated with poor antiretroviral adherence across multiple studies, which ultimately leads to worse HIV/AIDS treatment outcomes [42].

Unfortunately, similar to the shortage of trained medical providers in sub-Saharan Africa, there is also a shortage of trained mental health providers. In general, low income countries have between 0.05 psychiatrists and 0.16 psychiatric nurses per 100,000 people [13]. Only half of the countries in Africa have any type of community-based mental health care [13]. Countries with the largest shortage of mental health care workers in the world are Chad, Eritrea, and Liberia, each only have one psychiatrist in the entire country [13]. Much of sub-Saharan Africa has less than five mental health care workers per 100,000 individuals, and South Africa is the only country in sub-Saharan Africa with more than 25 mental health care workers per 100,000 people [13]. As such, there are clear needs for task shifting of mental health care for individuals with HIV/AIDS.

14.2.1   Task Shifting CBT in sub-Saharan Africa

Cognitive behavioral therapy (CBT) can be used to address a range of behavioral health needs among individuals living with HIV/AIDS, including to improve symptoms of depression, reduce HIV medication nonadherence, and reduce substance use [44, 45]. Although the majority of empirical support for CBT interventions among individuals living with HIV/AIDS is from the US and other developed countries, there is accumulating empirical support for CBT interventions in sub-Saharan Africa using task shifting models. In particular, CBT's structured, time limited approach has been viewed as particularly suitable for the demands of task shifting (i.e., to improve ease of training, supervision). See Table 14.1.

In this section, we will discuss examples of task shifting of evidence-based CBT interventions to address psychosocial and behavioral medicine issues among individuals living with HIV/AIDS in sub-Saharan Africa. These examples are highlighted in detail below in the Case Illustrations section. From these examples, we discuss considerations for future efforts when adapting and implementing CBT using a task shifting model in this population.

Table 14.1 Examples of task shifting cognitive behavioral therapy (CBT) for individuals living with HIV/AIDS in sub-Saharan Africa

Country	Intervention components	Number of sessions	Type of interventionist	Primary treatment outcomes
South Africa [46, 47]	Computer-delivered program to help counselors track delivery of specific intervention components and to explain complex concepts to patients in a straightforward, visual way; uses problem-solving strategies and follows social action theory (SAT [48])	6	Lay counselor	HIV medication adherence
Kenya [4, 5]	Cultural adaptation of group CBT to reduce alcohol use among HIV-infected outpatients	6	Lay counselor	Alcohol use
Zimbabwe [3]	Problem-solving therapy enhanced with a component of activity scheduling	6	Lay counselor	Depression
South Africa [49]	Blended motivational interviewing and problem-solving therapy to address risky substance abuse	4	Peer counselors	Substance abuse
Zimbabwe [50]	Problem-solving for HIV medication adherence	4	Lay adherence counselors	HIV medication adherence
South Africa [6]	Integrated CBT intervention of problem-solving for HIV medication adherence, CBT for depression	6–8	Lay adherence counselors/ nurses	HIV medication adherence, depression

14.3   Cognitive Behavioral Therapy for Adherence

As indicated above, although adherence counseling is routinely delivered in HIV clinic settings in South Africa it is not clear if this counseling is evidence-based, as there have been few efforts to describe or evaluate routine adherence counseling in this setting [51]. As such, despite efforts to use task shifting models to deliver adherence counseling in sub-Saharan Africa, continued efforts are needed to use task shifting to deliver evidence-based HIV medication adherence interventions in these settings. For instance, there is a substantial evidence base for cognitive behavioral interventions to improve HIV medication adherence, largely in developing countries. Simoni et al. [52] conducted a meta-analytic review of published randomized clinical trials (RCTs) that had evaluated a behavioral HIV medication adherence intervention. In this review (with most trials being US-based; 74 %), the majority of interventions (79 %) included CBT components, such as psychoeducation, motivational interviewing, healthy coping strategies, and some form of cognitive restructuring. Eighty-four percent of studies included behavioral CBT strategies (i.e., cue dosing, activity scheduling). The majority of studies (58 %) included three of the aforementioned CBT components. Further, interventions that included CBT components (compared to those that did not include CBT components) tended to show greater improvements in HIV medication nonadherence. Across studies, the most common providers were well-trained health care providers (i.e., physicians, nurses in 47 % of studies) or trained psychologists (in 26 % of studies). Over half of studies (53 %) used research staff (not clinic staff) to provide the intervention.

There are clear implications when we consider extending these research findings to LMICs, and sub-Saharan Africa in particular, where task shifting with other levels of providers is essential. There has been a similar review of RCTs of HIV medication adherence interventions in sub-Saharan Africa [53]. Although this review categorized interventions based on the use of behavioral and cognitive techniques, none of the identified interventions used a theory-driven CBT approach to address adherence, nor did the review discuss who was implementing the interventions to ascertain whether a task shifting model has been used to implement CBT for adherence in sub-Saharan Africa. Although there are few published examples of using task shifting to deliver CBT interventions for HIV medication adherence in HIV clinic settings, there are examples in progress that integrate evidence-based CBT interventions for adherence with other CBT interventions for co-occurring psychiatric symptoms that we discuss in more depth below.

14.4   Task Shifting of CBT for Co-occurring Psychiatric Symptoms Among HIV-Infected Individuals in sub-Saharan Africa

There have been few efforts to use task shifting models to deliver CBT specifically in sub-Saharan Africa for HIV populations; however, some preliminary work has been done to task shifting efficacious CBT interventions for depression and substance use among HIV-infected individuals in sub-Saharan Africa. The examples listed in this section are described in more detail in the Case Illustrations section, and then followed by specific considerations from this process that may affect future implementation and scalability.

14.4.1   CBT for Alcohol Use in HIV/AIDS

At the time of writing, perhaps the clearest example of systematically adapting and evaluating a task shifting delivery model of CBT in an HIV population in sub-Saharan Africa is that of Papas et al. [4, 5]. This team adapted CBT to reduce alcohol use among HIV-infected outpatients in Edloret, Kenya and conducted a preliminary pilot trial to examine initial feasibility and acceptability of paraprofessional delivery [5] and subsequently published a Stage 1 RCT evaluating its efficacy

[4]. CBT was initially selected for this work because of its strong empirical support in Western settings, and prior application in sub-Saharan Africa (i.e., Zambia [54]). Additionally, and central to task shifting models, it was also selected given its highly structured format, which was seen to be feasible for training paraprofessionals with limited formal education.

14.4.2   Integrated CBT Intervention for Alcohol Use and HIV Medication Adherence

One limitation of the work of Papas et al. [4, 5] in Kenya was a lack of a dual focus on HIV outcomes (e.g., HIV medication adherence). Given the prevalence of alcohol use disorders and its powerful effects on HIV medication adherence in sub-Saharan Africa [55], efforts to develop an integrated CBT intervention to address alcohol use and HIV medication adherence are also necessary. Preliminary work in this area has begun to be conducted in South Africa, where rates of alcohol consumption are also among the highest in the world [43]. This work in South Africa [56] is developing a lay adherence counselor-delivered CBT intervention to address hazardous alcohol use and HIV medication nonadherence in the public HIV clinic setting in South Africa.

14.4.3   CBT for Depression in HIV/AIDS

As an example of task shifting a CBT intervention for depression in HIV care in sub-Saharan Africa, Chibanda et al. [3] adapted problem-solving therapy for depression to be delivered by lay health workers in a Harare, Zimbabwe primary care setting. In this setting, lay health workers typically have at least primary school education, have lived locally for an extended period of time, and are intended to support HIV medication adherence and other psychological counseling in the HIV care setting. Although patients did not have to disclose their HIV status to enter into the trial, over half of all patients in the trial had an HIV-related problem, and the study was conducted at primary care clinic sites that see a large percentage of HIV-infected patients in this region. Up to six sessions of problem-solving therapy were offered either at the "Friendship bench," located adjacent to the HIV clinic setting, or in the patient's home.

14.4.4   Integrated CBT Intervention for Depression and HIV Medication Adherence

Although still in progress, there are initial efforts to integrate CBT for depression with an evidence-based CBT intervention for adherence (Life-Steps) [57, 58]. Andersen et al. [6] evaluated a nurse-delivered CBT intervention for depression and HIV medication adherence. The intervention was a six to eight session intervention based on cognitive behavioral therapy for adherence and depression [6]. Primary modifications to the original intervention included streamlining session content, and removing the cognitive restructuring module due to its complexity. Treatment modules included psychoeducation, motivational interviewing, problem-solving, activity scheduling, and relaxation training. Initial evidence suggests the intervention approach is acceptable to patients and associated with significant improvements in depression, functioning, and modest improvements in HIV medication adherence. Implementation was challenging, requiring extensive weekly supervision, initial training (88 h), supplemented with regular ongoing training. Additional research is needed in this area to determine whether a nurse- or lay counselor-delivered CBT intervention is feasible and sustainable for delivery in this setting, and whether the treatment is associated with long-term improvements in key health and psychological outcomes.

Bere and colleagues are evaluating a lay counselor-delivered CBT intervention for depression and HIV medication adherence in Zimbabwe [50]. The intervention combines Life-Steps for HIV medication adherence [57, 58] with an integrated behavioral activation and problem-solving therapy approach to depression, delivered in public HIV care in Harare, Zimbabwe by four trained lay adherence counselors. The study will determine whether the implementation strategy was feasible, acceptable, and associated with improvements in depression, HIV medication adherence, and HIV-related health outcomes. Descriptions of the formative qualitative work [59] and preliminary work to culturally adapt Life-Steps for this setting [50] provide important details regarding the necessary steps for adapting CBT for this resource-limited HIV care setting.

14.5 Case Illustrations of Task Shifting CBT in sub-Saharan Africa

14.5.1 Case 1: Task Shifting CBT for Alcohol Use Among HIV-Infected Patients in Kenya

As mentioned briefly above, Papas et al. [5] adapted CBT to be delivered by paraprofessionals in Kenya to address alcohol use among HIV-infected patients. The adaptation process began with initial formative qualitative work, followed by systematic treatment adaptation and pilot trial, and then a subsequent efficacy trial. Below the specific steps and details regarding the process of adaptation and implementation are highlighted.

14.5.1.1 Formative Phase

The first step in adapting CBT to address alcohol use among HIV-infected patients in Kenya consisted of formative qualitative work with patients, providers, and staff, as well as observation of local alcohol peer support groups [5]. Initial qualitative analysis found that the CBT model for alcohol use fit with the Kenyan culture; however, it was recommended in formative work that exercises be adapted to the local setting, for instance unique cultural contexts for drinking, as well as adapting language used to be appropriate for local idioms, and including culturally appropriate visual aids and metaphors. Cultural myths and misinformation about alcohol use and HIV outcomes in this population were incorporated into the CBT protocol. A focus on income-generating activities, particularly among female patients, was also incorporated. It was also decided that groups would be stratified by gender to allow for discussion of sensitive issues. Group format was selected given focus on social networks as key in Kenyan culture, and also because of implications for cost-effectiveness [60]. Selection of the primary treatment target—alcohol vs. other HIV-related behaviors—was decided upon locally. Assessments were also adapted to be fitting to local culture; for instance, breathalyzers were highly stigmatized given that they were used by Kenyan police and as such saliva tests were seen as more discrete and less stigmatized and thus were used instead to assess the primary outcome. Finally, the original CBT protocol was reduced to six sessions due to feasibility concerns.

14.5.1.2   Interventionist Selection, Training, and Supervision

Given the lack of trained mental health professionals providing substance use treatment in Kenya [60], two paraprofessionals with no prior CBT experience (one with a high school diploma and no counseling experience and one with a two-year post high school counseling diploma and minimal counseling experience) were hired to deliver the intervention. One of the providers was HIV-infected. Selection procedures included discussing case examples and conducting behavioral role plays, and the team aimed to select those with natural talents (empathy, emotional perceptiveness, good communication and analytical skills). The counselors received 175–300 h of training and supervision prior to the trial. Training in CBT included classroom work, role plays, videotaped feedback, and training in ethics and basic health education. Counselors conducted role plays with medical students as simulated patients, which were supervised and rated for use of CBT skills. Once counselors met a minimum threshold on adherence to the CBT manual, they then conducted pilot groups, which were videotaped.

14.5.1.3   Pilot Trial Results

Results from the initial pilot trial with 27 patients showed that the two lay providers were able to deliver CBT with modest fidelity and competence [5]. Pilot patient outcomes were favorable, including treatment attendance, acceptability, and reductions in alcohol use [5]. Additionally, although treatment attendance was fairly high (overall attendance was 77 %), numerous efforts were made to reduce barriers to attendance, such as text and phone call appointment reminders, reimbursement for transportation, and in some cases, transportation to the first CBT session [5].

14.5.1.4   Stage 1 Efficacy Trial

Subsequently, this team conducted a Stage 1 RCT to evaluate the efficacy of the adapted, paraprofessional intervention (delivered in Kiswahili) compared to usual care among HIV-infected HIV treatment eligible patients who reported hazardous/binge drinking ($n=75$) [4]. The primary outcome as indicated above was alcohol use (assessed using a timeline follow back and alcohol saliva tests). Results demonstrated large effect sizes between the conditions at the 30-day follow-up in reducing alcohol use ($d=0.95$). At a 90-day follow-up, abstinence from alcohol was 69 % in the CBT condition and 38 % in usual care. Participants randomized to CBT attended 93 % of the six sessions offered ($M=5.6$, SD$=0.66$). Ratings of counselor adherence and competence were conducted using a standardized rating scale [61]. Adherence and competence were found to be equivalent to bachelors-level therapists delivering CBT in the US. Although the results are promising, one noted limitation is the lack of attention to HIV outcomes in the trial, limiting the treatment to a single target. Although integrated CBT treatments have been developed and largely tested in the US to address HIV-related behaviors and co-occurring substance use [62, 63], it is unclear whether this is feasible for paraprofessional delivery in a resource constrained setting.

14.5.2   Case 2: Task Shifting an Integrated Intervention for Alcohol Use and HIV Medication Adherence in South Africa

To improve health outcomes alongside efforts to reduce alcohol use among HIV-infected patients, efforts are underway in South Africa to adapt an integrated CBT intervention for alcohol use and HIV medication adherence. The intervention was adapted for paraprofessional delivery in HIV care. Below the formative phase is described and the ongoing plan for evaluating the adapted intervention in an efficacy trial.

14.5.2.1   Formative Phase

Formative research was conducted in South Africa to examine the appropriateness and acceptability of an intervention delivered in HIV care to address both alcohol use and alcohol-related HIV medication nonadherence [55]. The formative phase was conducted at two HIV clinics in Tshwane, South Africa among 304 HIV-infected adults. Feedback was solicited on who would be optimal to deliver the intervention, the preferred quantity, duration, format, and settings of the sessions, specific skills to focus on, and potential involvement of friends and family. Regarding specific skills, patients were asked to assess the perceived utility of potential CBT skills (although not labeled as such), including non-alcohol related healthy coping strategies, relapse prevention, advantages and disadvantages of not drinking, and brainstorming ways to reduce frequency and quantity of alcohol consumption. Results from the formative work indicated that 95 % of patients surveyed felt there was a need for an intervention to address alcohol-related HIV medication adherence. Suggestions included two clinic-based sessions 1 h in length in a group format to be led by a peer (a fellow HIV treatment recipient) or an adherence counselor (typically a high school level paraprofessional trained to deliver standard adherence counseling in South Africa). Further, individuals with low levels of HIV medication adherence in particular strongly preferred paraprofessional interventionists. There was a strong preference for "strategies for coping that do not involve alcohol" to be a primary component of intervention, as well as discussing pros and cons of drinking. Authors suggested that this evidence points to the relevance of a CBT type intervention, including using motivational interviewing and relapse prevention strategies, to address alcohol-related nonadherence by paraprofessionals in the HIV clinic setting [55].

14.5.2.2 Protocol for Evaluating Intervention Delivery and Patient Outcomes

In response [56], this team has developed a protocol to evaluate a CBT intervention to address alcohol and HIV medication nonadherence in the HIV clinic setting in South Africa. This team is adapting a blended motivational interviewing/problem-solving therapy intervention that has been developed to address alcohol use among individuals in South Africa [49] for the needs of HIV-positive alcohol using patients. The blended motivational interviewing/problem intervention for adherence/alcohol use aims to increase motivation to reduce alcohol use and promote HIV medication adherence. Feedback will be provided on levels of substance use, and psychoeducation will be provided on how alcohol use impacts HIV treatment outcomes. Motivational interviewing strategies will increase readiness to change and build rapport, and readiness change will be assessed using a "readiness ruler." Other CBT techniques include a motivational interviewing decisional balance exercise, problem-solving skills to cope with triggers, acceptance, and coping with negative thoughts. A motivational interviewing style is emphasized throughout the intervention.

Adaptation of the intervention followed four initial focus groups and results of the formative phase [55]. Lay adherence counselors (i.e., high school diploma level, often HIV positive) are being trained to deliver the intervention. Patients are being recruited from the public hospital-based HIV clinics in Tshwane, South Africa where the pilot work took place, specifically patients who are HIV positive, on HIV medication, and categorized as "harmful/hazardous drinkers" using the Alcohol Use Disorders Identification Test (AUDIT) [64]. Participants are randomized to one of three conditions, a motivational interviewing/problem-solving alcohol and adherence intervention, a time matched motivational interviewing/problem-solving "wellness" intervention, and treatment as usual. Alcohol use and HIV medication adherence will be assessed at baseline, three-, six-, and 12 months using interviews and biological specimens. Finally, a process evaluation will assess counselors' and participants' perceptions of acceptability and effectiveness.

This trial will provide important evidence regarding the effectiveness and feasibility of using a lay counselor-delivered integrated intervention to address alcohol use and HIV medication nonadherence. Additionally, if the intervention is effective, authors indicate they will offer training to other staff at the clinics and other interested health workers on how to screen and deliver the intervention. This has important implications for sustainability of the intervention. When this stage of implementation is reached, ongoing evaluation is needed as to when clinic-based counselors, as opposed to lay counselors hired for research purposes, are feasibly and competently able to deliver the CBT intervention.

14.5.3   Case 3: Task Shifting CBT for Depression in HIV Primary Care in Zimbabwe—the "Friendship Bench"

Chibanda et al. [3] trained lay health workers in HIV primary care in Harare, Zimbabwe in problem-solving therapy for depression. Although not focused on HIV specifically, over half of all patients in the trial (52 %) presented with an HIV-related problem, and the treatment was implemented at primary care clinic sites that treat a large percentage of HIV-infected patients in this region. This case illustration describes the process of training and supervising the lay health workers and implementing the "Friendship Bench" intervention in Harare, Zimbabwe. We present results from the initial implementation trial for the Case Illustration, although the Friendship bench continues to be ongoing in these clinic settings. Current priorities include scaling up the Friendship bench to other clinic settings, particularly in rural Zimbabwe, and integrating with evidence-based ART adherence counseling [50].

14.5.3.1   Interventionist Training

In the pilot implementation trial (Chibanda et al. [3]), 20 lay health workers were trained in a locally adapted problem-solving therapy intervention. Lay health workers in this setting are intended to support nurses in primary care and are locally called "ambuya utano" or "grandmother health provider." The lay health workers support individuals living with HIV/AIDS and TB, provide psychological counseling and HIV medication adherence counseling, and promote community health education in designated geographic areas. In the setting where the trial took place, the lay workers were female, literate, had at least primary school education, and had lived locally for at least 15 years. An eight-day training was conducted by two psychologists with expertise in problem-solving therapy, a general nurse, and a psychiatrist. The training included education on common mental disorders, including a locally defined depressive disorder ("kufungisisa," or thinking too much; [65]), skills to identify common mental disorders using a local, standardized screener (Shona Symptom Questionnaire; [66]), and how to deliver the locally adapted problem-solving therapy. For the study, 10 lay health workers were randomly selected to participate in the pilot trial. These individuals received ongoing training every two weeks for the first six months and then monthly.

14.5.3.2   Interventionist Supervision

Supervision for the lay health workers included a weekly, one hour long group supervision led by a general nurse with prior counseling training. Group supervision was also conducted by a clinical psychologist one hour every two weeks, and by a psychiatrist monthly for 45 minutes. The lay workers also participated in a daily peer support group facilitated by one of the lay health workers.

14.5.3.3   Friendship Bench Approach

At the clinic settings, clients can be referred or can self-refer to the "Friendship bench"—a large wooden bench located under a tree adjacent to the clinic setting—which was available daily from 9 am to 12 pm. During the implementation trial, one lay worker was responsible for the bench daily and would approach the bench after a client sat on it to deliver a problem-solving therapy session. The problem-solving therapy intervention included basic problem-solving strategies (i.e., identifying problems, brainstorming practical and feasible solutions, and selecting and implementing a solution). Patients received feedback on their symptoms on the Shona Symptom Questionnaire, including psychoeducation on kufungisisa. The intervention was locally adapted for lay health worker delivery. Up to six sessions of problem-solving therapy were offered either at the Friendship bench or in the patient's home. Home visits included prayer with family, which was seen as an essential component for appropriateness of the intervention in the local Zimbabwean culture. For patients with kufungisisa or extreme poverty, problem-solving therapy was also enhanced with activity scheduling and local income-generating activities (peanut butter making, recycling).

14.5.3.4   Implementation Trial Results

The lay health workers evaluated the problem-solving therapy intervention (i.e., rated the "ease with which they learned the problem-solving therapy approach, delivered it, and proportion of patients who appeared to benefit from it"). Focus groups were also conducted following implementation of the Friendship Bench. These groups pointed to successes of the program, including a view that the providers were trustworthy and wise, that patients received motivation and support from home visits, and that the approach minimized stigma associated with mental health treatment. The lay health workers also reported that the structure of the therapy approach supported them in monitoring progress, in particular the step of problem-solving therapy of breaking down problems into specific/manageable steps. Over the course of the research study, 320 patients used the Friendship bench. All patients completed a minimum of three sessions over six weeks, with 30 % completing all six sessions. After a minimum of three sessions, there was a meaningful clinical reduction in clinical symptoms (on the SSQ). This approach using peer- and nurse-led supervision, with an option for specialist referral, which was utilized very infrequently, was seen as a potentially sustainable model for task shifting in this community, and continues to be ongoing, with intended efforts for larger scale-up in rural areas.

14.6 Summary and Considerations for Task Shifting CBT in Resource-Poor Settings

Across these examples of task shifting CBT for behavioral health needs among HIV-infected individuals in sub-Saharan Africa, although still in early phases, it seems that task shifting CBT across the examples provided was feasible, appropriate, and acceptable to patients. In some cases, paraprofessional delivery, as illustrated in formative qualitative work in South Africa to develop an alcohol/adherence intervention [55], may even be preferable (i.e., using a peer or fellow HIV treatment recipient as the provider). This may not be so surprising considering the leading addiction programs across the world are peer-led [67]. Whether lay counselors are able to deliver a more complicated integrated intervention [51, 56] will answer important questions on the types of interventions paraprofessionals are most well suited to deliver. These decisions will likely need to consider the advantages and disadvantages of incorporating multiple treatment targets in an integrated treatment protocol (i.e., improved efficiency yet also potentially added complexity that may reduce feasibility or acceptability for training, supervision, and long-term therapist skill acquisition).

As indicated above, the primary CBT techniques that have been used in sub-Saharan Africa among HIV-infected patients have been problem-solving therapy, motivational interviewing, and activity scheduling. Although a bit outside the scope of this chapter, there has also been extensive work evaluating trauma focused CBT (TF-CBT) in Zambia and Tanzania [68, 69] among youth, as well as adapting interpersonal psychotherapy to treat depression in Uganda [70]. Interpersonal psychotherapy has also been delivered by lay counselors to address depression among HIV-infected individuals in South Africa [71].

Across these studies, when adapting CBT techniques for resource-limited settings, often the key consideration in the adaptation is cultural modification and adapting for paraprofessional delivery while also maintaining the core components of the intervention. Given that many CBT manuals are initially tested and developed using masters- or doctoral-level therapists in high income countries, considering changes to the treatment manual and training procedures for lay counselors or health care workers with no background in psychology or counseling is essential. Often these modifications include (1) focusing on *how* training is conducted; (2) simplifying terms and avoiding clinical jargon; and (3) adapting the structure of supervision. Regarding cultural adaptations, changes may include ensuring appropriate delivery within a local context, linguistic modifications, and including local idioms, metaphors, and stories, as well as adapting for low literacy populations. For instance, while there is no empirical support for home-based prayer with family in the treatment of depression, providers in Zimbabwe felt that it was inappropriate to remove, and that the treatment would no longer be acceptable to patients or families if not included [3]. Another example of the importance of community buy-in when selecting and adapting the intervention approach was in Papas et al. [5] in which the primary treatment target (alcohol as opposed to other HIV-related health behaviors) was decided upon locally and that the community urged for this to be the focus. These adaptations reflect a larger literature on community-based participatory research (CBPR) that identifies the need to have the community dictate research and clinical priorities [72, 73].

It is interesting to note that across the aforementioned clinical examples of task shifting, CBT was selected or deemed to be appropriate in process evaluations for paraprofessional delivery given its structured format. Although easier for training purposes, the structured format may be challenging at times for lay counselor providers not familiar with structured CBT type approaches in learning how to maintain a primary focus on the key intervention target (e.g., adherence), particularly when patients may also request addressing other health behaviors in the context of the intervention. Ongoing considerations when adapting CBT in this type of setting should consider maintaining a structured, manual format and assessing what types of manuals are most easy to use by counselors (e.g., workbooks, flip manuals; [6, 74]). That being said, dissemination and implementation research models have indicated that the more flexible the delivery of an intervention the greater the likelihood for ultimate adoption in clinical settings [75–77]. As such, finding a balance between providing structure and allowing for some flexibility in delivery, for instance using a modular approach [78, 79], may be necessary.

14.7   Novel Approaches Using Technology

Technology-based platforms to support the delivery of evidence-based behavioral HIV care have emerged in resource-limited settings, for instance using text messaging (SMS) reminders support for adherence [80] and using multimedia-based interventions to standardize the delivery of evidence-based interventions. One example of using a computer-, multimedia-based intervention as a means to support task shifting of adherence counseling in South Africa is the "Masivukeni" ("let's wake up") intervention. Currently being evaluated in a randomized clinical trial in South

Africa [46], the intervention is a six-session lay counselor-delivered intervention that uses multimedia to help counselors track delivery of specific intervention components and to explain complex concepts to patients in a straightforward, visual way. The computer program includes scripted text, imagery, animations, audio, and video to delivery information and provides a structured agenda for each session. The intervention program only requires basic computer familiarity (e.g., how to use a mouse and keyboard, open and close programs). The intervention is based on social action theory (SAT; [48]) and utilizes some CBT strategies (i.e., problem-solving barriers to adherence, social support). Each 45 min session includes interactive multimedia components to provide psychoeducation on HIV medication adherence and problem solve barriers to adherence (for greater description of the intervention, see Remien et al. [46]). The program tracks activities, time spent on activities and sessions, and patient responses. These built-in features of activity tracking allow for supervision that is not human resource-intensive and thereby addresses the problem of limited resources for supervision. The program also allows for easy printing of personalized patient data that can be used by counselors and patients, and can save information/questions session to session to enable reviewing at subsequent sessions. A screener for mental health and substance use is incorporated in the program and gives automated scoring and referral scripts to the counselor, enabling counselors with modest training to make critical referral for mental health and substance use problems that may compromise medical adherence [46]. Although the intervention is still being tested, recently published pilot data ($n=55$) indicate that the Masivukeni intervention was associated with improvements in HIV medication adherence (measured as clinic-based pill count data), more positive attitudes towards disclosure and medication social support, and better clinic–patient relationships compared to treatment as usual adherence counseling [47]. In formative work, the intervention was also found to be feasible and acceptable for lay counselor delivery [46]. If it proves effective, feasible, and acceptable in the larger trial, multimedia-based platforms may be a potentially useful strategy to promote sustainable implementation of task shifting models delivering CBT in HIV care in sub-Saharan Africa.

14.8 Moving from Effectiveness to Implementation Research for Task Shifting CBT

Alongside the promising results of effectiveness trials of CBT using task shifting models, clear implementation challenges emerge from these examples of task shifting CBT in this setting. Primary implementation challenges include poor role definition or clarity on scope of work for lay counselors, lack of standardized training, and inadequate supervision, support, and compensation. For long-term sustainability, a primary consideration is whether activities would be feasible if conducted in a clinic-based setting without any additional research resources. For instance, the amount of training and supervision described in each of the examples may likely not be sustainable in a real-world clinical setting. For instance, in the Papas et al. [4, 5] studies, counselors received 175–300 h of training and supervision prior to starting to see patients for the trial that included not only didactics, but also role plays, videotaped feedback, and supervised sessions with rated CBT skill use. Indeed, in that study, transitioning supervision and training to local supervisors was not attained, and the US-based lead investigator remained on-site throughout the course of the study to maintain her responsibilities of in-person supervision.

The model for supervision seemed to fully embody a task shifting approach in the Friendship Bench, as it was a tiered approach using daily peer supervision, weekly nurse-led supervision, and supervision with a clinical psychologist and psychiatrist once every two weeks and monthly, respectively [3]. Although this is likely also more intensive than would be feasible in a non-research context, it is a good example of a task shifting model of supervision for this intervention. Additionally, in one study [5], numerous efforts were made to reduce barriers to attendance that may not be feasible in non-research contexts, such as text and phone call appointment reminders, reimbursement for transportation, and in some cases, transportation to the first CBT session. When a later stage of implementation is reached outside the context of a research study, ongoing evaluation is needed as to when clinic-based counselors, as opposed to lay counselors hired for research purposes, are feasibly and competently able to deliver the CBT intervention. Another important consideration when considering efforts to implement CBT in clinical settings outside of a research context will be how to standardize selection of paraprofessional counselors. Papas et al. [4, 5] aimed to hire for natural talents (empathy, emotional perceptiveness, good communication and analytical skills) assessed using case conceptualizations and behavioral role plays. It remains an empirical question whether this selection approach is effective and feasible in a real-world clinical setting. If task shifting CBT for behavioral medicine conditions proves to be feasible and effective in the ongoing work, it may be a particularly appealing approach to meet the needs for integrating behavioral health interventions into HIV care in sub-Saharan Africa [81].

14.9   Conclusions and Resources

In conclusion, task shifting behavioral medicine CBT interventions for ART adherence and co-occurring mental health problems for individuals living with HIV/AIDS is a promising and essential strategy for meeting the treatment needs in the context of a specialized provider shortage in sub-Saharan Africa. Addressing ART adherence concerns and the co-occurring mental health problems which disrupt ART adherence are key to the success of biomedical treatment as prevention efforts to curbing the HIV/AIDS epidemic in sub-Saharan Africa. In many ways task shifting of biomedical ART programs can only succeed in the context of also task shifting evidence-based CBT interventions to promote ART adherence and viral suppression. For readers interested in more details on task shifting efforts for behavioral medicine in sub-Saharan Africa, please visit these resources:

1. Africa Focus on Intervention Research for Mental Health (AFFIRM) http://www.affirm.uct.ac.za/affirm-aims: A research and capacity development hub in six sub-Saharan African countries: Ethiopia, Ghana, Malawi, South Africa, Uganda, and Zimbabwe—evaluating task shifting/sharing interventions for mental health disorders delivered by community health workers in South Africa and Ethiopia.
2. Programme for Improving Mental health carE (PRIME) http://www.prime.uct. ac.za/: An initiative focused on implementing and scaling up of treatment programs for mental disorders, with a focus on community involvement, and health service and system strengthening.
3. Emerging Mental Health Systems in Low- and Middle-Income Countries (EMERALD) http://www.emerald-project.eu: An initiative focused on strengthening the health system (training/resources/infrastructure etc.) to lay the groundwork for universal mental health care coverage at the primary care level.

References

1. World Health Organization. Task shifting: Rational redistribution of tasks among health workforce teams: global recommendations and guidelines. Geneva, Switzerland: WHO Press; 2008.
2. Padmanathan P, De Silva MJ. The acceptability and feasibility of task-sharing for mental healthcare in low and middle income countries: a systematic review. Soc Sci Med. 2013;97:82–6.
3. Chibanda D, Mesu P, Kajawu L, Cowan F, Araya R, Abas MA. Problem-solving therapy for depression and common mental disorders in Zimbabwe: piloting a task-shifting primary mental health care intervention in a population with a high prevalence of people living with HIV. BMC Public Health. 2011;11:828. doi:10.1186/1471-2458-11-828.
4. Papas RK, Sidle JE, Gakinya BN, et al. Treatment outcomes of a stage 1 cognitive-behavioral trial to reduce alcohol use among human immunodeficiency virus-infected out-patients in western Kenya. Addiction. 2011;106(12):2156–66. doi:10.1111/j.1360-0443.2011.03518.x.
5. Papas RK, Sidle JE, Martino S, et al. Systematic cultural adaptation of cognitive-behavioral therapy to reduce alcohol use among HIV-infected outpatients in western Kenya. AIDS Behav. 2010;14(3):669–78. doi:10.1007/s10461-009-9647-6.
6. Andersen LS, Magidson JF, O'Cleirigh C, Remmert JE, Kagee A, Leaver M, Stein DJ, Safren SA, Joska J. A pilot study of a nurse-delivered cognitive behavioral therapy intervention (Ziphamandla) for adherence and depression in HIV in South Africa. Journal of Health Psychology. 2016.
7. American Cancer Society. Cancer in Africa. Atlanta: American Cancer Society Inc; 2011.
8. Diabetes Leadership Forum. Diabetes: the hidden pandemic and its impact on Sub-Saharan Africa. 2010. http://www.changingdiabetesbarometer.com/docs/Diabetes%20in%20sub-saharan%20Africa.pdf.
9. UNAIDS. The Gap report. 2014. http://www.unaids.org/sites/default/files/en/media/unaids/contentassets/documents/unaidspublication/2014/UNAIDS_Gap_report_en.pdf.
10. Ahmat A, Bilal N, Herbst H, Weber S. How many health workers? In: Soucat A, Scheffler R, Ghebreyesus TA, editors. The labor market for health workers in Africa: a new look at the crisis. Washington, DC: World Bank; 2013.

11. Maddison AR, Schlech WF. Will universal access to antiretroviral therapy ever be possible? The health care worker challenge. Can J Infect Dis Med Microbiol. 2010;21(1):e64–9.
12. World Health Organization. Achieving the health-related MDGs. It takes a workforce! Geneva: World Health Organization; 2015.
13. Saxena S, Thornicroft G, Knapp M, Whiteford H. Resources for mental health: scarcity, inequity, and inefficiency. Lancet. 2007;370(9590):878–89. doi:10.1016/S0140-6736(07)61239-2.
14. WHO Int. Taking Stock. Task shifting to tackle health worker shortages. 2006. http://www.who.int/healthsystems/task_shifting_booklet.pdf.
15. Harries AD, Hargreaves NJ, Gausi F, Kwanjana JH, Salaniponi FM. High death rates in health care workers and teachers in Malawi. Trans R Soc Trop Med Hyg. 2002;96(1):34–7.
16. Huddart J, Picazo O. The health sector human resource crisis in Africa: an issues paper. Washington, DC: United States Agency for International Development; 2003.
17. Naicker S, Eastwood JB, Plange-Rhule J, Tutt RC. Shortage of healthcare workers in Sub-Saharan Africa: a nephrological perspective. Clin Nephrol. 2010;74 Suppl 1:S129–33.
18. Mills EJ, Kanters S, Hagopian A, et al. The financial cost of doctors emigrating from Sub-Saharan Africa: human capital analysis. BMJ. 2011;343, d7031.
19. Mullan F, Frehywot S, Omaswa F, et al. Medical schools in Sub-Saharan Africa. Lancet. 2011;377(9771):1113–21. doi:10.1016/S0140-6736(10)61961-7.
20. WHO. Working together for health: the world health report 2006. 2006. http://www.who.int/whr/2006/whr06_en.pdf?ua=1.
21. Mdege ND, Chindove S, Ali S. The effectiveness and cost implications of task-shifting in the delivery of antiretroviral therapy to HIV-infected patients: a systematic review. Health Policy Plan. 2013;28(3):223–36. doi:10.1093/heapol/czs058.
22. Callaghan M, Ford N, Schneider H. A systematic review of task- shifting for HIV treatment and care in Africa. Hum Resour Health. 2010;8:8. doi:10.1186/1478-4491-8-8.
23. Mwai GW, Mburu G, Torpey K, Frost P, Ford N, Seeley J. Role and outcomes of community health workers in HIV care in Sub-Saharan Africa: a systematic review. J Int AIDS Soc. 2013;16:18586.
24. Gimbel-Sherr SO, Micek MA, Gimbel-Sherr KH, et al. Using nurses to identify HAART eligible patients in the Republic of Mozambique: results of a time series analysis. Hum Resour Health. 2007;5:7. doi:10.1186/1478-4491-5-7.
25. Bangsberg DR, Perry S, Charlebois ED, Clark RA, Roberston M, Zolopa AR, Moss A. Non-adherence to highly active antiretroviral therapy predicts progression to AIDS. Aids. 2001;15(9):1181–3.
26. Mills EJ, Nachega JB, Buchan I, et al. Adherence to antiretroviral therapy in Sub-Saharan Africa and North America: a meta-analysis. JAMA. 2006;296(6):679–90. doi:10.1001/jama.296.6.679.
27. Palombi L, Marazzi MC, Guidotti G, et al. Incidence and predictors of death, retention, and switch to second-line regimens in antiretroviral- treated patients in Sub-Saharan African Sites with comprehensive monitoring availability. Clin Infect Dis. 2009;48(1):115–22.
28. Schneider H, Hlophe H, van Rensburg D. Community health workers and the response to HIV/AIDS in South Africa: tensions and prospects. Health Policy Plan. 2008;23(3):179–87. doi:10.1093/heapol/czn006.
29. Schneider H, Lehmann U. Lay health workers and HIV programmes: implications for health systems. AIDS Care. 2010;22 Suppl 1:60–7. doi:10.1080/09540120903483042.
30. Lewin SA, Dick J, Pond P, et al. Lay health workers in primary and community health care. Cochrane Database Syst Rev. 2005;1, CD004015. doi:10.1002/14651858.CD004015.pub2.
31. Price J, Binagwaho A. From medical rationing to rationalizing the use of human resources for AIDS care and treatment in Africa: a case for task shifting. Dev World Bioeth. 2010;10(2):99–103. doi:10.1111/j.1471-8847.2010.00281.x.
32. Iwu EN, Holzemer WL. Task shifting of HIV management from doctors to nurses in Africa: clinical outcomes and evidence on nurse self-efficacy and job satisfaction. AIDS Care. 2014;26(1):42–52. doi:10.1080/09540121.2013.793278.

33. Mukora R, Charalambous S, Dahab M, Hamilton R, Karstaedt A. A study of patient attitudes towards decentralisation of HIV care in an urban clinic in South Africa. BMC Health Serv Res. 2011;11:205. doi:10.1186/1472-6963-11-205.

34. Assefa Y, Kiflie A, Tekle B, Mariam DH, Laga M, Van Damme W. Effectiveness and acceptability of delivery of antiretroviral treatment in health centres by health officers and nurses in Ethiopia. J Health Serv Res Policy. 2012;17(1):24–9. doi:10.1258/jhsrp.2011.010135.

35. Boyer S, Protopopescu C, Marcellin F, et al. Performance of HIV care decentralization from the patient's perspective: health-related quality of life and perceived quality of services in Cameroon. Health Policy Plan. 2012;27(4):301–15. doi:10.1093/heapol/czr039.

36. Ledikwe JH, Kejelepula M, Maupo K, et al. Evaluation of a well-established task-shifting initiative: the lay counselor cadre in Botswana. PLoS One. 2013;8(4), e61601. doi:10.1371/journal.pone.0061601.

37. Hermann K, Van Damme W, Pariyo GW, et al. Community health workers for ART in Sub-Saharan Africa: learning from experience—capitalizing on new opportunities. Hum Resour Health. 2009;7:31. doi:10.1186/1478-4491-7-31.

38. Berman PA, Gwatkin DR, Burger SE. Community-based health workers: head start or false start towards health for all? Soc Sci Med. 1987;25(5):443–59.

39. Gilson L, Walt G, Heggenhougen K, et al. National community health worker programs: how can they be strengthened? J Public Health Policy. 1989;10(4):518–32.

40. Igumbor JO, Scheepers E, Ebrahim R, Jason A, Grimwood A. An evaluation of the impact of a community-based adherence support programme on ART outcomes in selected government HIV treatment sites in South Africa. AIDS Care. 2011;23(2):231–6. doi:10.1080/09540121.2010.498909.

41. Rabkin M, El-Sadr WM. Why reinvent the wheel? Leveraging the lessons of HIV scale-up to confront non-communicable diseases. Glob Public Health. 2011;6(3):247–56. doi:10.1080/17441692.2011.552068.

42. Nakimuli-Mpungu E, Bass JK, Alexandre P, et al. Depression, alcohol use and adherence to antiretroviral therapy in Sub-Saharan Africa: a systematic review. AIDS Behav. 2012;16(8):2101–18. doi:10.1007/s10461-011-0087-8.

43. Shield KD, Rylett M, Gmel G, Gmel G, Kehoe-Chan TAK, Rehm J. Global alcohol exposure estimates by country, territory and region for 2005—a contribution to the comparative risk assessment for the 2010 global burden of disease study. Addiction. 2013;108(5):912–22. doi:10.1111/add.12112.

44. Labbe A, Yeterian J, Wilner J, Kelly J. Cognitive and behavioral approaches for treating substance use disorders among behavioral medicine patients. In: Vranceau A, Safren S, Greer J, editors. Massachusetts general hospital handbook of behavioral medicine. New York: Springer; 2016.

45. Blashill A, Dale S, Jampel J, Safren S. HIV. In: Vranceaunu A, Greer J, Safren S, editors. Massachusetts general hospital handbook of behavioral medicine. New York: Springer; 2016.

46. Remien RH, Mellins CA, Robbins RN, et al. Masivukeni: development of a multimedia based antiretroviral therapy adherence intervention for counselors and patients in South Africa. AIDS Behav. 2013;17(6):1979–91. doi:10.1007/s10461-013-0438-8.

47. Robbins RN, Mellins CA, Leu C-S, et al. Enhancing lay counselor capacity to improve patient outcomes with multimedia technology. AIDS Behav. 2015;19:163–76. doi:10.1007/s10461-014-0988-4.

48. Ewart CK. Social action theory for a public health psychology. Am Psychol. 1991;46(9):931–46.

49. Sorsdahl K, Myers B, Ward CL, et al. Adapting a blended motivational interviewing and problem-solving intervention to address risky substance use amongst South Africans. Psychother Res. 2014;25:435–44. doi:10.1080/10503307.2014.897770.

50. Bere T, Nyamayaro P, Magidson J, et al. Cultural adaptation of a cognitive-behavioral intervention to improve adherence to antiretroviral therapy among people living with HIV/AIDS in Zimbabwe: "Nzira Itsva." J Health Psychol. In press.

51. Dewing S, Mathews C, Schaay N, Cloete A, Louw J, Simbayi L. "It's important to take your medication everyday okay?" An evaluation of counselling by lay counsellors for ARV adherence support in the Western Cape, South Africa. AIDS Behav. 2013;17(1):203–12. doi:10.1007/s10461-012-0211-4.

52. Simoni JM, Pearson CR, Pantalone DW, Marks G, Crepaz N. Efficacy of interventions in improving highly active antiretroviral therapy adherence and HIV-1 RNA viral load. J Acquir Immune Defic Syndr. 2006;43 Suppl 1:S23–35. doi:10.1097/01.qai.0000248342.05438.52.

53. Bärnighausen T, Chaiyachati K, Chimbindi N, Peoples A, Haberer J, Newell M-L. Interventions to increase antiretroviral adherence in Sub-Saharan Africa: a systematic review of evaluation studies. Lancet Infect Dis. 2011;11(12):942–51. doi:10.1016/S1473-3099(11)70181-5.

54. Jones DL, Ross D, Weiss SM, Bhat G, Chitalu N. Influence of partner participation on sexual risk behavior reduction among HIV-positive Zambian women. J Urban Health 2005;82 (3 Suppl 4):iv92–iv100.

55. Kekwaletswe CT, Morojele NK. Alcohol use, antiretroviral therapy adherence, and preferences regarding an alcohol-focused adherence intervention in patients with human immunodeficiency virus. Patient Prefer Adherence. 2014;8:401–13. doi:10.2147/PPA.S55547.

56. Parry CD, Morojele NK, Myers BJ, et al. Efficacy of an alcohol-focused intervention for improving adherence to antiretroviral therapy (ART) and HIV treatment outcomes—a randomised controlled trial protocol. BMC Infect Dis. 2014;14:500. doi:10.1186/1471-2334-14-500.

57. Safren SA, Otto MW, Worth JL. Life-steps: applying cognitive-behavioral therapy to patient adherence in HIV medication treatment. Cogn Behav Pract. 1999;6:332–41.

58. Safren S, Gonzalez J, Soroudi N. Coping with chronic illness: a cognitive-behavioral therapy approach for adherence and depression. Therapist guide. New York: Oxford University Press; 2008.

59. Kidia K, Machando D, Bere T, et al. "I was thinking too much": experiences of HIV-positive adults with common mental disorders and poor adherence to antiretroviral therapy in Zimbabwe. Trop Med Int Health. 2015;20(7):903–13. doi:10.1111/tmi.12502.

60. Braithwaite RS, Nucifora KA, Kessler J, et al. Impact of interventions targeting unhealthy alcohol use in Kenya on HIV transmission and AIDS-related deaths. Alcohol Clin Exp Res. 2014;38(4):1059–67. doi:10.1111/acer.12332.

61. Carroll KM, Nich C, Sifry RL, et al. A general system for evaluating therapist adherence and competence in psychotherapy research in the addictions. Drug Alcohol Depend. 2000;57(3):225–38.

62. Parsons JT, Rosof E, Punzalan JC, Maria LD. Integration of motivational interviewing and cognitive behavioral therapy to improve HIV medication adherence and reduce substance use among HIV-positive men and women: Results of a pilot project. AIDS Patient Care STDS. 2005;19(1):31–9. doi:10.1089/apc.2005.19.31.

63. Mimiaga MJ, Reisner SL, Pantalone DW, O'Cleirigh C, Mayer KH, Safren SA. A pilot trial of integrated behavioral activation and sexual risk reduction counseling for HIV-uninfected men who have sex with men abusing crystal methamphetamine. AIDS Patient Care STDS. 2012;26(11):681–93. doi:10.1089/apc.2012.0216.

64. Barbor TF, de la Fuente JR, Sunder J, Grant M. AUDIT: the alcohol use disorders identification test. Guidelines for use in primary health care. Geneva: World Health Organization; 1992.

65. Patel V, Araya R, Bolton P. Treating depression in the developing world. Trop Med Int Health. 2004;9(5):539–41. doi:10.1111/j.1365-3156.2004.01243.x.

66. Patel V, Simunyu E, Gwanzura F, Lewis G, Mann A. The Shona symptom questionnaire: the development of an indigenous measure of common mental disorders in Harare. Acta Psychiatr Scand. 1997;95(6):469–75.

67. Alcoholics anonymous. 2001. http://www.aa.org/.

68. O'Donnell K, Dorsey S, Gong W, Ostermann J, Whetten R, Cohen JA, Itemba D, Manongi R, Whetten K. Treating maladaptive grief and posttraumatic stress symptoms in orphaned children in Tanzania: Group-based trauma-focused cognitive–behavioral therapy. Journal of traumatic stress. 2014;27(6):664–71.

69. Murray LK, Familiar I, Skavenski S, et al. An evaluation of trauma focused cognitive behavioral therapy for children in Zambia. Child Abuse Negl. 2013;37(12):1175–85. doi:10.1016/j.chiabu.2013.04.017.

70. Bolton P, Bass J, Neugebauer R, et al. Group interpersonal psychotherapy for depression in rural Uganda: a randomized controlled trial. JAMA. 2003;289(23):3117–24. doi:10.1001/jama.289.23.3117.

71. Petersen I, Bhana A, Baillie K, MhaPP Research Programme Consortium. The feasibility of adapted group-based interpersonal therapy (IPT) for the treatment of depression by community health workers within the context of task shifting in South Africa. Community Mental Health J. 2012;48(3):336–41.

72. Tapp H, White L, Steuerwald M, Dulin M. Use of community-based participatory research in primary care to improve healthcare outcomes and disparities in care. J Comp Eff Res. 2013;2(4):405–19. doi:10.2217/cer.13.45.

73. Stacciarini J-MR, Shattell MM, Coady M, Wiens B. Review: community-based participatory research approach to address mental health in minority populations. Community Ment Health J. 2011;47(5):489–97. doi:10.1007/s10597-010-9319-z.

74. Andersen L, Joska J, Safren S. Life steps for ART adherence. 2013. http://hivmentalhealth.co.za/wp-content/uploads/2013/05/Life-Steps-ART-Adherence1.pdf.

75. Glasgow RE, Vogt TM, Boles SM. Evaluating the public health impact of health promotion interventions: the RE-AIM framework. Am J Public Health. 1999;89(9):1322–7.

76. Thorpe KE, Zwarenstein M, Oxman AD, et al. A pragmatic–explanatory continuum indicator summary (PRECIS): a tool to help trial designers. CMAJ. 2009;180(10):E47–57. doi:10.1503/cmaj.090523.

77. Damschroder LJ, Aron DC, Keith RE, Kirsh SR, Alexander JA, Lowery JC. Fostering implementation of health services research findings into practice: a consolidated framework for advancing implementation science. Implement Sci. 2009;4:50. doi:10.1186/1748-5908-4-50.

78. Safren S, O'Cleirigh C, Tan JY, et al. A randomized controlled trial of cognitive behavioral therapy for adherence and depression (CBT-AD) in HIV-infected individuals. Health Psychol. 2009;28(1):1–10. doi:10.1037/a0012715.

79. Safren S, O'Cleirigh CM, Bullis JR, Otto MW, Stein MD, Pollack MH. Cognitive behavioral therapy for adherence and depression (CBT-AD) in HIV-infected injection drug users: a randomized controlled trial. J Consult Clin Psychol. 2012;80(3):404–15. doi:10.1037/a0028208.

80. Pop-Eleches C, Thirumurthy H, Habyarimana JP, et al. Mobile phone technologies improve adherence to antiretroviral treatment in a resource-limited setting: a randomized controlled trial of text message reminders. AIDS. 2011;25(6):825–34. doi:10.1097/QAD.0b013e32834380c1.

81. Kaaya S, Eustache E, Lapidos-Salaiz I, Musisi S, Psaros C, Wissow L. Grand challenges: improving HIV treatment outcomes by integrating interventions for co-morbid mental illness. PLoS Med. 2013;10(5), e1001447. doi:10.1371/journal.pmed.1001447.

Chapter 15
Cultural Competence Within Behavioral Medicine: Culturally Competent CBT with Diverse Medical Populations

C. Andres Bedoya, Sannisha K. Dale, and Peter P. Ehlinger

15.1 Introduction

Behavioral medicine, as a field, has made significant advances providing interdisciplinary evidence and theory in support of promoting health and the prevention of illness [1, 2]. As with the overall field of medicine, however, the majority of these advances within practice and research have centered on the experience of a select subset of the US population (i.e., middle-class White men) in spite of ever growing demographic diversity within the country [3, 4]. Such demographic diversity is a salient issue for the field of behavioral medicine as it has implications for health promotion, disease prevalence, and health disparities [5].

Various organizations have called for the inclusion of cultural competence in psychological treatment and research with diverse groups (e.g., [5, 6]). For example, the Health Disparities Strategic Plan developed by the National Institute on Drug Abuse [7] highlights the need for clinical research with ethnic minorities, including appropriate operationalization of the term *culture* and adjusting current methodologies to meet the needs of minorities. Healthy People 2020 [5], the federal initiative to reduce health disparities and increase the quality and years of healthy life, similarly highlights the need to conduct clinical research with diverse populations.

Despite advocacy for cultural competence in clinical care and research, there has been limited empirical examination of cultural competence within behavioral medicine. Reported barriers to examining cultural competence within psychosocial intervention research have included variability in how cultural competence is defined

C.A. Bedoya, Ph.D. (✉) • S.K. Dale, Ph.D., Ed.M. • P.P. Ehlinger, B.A.
Behavioral Medicine Service, Department of Psychiatry, Massachusetts General Hospital, Harvard Medical School, Boston, MA, USA
e-mail: abedoya@mgh.harvard.edu; skdale@mgh.harvard.edu; pehlinger@mgh.harvard.edu

© Springer Science+Business Media New York 2017
A.-M. Vranceanu et al. (eds.), *The Massachusetts General Hospital Handbook of Behavioral Medicine*, Current Clinical Psychiatry,
DOI 10.1007/978-3-319-29294-6_15

(e.g., [8]), misperception that cultural competence methods are ill-suited for use with evidence-based research [9], and lack of methodologies to guide and communicate steps taken in tailoring an intervention for specific populations [10]. Yet, there is growing empirical support both for differentiating general competence from cultural competence (e.g., [11]) and for the positive impact of cultural competence on therapeutic processes and outcomes [12].

15.2   Cultural Groups

The importance of cultural competency in behavioral medicine treatment approaches is echoed by the diversity among individuals in the USA as well as the large disparities in health conditions between some groups. For instance, according to the 2010 US census, the population consisted of 16.3 % Latino, 14 % Black, 6 % Asian, 2 % American Indian and Alaska Native, and 7 % some other race [13]. Furthermore, these numbers do not begin to reflect the diversity of the US population in terms of gender, religion, sexual orientation, socioeconomic class, and other areas of diversity. Such diversity can be based on differences between an individual and group in comparison to an established norm [14]. What is considered diverse may be influenced by context and a number of other factors—such as ethnicity, race, and gender—that are not mutually exclusive and can occur in combination [15].

15.3   Prevalence of Health Disparities

In the USA, there are clear differences in the prevalence of health conditions between groups, with some groups having higher prevalence for certain conditions [16]. Current smoking is highest among adults who did not complete high school (34.6%), fall below the federal poverty line (37.9%), and identify as American Indian or Alaskan Native (34.4 %) [16]. The prevalence of binge drinking is highest among men (24.6%), 18–34-year-olds (59.7), and White non-Hispanics (21.1%) [16]. Diabetes is more prevalent amongst individuals above age 65 (43.5 %), identifying as multiracial (14%), and having less than a high school education (11.6%) [16]. Among adults who rated their health as poor or fair in a national survey, 37.6 % spoke Spanish at home, 40.7 % had another language spoken at home, 39.4 % had a disability, and a combined 82.2 % were Black (non-Latino), Latino, or American Indian/Alaskan Native [16]. In addition, the rate of HIV infection among racial/ethnic minorities (e.g., Blacks 84.0 %, Latinos 30.9 %) and men who have sex with men (MSM, 382.6%) is alarmingly high compared to Whites (9.1 %) and other men (8.2%) [16]. The prevalence of obesity is 53 % among Black females (versus 37 % for males), 44 % among Mexican-American females (versus 35 % for males), and 50–60 % among persons with disabilities [16]. In terms of women's reproductive health, Black women have a higher rate (17.1 %) of preterm (<37 weeks) births compared to Latinos (11.8 %) and Whites (10.8 %) [16].

Beyond physical health conditions, there are also disparities in terms of comorbid mental health issues. For instance, women are more likely to be diagnosed with depression and anxiety than men [17]; men tend to be diagnosed with substance abuse and antisocial disorders compared to women [17]; LGBTQ persons struggle with high rates of trauma histories, substance use disorders, and suicide attempts and completions [18, 19]. Also racial/ethnic minorities lack access to mental health care that has been linked to income, health insurance, and language barriers [20] and they receive poor quality of mental health care when dealing with mental health issues [20]. In addition, racial/ethnic minorities may not seek out or remain engaged with mental health services due to stigma and discrimination [21].

With the noted disparities in the prevalence of health conditions and comorbid mental health issues between diverse groups in the USA, patients seen by behavioral medicine service providers will encapsulate and represent a broad range of cultural identities. Therefore having the appropriate tools to deliver appropriate quality care in a culturally competent manner that attract, engage, and retain diverse patients is essential.

15.4   Evidence Base for Cognitive Behavioral Interventions with Diverse Cultural Groups with Medical Conditions

Available evidence from a meta-analytic review of 76 studies supports that culturally adapted mental health interventions result in therapeutic benefits among racial/ethnic minority adults across a variety of psychiatric conditions [22], in particular for adapted CBT treatment of depression among Latinos and African-Americans [23, 24]. Though there is limited evidence, existing data indicate the potential efficacy of cognitive behavioral interventions and approaches across diverse groups for common medical and mental health issues seen in behavioral medicine settings, with the evidence for efficacy in some diverse populations (e.g., racial/ethnic minority groups) still lacking [25–28].

The evidence for the use and efficacy of CBT strategies in behavioral medicine approaches among ethnic/racial minorities is indicated by several studies on CBT for depression and stress management, medication adherence, and pain management. Rosselló and Bernal [26] evaluated the efficacy of Cognitive Behavioral Therapy (CBT) and Interpersonal Psychotherapy (IPT) in treating depression among adolescents in Puerto Rico and found that both CBT and IPT significantly reduced depressive symptoms. In a study with depressed Latino primary care patients, in comparison to those in enhanced usual care, Latino adults who received a culturally focused psychiatric consultation reported significant improvements on depression [29]. Safren and colleagues [30] found that, in an HIV-positive sample consisting of 49 % racial/ethnic minorities, CBT targeting depression and poor adherence (CBT-AD) was effective in increasing medication adherence and reducing depression, although race/ethnicity was not examined as a moderator of study outcomes. A culturally adapted version of the CBT-AD intervention was found effective for both depression and medication adherence, compared to standard care, among HIV-positive Mexican/Mexican-American adults in a study conducted at a community-based HIV clinic [31]. Similarly, in a study of CBT for stress management and positive psychological well-being among HIV-positive racial/ethnic minority women with human papillomavirus, researchers found that group CBT resulted in significant increases in positive well-being, while a psychoeducational seminar did not [32]. Beissner and colleagues [25] assessed the feasibility and potential efficacy of a CBT- and exercise-based intervention for a diverse group (African-American, Latino, and White) of senior citizens with chronic back pain and found similar significant decreases in pain-related disability for all groups; however significant gains in other outcomes (pain intensity, social activity, activities of daily living, depressive symptoms) were only observed for Latino participants.

The efficacy of CBT strategies in behavioral medicine approaches among ethnic/racial minorities has also been demonstrated in studies addressing smoking, substance use, and binge eating. A meta-analysis by Windsor and colleagues [28] assessed the impact of CBT in reducing substance use comparing studies with a predominantly non-Hispanic White (NHW) sample and studies with a predominantly Black and/or Hispanic (B/H) sample. They found that while CBT had similar effects on substance use for NHW and B/H studies, the impact of CBT was stronger in NHW than B/H studies and there was lower retention and engagement in B/H studies. Webb and colleagues [27] found that a group CBT intervention was efficacious for smoking cessation in an African-American sample and her research group is currently conducting an RCT to compare standard CBT with culturally tailored CBT (i.e., incorporating factors such as spirituality and discrimination) for smoking cessation among African-Americans. Researchers [33] also compared treatments (self-help CBT vs. an anti-obesity medication) for binge eating disorder in a sample of majority racial/ethnic participants (55 %) and treatment outcomes differed significantly at 6 months with the self-help CBT group reporting lower binge-eating frequency; however, race/ethnicity did not significantly predict or moderate outcomes.

Though the empirical evidence supports applying cultural competence within mental health interventions with medically ill populations, there are few guides on how to do so within one's own practice (see [8]). Miranda and colleagues [10] indicated a lack of methodologies available to guide tailoring evidence-based interventions for specific populations. A difficulty in illustrating cultural competence in clinical research is that the decisions and decision-making process of ensuring cultural competence are often part of the unspoken portions of published research [34].

15.5   Cultural Competence Defined

To address cultural competence in clinical care and research with diverse groups, the meaning of *culture* should be clearly defined [35]. Common components to culture include having shared ideas, meanings, and values that guide patterns of behavior, and these may exist at an unconscious level and change based on experience of the individual or group [36]. Culture may also be transmitted in a variety of ways, including (a) vertical transmission from parent to child, (b) horizontal transmission from peers, and (c) oblique transmission through adults and institutions of the majority culture [37].

Similarly, the construct of cultural competence has been defined in various ways. Though there is no singular definition, a generally accepted definition is that cultural competence involves the necessary understanding of cultural influences to provide appropriate care for patients from a diverse cultural group (see [8, 38]). It involves the ability to incorporate a respect and understanding of participants' sociocultural context [34, 39–41], as well as behaviors and skills that a cultural group would perceive as culturally competent [42]. Cultural competence can be composed of culture-specific components that are unique to a cultural group and culture-universal components that may apply to more than one cultural group [42]. It involves taking into account individual difference within cultural groups and the extent, if any, that culture is a salient issue for the individual seeking treatment [8]. Cultural competence also involves continuous learning and experience as cultural groups and contexts are continuously changing.

15.6   Cultural Competence Framework

There also are a myriad of models and tools for conceptualizing areas of cultural competence and communicating the process of working towards cultural competence. Though there are some ways that these differ, generally agreed upon components involve having knowledge, skills, and a problem-solving approach [8, 9]. One of the most commonly recognized frameworks is the tripartite model of multicultural competence (see [8, 43]). Within this framework, cultural competence involves a set of characteristics the provider may develop including: (a) awareness of one's own beliefs, biases, and attitudes; (b) knowledge and understanding of the cultural group; and (c) skills and tools to provide culturally sensitive assessment and intervention. Each of these components holds equal importance and should be addressed for each cultural group one is attempting to provide culturally competent care.

15.7   Applying Cultural Competence to Enhance Care

Within this tripartite framework, building cultural competence involves developing these characteristics and skill set across all three components. For behavioral medicine it also involves considering, across each of these components, the extent that a patient's physical and mental health are influenced by their cultural background.

As depicted above, an initial component of working towards cultural competence involves increasing awareness of one's beliefs, biases, and attitudes. This component can be described as "knowing oneself" and may involve exploring the impact of one's life experiences (e.g., migration, privilege, marginalization), family of origin, worldview, sociopolitical context and other factors have shaped one's view of self and others. This self-reflection may also be applied to one's views, biases, and attitudes about physical and mental illness. It also involves consideration of one's view of diverse groups, including those that one is a part of, and may involve evaluation of how this has changed across time or differs by day-to-day context. A number of tools are available to help providers on the course of self-awareness (e.g., [44, 45]). For example, the Cultural Self-Awareness Assessment [45] is one tool for examining the subjectivity a provider brings to the therapeutic encounter. As with each of the tripartite domains, getting to "knowing oneself" from a cultural competence standpoint is a continuous and lifelong process.

A second component involves having the knowledge and understanding of the cultural group. This may involve gaining an understanding specific to a population (e.g., Native Americans) or gaining an understanding that may apply across cultural groups. Group-specific tools are available that describe cultural factors that may be considered, for example in mental health treatment with Latinos, African-Americans, Asian-Americans, and Native Americans [46] as well as LGBT individuals [47, 48]). Increased cultural competence through knowledge of a specific group also involves having skills to examine the extent that individual difference is at play.

Finally, developing cultural competence also involves having the skills and tools needed to provide effective care across various aspects of the therapeutic encounter. This may involve tools that can be applied at specific points of treatment (e.g., [49–51]). For example, the Engagement Interview Protocol (EIP; [51])—a tool that incorporates both standard psychiatric assessment and other culturally relevant assessments (e.g., [52])—is meant to engage patients into care through the inclusion of culture within assessment, diagnosis, and treatment planning. Applying tools such as the EIP involves assessing the patient's worldview and understanding of their symptoms and tailoring care accordingly. This work is also in line with a culturally sensitive framework aimed to adapt interventions for cultural groups (e.g., [50, 53]). Hays [53] provides a framework (i.e., represented by the pneumonic, ADDRESSING)—informed by the American Psychological Association's [6] multicultural guidelines—specifically for conducting culturally responsive CBT that considers both strengths and potential limits of CBT with diverse groups and applies this framework in assessment, an approach with which to engage the patient and consider adaptations to treatment. The latter involves considering the possible influence of culture on such areas as use of culturally respectful behavior, assessment of the patient's strengths and support, validating the patient's cultural beliefs and experience with oppression, while utilizing this information to inform application of cognitive behavioral tools themselves. Similarly, Bernal and Saez-Santiago [50] have proposed that an intervention can be culturally centered through considering eight elements including language; persons; metaphors; content; concepts; goals; methods; and context. See Table 15.1.

15.8   Case Example

Gloria is a 34-year-old divorced Latina mother of two young children, 3- and 5-year-old sons. She is a college graduate working full-time in a management level position at a local bank branch. Gloria was exposed to HIV approximately 8 months ago from her husband of 10 years who, unbeknownst to her, had begun using injection drugs and had contracted HIV. At the time of his diagnosis, Gloria's husband disclosed his HIV status and they both agreed that she should also be tested for HIV. After testing positive for the HIV virus, Gloria has focused on separating from her husband. She continued to work full-time and, with her two sons, has been living with her parents. She has begun proceeding for divorce, has temporary full custody of her children, and has limited contact with her husband.

At her most recent medical appointment—only her second since diagnosis—Gloria spoke with her infectious disease provider about her mental health symptoms and was referred for therapy for depression in response to contracting HIV. During the first session, the therapist utilized the Engagement Interview Protocol to both conduct a standard psychiatric assessment and engage her in therapy through culturally sensitive treatment negotiation. Through standard assessment questions Gloria indicated that she had never had a significant period of depression beyond some challenges during adolescence after her parents' temporary separation. After finding out she was HIV-positive and during the separation from her husband, she felt that she alternated between feeling numb and angry. Over the past 2 months she has been more aware of a number of symptoms including sleeping excessively, difficulty concentrating, and easily being brought to tears. Gloria did not believe that anyone in her family had ever been diagnosed with a psychiatric illness, but she did suspect that a paternal aunt and cousin had dealt with depression. Gloria's medical history was unremarkable except for HIV diagnosis 8 months ago; she has an infectious disease provider who she met with once after the initial diagnosis but she has not followed the provider's recommendation to begin medications for HIV and is unsure about continuing care. She is also the youngest of three, with a sister and brother. She has a small but close group of friends, with Gloria spending the majority of her time with her extended family who she sees as her strongest supporters. Gloria's mother was born in Mexico, with the family strongly identifying with their Mexican-American cultural background. She enjoys spending time with her children and finds strength from both her family and Catholic religious beliefs.

Through application of the EIP, the therapist also aimed to gauge Gloria's view of her symptoms and the treatments she believed would be most useful for her. Through questions meant to assess the patient's explanatory model of her illness the therapist found that rather than describe her symptoms as "depression," Gloria tended to group her symptoms under the umbrella of "not feeling like myself" and to emphasize her physical symptoms such as sleeping excessively and having to push herself to do things, as well as trouble concentrating and planning. Gloria also indicated her belief that the separation served as the primary cause of her symptoms since she felt she had tried to make the marriage work and that in some way she

Table 15.1 Examples of measures and tools in cultural competence

Measure/tool	Description	Goal	References
Cultural formulation interview	A brief semi-structured interview consisting of 16 questions that can be used within the initial assessment to gauge the impact of culture on mental health. An informant version and supplementary modules for specific patient populations are also available.	Assessing the extent that social and cultural features influence clinical presentation and treatment.	[49]
Culturally responsive cognitive behavioral therapy	An approach for integrating an understanding of cultural influences within cognitive behavioral therapy (CBT). Considers the possible advantages and limitations of incorporating a multicultural view within CBT, across a broad range of diverse patient groups.	To increase the effectiveness of CBT with diverse patients. The tool provides general considerations for conducting culturally responsive CBT as well as examines its application across specific cultural groups.	[39, 53]
Cultural self-awareness assessment	A guide for clinicians' development of cultural competence with diverse patients. Presented primarily as a tool within clinical psychology training, it provides a guideline for development of competence.	A tool that can be applied to increase competence with diverse groups through development of greater cultural self-awareness. This involves assessment of critical self-awareness characteristics such as defensiveness, openness to individual differences and awareness of one's own racial identity attitutes and privelege.	[45]
Engagement interview protocol	A semi-structured interview that can be applied with patients to improve clinical and cultural sensitivity. The tool incorporates both standard psychiatric and culturally relevant assessments.	A tool that can be used to gauge the patients' illness narratives and explanatory models in order to engage patients in mental health care.	[51, 52]
Social matrix	A visual tool developed for exploring subjective sense of privilege and marginalization across multiple intersecting domains. Intended for use within supervision, training and academic settings, the social matrix can be filled out by the therapist for themself, the patient and the patient's family.	A tool for informing one's clinical work through exploring privilege and marginalization within the therapist's life experience and how this maps onto the life experience of the patient and the patient's family.	[44]

failed both because her soon-to-be ex-husband had continued using drugs and that they ultimately separated. She also noted, less clearly, that contracting HIV as having a role. By asking Gloria about the cause of her symptoms, she also shared that she had not disclosed her HIV status to anyone (i.e., parents, family, friends) and felt very ashamed and guilty for what she perceives as her role in contracting HIV. The EIP assessment also allowed Gloria to share that she does not know how long her symptoms are going to last but that she fears these will last a long time and may ultimately result in her losing her job and not being able to care for her children. Gloria hoped that individual therapy would help her to "feel more like myself again." She does not believe that psychiatric medications would be helpful for her, as she feels this would indicate that she "is really crazy." Additionally, she was interested in possible resources for helping her to get housing near her parents' home and support for childcare. With further probing that aimed to elicit specific short-term goals, the therapist worked with Gloria to establish more explicit goals that address her chief fears and problems. Potential goals included tackling her fears about losing her job and feeling better about herself, in particular less guilt and shame around her divorce, contracting HIV, and her fear that her two boys, who have tested HIV-negative, will contract HIV.

An additional goal of the initial sessions is to provide a culturally sensitive disclosure of diagnosis and treatment planning. In Gloria's case, the therapist was attentive to Gloria's discomfort with labeling her symptoms as depression and thus was sensitive not to provide a diagnostic label too quickly. In this sense, the patient is seen as the expert on their own symptoms and the therapist is available to provide their view and professional opinion. The therapist initially used Gloria's terminology in summarizing her symptoms and their impact, linking these with the goals she would like to achieve through treatment. Given the patient's level of acculturation (i.e., bicultural), the therapist provided feedback on diagnosis in line with the Western belief system regarding her psychiatric symptoms while also being flexible to accept that other explanatory models may also be valid. The therapist also clarified discrepancies between the patient's stated goals and the therapist's role, for example by providing appropriate referrals for addressing her housing and childcare needs. Throughout the course of treatment, the provider was also careful to continuously examine his own cultural values and biases across the multiple issues at play in the case.

The therapist and patient worked collaboratively to clarify the focus of treatment and potential tools that could be applied to reach Gloria's goals. In line with this, the therapist applied a cognitive behavioral intervention for treatment of depression and adherence among HIV-positive adults (i.e., CBT-AD; [30, 54]) with the plan to conduct weekly outpatient sessions over the course of 12–16 weeks. The therapist considered potential ways to culturally tailor the intervention for Gloria based on the available literature for providing culturally appropriate CBT for Latinos (e.g., [55]) and in particular examples of culturally adapted CBT-AD for HIV-positive Mexican Americans [31]. Potential Latino cultural values were examined with the patient and, when found applicable, incorporated within treatment. For example, as Gloria had strongly indicated family as an important part of her life (i.e., *familismo*), initial behavioral activation exercises focused on engaging in activities with her children, as well as supportive extended family members. Similarly, over the course of therapy, the therapist and patient considered the extent that Gloria adhered to cultural beliefs such as women must be self-sacrificing for the good of the family regardless of the husband's behavior (i.e., *marianismo*) and the extent she believed she should feel a sense of shame (i.e., *vergüenza*) over negative outcomes to herself, her children, and the extended family (e.g., upcoming divorce). These beliefs were normalized within its sociopolitical context, were examined to the extent that Gloria was aware of holding them, and, as appropriate, were addressed within cognitive restructuring exercises as part of challenging depressogenic thinking patterns about self.

In addition, cultural values and beliefs were examined to address thoughts, feelings, and behavior that negatively impacted her reaction to her HIV diagnosis and adherence to HIV treatment recommendations. A number of sessions focused on the extent that fears (e.g., impact of HIV disease progression; people in her community learning of her HIV status; discrimination to herself or family) served as barriers to fully engaging in HIV care. For example, Gloria indicated that she was concerned about taking HIV medications as these served as a shameful reminder of her illness and, instead, she believed that the biggest priority was that her children would be best served by focusing on maintaining her position as a bank manager and working hard to ensure their financial independence. Treatment incorporated cultural values and beliefs that were salient to Gloria to normalize her response to diagnosis of a chronic and stigmatized illness, highlighted areas of strength, and helped her develop more adaptive thinking patterns and coping tools.

15.9   Future Directions

Throughout this chapter we have highlighted the importance of providing culturally competent care to patients served in behavioral medicine settings especially given the health disparities faced by diverse groups within the USA. We have also reviewed the definition and theoretical framework for cultural competency and discussed specific tools that can be utilized by clinicians in behavioral medicine settings. Tailored and adapted CBT has shown promise in effectively addressing mental health conditions among diverse groups and we have outlined the ways in which tools to enhance cultural competency can be utilized in delivering CBT in medical populations. However, there are still areas for further research and clinical application of culturally competent CBT in behavioral medicine settings. First, cultural competency is often mistakenly conceptualized as a knowledge base and set of tools/skills that once learned are sufficient to effectively work across diverse populations. However, cultural competency is a process that never ends and at its core requires ongoing curiosity and genuine interest in the ways in which patients' multiple identities intersect with their medical conditions and how this intersection impacts patients in reaching their health goals. Second, while the evidence for the efficacy of culturally tailored or adapted CBT is growing, there is still a need for additional research on culturally tailored CBT for diverse patients suffering from many health conditions such as HIV, cancer, obesity, and substance use. Third, for existing evidence-based culturally tailored CBT interventions among medical populations, research is needed that examines the added benefit of each intervention component to better inform what tools for enhancing culturally competent care should be disseminated in behavioral medicine settings. Lastly, while cognitive behavioral therapy is an evidence-based and commonly used psychotherapeutic model in behavioral medicine settings, elements of other psychotherapeutic models may be beneficial in delivering culturally competent care. For instance, interpersonal therapy [56], mindfulness techniques [57], motivational interviewing [58], and dialectical behavioral therapy [59] offer tools for (a) validating patients' illnesses and struggles associated with their diverse identities and (b) enhancing acceptance, distress tolerance, and behavior change.

References

1. Belar CD, Deardorff WW. Intervention strategies in clinical health psychology. In: Belar CD, Deardorff WW, editors. Clinical health psychology in medical settings: a practitioner's guidebook. 2nd ed. Washington, DC: American Psychological Association; 2009. p. 81–110.
2. Smith TW, Suls J. Introduction to the special section on the future of health psychology. Health Psychol. 2004;23(2):115–8.
3. Kazarian S, Evans D. Handbook of cultural health psychology. San Diego: Academic; 2001.
4. Smith TW, Kendall PC, Keefe FJ. Behavioral medicine and clinical health psychology: introduction to the special issue, a view from the decade of behavior. J Consult Clin Psychol. 2002;70(3):459–62.
5. US Department of Health and Human Services. 2012. Rockville: Agency for healthcare research and quality.
6. American Psychological Association. Guidelines on multicultural education, training, research, practice, and organizational change for psychologists. Am Psychol. 2003;58:377–402.
7. Health Disparities Strategic Plan. National Institute on Drug Abuse (NIDA). 2013. http://www.drugabuse.gov/health-disparities-strategic-plan-fy2009-2013. Accessed 12 Aug 2015.
8. Sue S, Zane N, Nagayama Hall GC, Berger LK. The case for cultural competency in psychotherapeutic interventions. Annu Rev Psychol. 2009;60(1):525–48.
9. Whaley AL, Davis KE. Cultural competence and evidence-based practice in mental health services: a complementary perspective. Am Psychol. 2007;62(6):563–74.
10. Miranda J, Bernal G, Lau A, Kohn L, Hwang W-C, LaFromboise T. State of the science on psychosocial interventions for ethnic minorities. Annu Rev Clin Psychol. 2005;1(1):113–42.
11. Imel ZE, Baldwin S, Atkins DC, Owen J, Baardseth T, Wampold BE. Racial/ethnic disparities in therapist effectiveness: a conceptualization and initial study of cultural competence. J Couns Psychol. 2011;58(3):290–8.
12. Tao KW, Owen J, Pace BT, Imel ZE. A meta-analysis of multicultural competencies and psychotherapy process and outcome. J Couns Psychol. 2015;62(3):337–50.
13. United States Census Bureau. Overview of race and Hispanic origin. Washington, DC: US Department of Commerce; 2010.
14. Kato P, Mann T. Handbook of diversity issues in health psychology, vol. 1. New York: Springer; 1996.
15. Jackson PB, Williams DR. The intersection of race, gender, and SES: health paradoxes. In: Schulz AJ, Mullings L, editors. Gender, race, class, & health: intersectional approaches. San Francisco: Jossey-Bass; 2006. p. 131–62.

16. Centers for Disease Control. CDC health disparities and inequalities report—United States. Atlanta: Centers for Disease Control and Prevention; 2013. p. 1–189.
17. Eaton NR, Keyes KM, Krueger RF, Balsis S, Skodol AE, Markon KE, et al. An invariant dimensional liability model of gender differences in mental disorder prevalence: evidence from a national sample. J Abnorm Psychol. 2012;121(1):282–8.
18. Brown LS, Pantalone D. Lesbian, gay, bisexual, and transgender issues in trauma psychology: a topic comes out of the closet. Traumatology. 2011;17(2):1–3.
19. King M, Semlyen J, Tai S, Killaspy H, Osborn D, Popelyuk D, Nazareth I. A systematic review of mental disorder, suicide, and deliberate self harm in lesbian, gay and bisexual people. BMC Psychiatry. 2008;8(1):70.
20. National Alliance on Mental Illness (2006). Evidence-Based Practices and Multicultural Mental Health. Arlington, VA: NAMI Multicultural Action Center.
21. Gary F. Stigma: barrier to mental health care among ethnic minorities. Issues Ment Health Nurs. 2005;26(10):979–99.
22. Griner D, Smith TB. Culturally adapted mental health intervention: a meta-analytic review. Psychother Theory Res Pract Train. 2006;43(4):531–48.
23. Kohn LP, Oden T, Muñoz RF, Robinson A, Leavitt D. Brief report: adapted cognitive behavioral group therapy for depressed low-income African American women. Community Ment Health J. 2002;38(6):497–504.
24. Miranda J, Chung JY, Green BL, et al. Treating depression in predominantly low-income young minority women: a randomized controlled trial. JAMA. 2003;290(1):57–65.
25. Beissner K, Parker S, Henderson Jr CR, Pal A, Papaleontiou M, Reid MC. Implementing a combined cognitive-behavioral + exercise therapy protocol for use by older adults with chronic back pain: evidence for a possible race/ethnicity effect. J Aging Phys Act. 2012;20(2):246.
26. Rosselló J, Bernal G. The efficacy of cognitive-behavioral and interpersonal treatments for depression in Puerto Rican adolescents. J Consult Clin Psychol. 1999;67(5):734–45.
27. Webb MS, de Ybarra DR, Baker EA, Reis IM, Carey MP. Cognitive–behavioral therapy to promote smoking cessation among African American smokers: a randomized clinical trial. J Consult Clin Psychol. 2010;78(1):24–33.
28. Windsor LC, Jemal A, Alessi EJ. Cognitive behavioral therapy: a meta-analysis of race and substance use outcomes. Cultur Divers Ethnic Minor Psychol. 2015;21(2):300–13.
29. Bedoya CA, Traeger L, Trinh N-HT, Chang TE, Brill CD, Hails K, et al. Impact of a culturally focused psychiatric consultation on depressive symptoms among Latinos in primary care. Psychiatr Serv. 2014;65(10):1256–62.
30. Safren SA, O'Cleirigh C, Tan JY, Raminani SR, Reilly LC, Otto MW, Mayer KH. A randomized controlled trial of cognitive behavioral therapy for adherence and depression (CBT-AD) in HIV-infected individuals. Health Psychol. 2009;28(1):1–10.
31. Simoni JM, Wiebe JS, Sauceda JA, Huh D, Sanchez G, Longoria V, et al. A preliminary RCT of CBT-AD for adherence and depression among HIV-positive Latinos on the U.S.-Mexico border: the Nuevo Día STUDY. AIDS Behav. 2013;17(8):2816–29.
32. Jensen SE, Pereira DB, Whitehead N, Buscher I, McCalla J, Andrasik M, et al. Cognitive–behavioral stress management and psychological well-being in HIV+ racial/ethnic minority women with human papillomavirus. Health Psychol. 2013;32(2):227–30.
33. Grilo CM, Masheb RM, White MA, Gueorguieva R, Barnes RD, Walsh BT, et al. Treatment of binge eating disorder in racially and ethnically diverse obese patients in primary care: randomized placebo-controlled clinical trial of self-help and medication. Behav Res Ther. 2014;58:1–9.
34. Rogler LH, Malgady RG, Rodriguez O. Hispanics and mental health: a framework for research. Malabar: Krieger; 1989.
35. Guarnaccia PJ, Rodriguez O. Concepts of culture and their role in the development of culturally competent mental health services. Hisp J Behav Sci. 1996;18(4):419–43.
36. Institute of Medicine. Unequal treatment: confronting racial and ethnic disparities in health care. Washington, DC: National Academic Press; 2002.
37. Berry JW. Cross-cultural psychology: research and applications. Cambridge: Cambridge University Press; 2002.

38. Hays P. Addressing cultural complexities in practice: a framework for clinicians and counselors. Washington, DC: American Psychological Association; 2001.
39. Hays PA, Iwamasa GY. Culturally responsive cognitive-behavioral therapy: assessment, practice, and supervision. Washington, DC: American Psychological Association; 2006.
40. Resnicow K, Yaroch AL, Davis A, Wang DT, Carter S, Slaughter L, et al. Go girls! Results from a nutrition and physical activity program for low-income, overweight African American adolescent females. Health Educ Behav. 2000;27(5):616–31.
41. Vega WA, Lopez SR. Priority issues in Latino mental health services research. Ment Health Serv Res. 2001;3(4):189–200.
42. Sue DW. Multidimensional facets of cultural competence. Couns Psychol. 2001;29(6):790–821.
43. Sue DW, Bernier JE, Durran A, Feinberg L, Pedersen P, Smith EJ, Vasquez-Nuttall E. Position paper: cross-cultural counseling competencies. Couns Psychol. 1982;10(2):45–52.
44. Kliman, J. Intersections of social privilege and marginalization: a visual teaching tool. In: Ariel J, Hernández-Wolfe P, Stearns S, editors. Expanding our social justice practices: advances in theory and training. Washington, DC: American Family Therapy Academy; 2010 Winter. pp. 39–48.
45. Roysircar G. Cultural self-awareness assessment: Practice examples from psychology training. Prof Psychol Res Pract. 2004;35(6):658–66.
46. American Psychological Association. Guidelines on multicultural education, training, research, practice, and organizational change for psychologists. Washington, DC: American Psychological Association; 2009.
47. Boroughs MS, Bedoya CA, O'Cleirigh C, Safren SA. Toward defining, measuring, and evaluating LGBT cultural competence for psychologists. Clin Psychol Sci Pract. 2015;22(2):151–71. doi:10.1111/cpsp.12098.
48. American Psychological Association (2012). Guidelines for psychological practice with lesbian, gay, and bisexual clients. American Psychologist, 67, 10–42.
49. American Psychiatric Association. Diagnostic and statistical manual of mental disorders. 5th ed. Arlington: American Psychiatric; 2013.
50. Bernal G, Sáez-Santiago E. Culturally centered psychosocial interventions. J Community Psychol. 2006;34(2):121–32.
51. Yeung A, Yu S-C, Fung F, Vorono S, Fava M. Recognizing and engaging depressed Chinese Americans in treatment in a primary care setting. Int J Geriatr Psychiatry. 2006;21(9):819–23.
52. Kleinman A. Patients and healers in the context of culture: an exploration of the borderland between anthropology, medicine, and psychiatry, vol. 3. Berkeley: University of California Press; 1980.
53. Hays PA. Integrating evidence-based practice, cognitive–behavior therapy, and multicultural therapy: ten steps for culturally competent practice. Prof Psychol Res Pract. 2009;40(4):354–60. doi:10.1037/a0016250.
54. Newcomb ME, Bedoya CA, Blashill AJ, Lerner JA, O'Cleirigh C, Pinkston MM, Safren SA. Description and demonstration of cognitive behavioral therapy to enhance antiretroviral therapy adherence and treat depression in HIV-infected adults. Cogn Behav Pract. 2014;22(4):430–8.
55. Organista KC. Cognitive-behavioral therapy with Latinos and Latinas. In: Hays PA, Iwamasa GY, editors. Culturally responsive cognitive-behavior therapy: assessment, practice, and supervision. Washington, DC: American Psychological Association; 2006. p. 73–96.
56. Klerman GL, Weissman MM, Rounsaville BJ, Chevron ES. Interpersonal psychotherapy of depression. New York: Basic Books; 1984.
57. Bauer-Wu S. Leaves falling gently: Living fully with serious and life-limiting illness through mindfulness, compassion, and connectedness. New York: Harbinger; 2011.
58. Miller W, Rollnick S. Motivational interviewing: Helping people change. 3rd ed. New York: Guilford Press; 2013.
59. Linehan MM. Skills training manual for treating borderline personality disorder. Vol. xii. New York: Guilford Press; 1993.

Resources

Cultural Competence Guidelines

American Psychological Association. Mental health: a guide for Latinos and their families. 2008. Retrieved from www.psychiatry.org/practice/professional-interests/diversityomna/diversity-resources/diversity-resources.

American Psychological Association. Guidelines for psychological practice with lesbian, gay, and bisexual clients. Am Psychol. 2012;67(1):10–42.

American Psychological Association. Mental health: a guide for African Americans and their families. 2012b. Retrieved from www.psychiatry.org/practice/professional-interests/diversityomna/diversity-resources.

American Psychological Association. Working with immigrant-origin clients. 2013. http://www.apa.org/topics/immigration/immigration-report-professionals.pdf.

American Psychological Association. Guidelines for psychological practice with older adults. Am Psychol. 2014;69:34–65. http://www.apa.org/practice/guidelines/older-adults.pdf.

Council of National Psychological Associations for the Advancement of Ethnic Minority Interests. Psychology education and training from culture-specific and multiracial perspectives: critical issues and recommendations. Washington, DC: American Psychological Association; 2009. Retrieved from http://www.apa.org/pi/oema.

National Societies and Professional Associations

Adult development and aging—Division 20 of the APA. http://www.apadivisions.org/division-20/.

Asian American Psychological Association. http://www.aapaonline.org.

Association of Black Psychologists. http://www.abpsi.org/.

International Association for Cross-Cultural Psychology. http://www.iaccp.org.

International Psychology—Division 52 of the APA. http://div52.org/.

National Latina/o Psychological Association. http://www.nlpa.ws/.

Office of Ethnic Minority Affairs, American Psychological Association. http://www.apa.org/pi/oema/.

Society for Community Research and Action: Division of Community Psychology—Division 27 of the APA. http://www.scra27.org/.

Society for the Psychological Study of Culture, Ethnicity and Race—Division 45 of the APA. http://www.apa.org/about/division/div45.aspx.

Society for the Psychological Study of Lesbian, Gay, Bisexual, and Transgender Issues—Division 44 of the APA. http://www.apa.org/about/division/div44.aspx.

Society for the Psychological Study of Men and Masculinity—Division 51 of the APA. http://www.apa.org/about/division/div51.aspx.

Society for the Psychology of Religion and Spirituality—Division 36 of the APA. http://www.apa.org/about/division/div36.aspx.

Society for the Psychology of Women—Division 35 of the APA. http://www.apa.org/divisions/div35/.

Society of Indian Psychologists. http://aiansip.org/.

General Resources

Disparities Solution Center. https://www2.massgeneral.org/disparitiessolutions/.

National Center for Cultural Competence. http://nccc.georgetown.edu/.

Index

© Springer Science+Business Media New York 2017
A.-M. Vranceanu et al. (eds.), *The Massachusetts General Hospital Handbook of Behavioral Medicine*, Current Clinical Psychiatry,
DOI 10.1007/978-3-319-29294-6